T0250262

PRACTICAL
STATISTICAL
METHODS

A SAS PROGRAMMING APPROACH

PRACTICAL STATISTICAL METHODS

A SAS PROGRAMMING APPROACH

Lakshmi V. Padgett

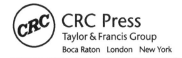

CRC Press
Taylor & Francis Group
Boca Raton London New York

CRC Press is an imprint of the
Taylor & Francis Group an **informa** business

A CHAPMAN & HALL BOOK

CRC Press
Taylor & Francis Group
6000 Broken Sound Parkway NW, Suite 300
Boca Raton, FL 33487-2742

© 2011 by Taylor & Francis Group, LLC
CRC Press is an imprint of Taylor & Francis Group, an Informa business

No claim to original U.S. Government works

Printed in the United States of America on acid-free paper
Version Date: 20110701

International Standard Book Number: 978-1-4398-1282-2 (Hardback)

Library of Congress Cataloging-in-Publication Data

Padgett, Lakshmi V.
  Practical statistical methods : a SAS programming approach / Lakshmi V. Padgett.
    p. cm.
  Includes bibliographical references and index.
  ISBN 978-1-4398-1282-2 (hardcover : alk. paper)
  1. SAS (Computer program language) 2. Mathematical statistics--Data processing. 3. Probabilities--Data processing. I. Title.

QA276.45.S27P33 2011
519.50285--dc23   2011019323

Visit the Taylor & Francis Web site at
http://www.taylorandfrancis.com

and the CRC Press Web site at
http://www.crcpress.com

To my father and

in loving memory of my mother

Contents

Preface

This book discusses various statistical methods aimed at a diverse audience. A broad spectrum of methods is given that will be useful for researchers without much statistical background. Omitting mathematical details and complicated formulae, SAS programs are provided to carry out the necessary analyses and draw appropriate inferences for statistical problems that are widely used by most researchers. Similar types of programs can be used with other statistical packages, drawing similar conclusions. The book emphasizes the different, commonly used methodologies and interpretation of the data using SAS version 9.1.

Practical Statistical Methods: A SAS Programming Approach will assist researchers in all fields, including those in the pharmaceutical industry, the biological sciences, physical sciences, social sciences, market research, and psychology. Additionally, it will be a reference book for applied statisticians working with researchers in the fields indicated above. It will also be helpful as supplemental reading material for graduate students taking a statistical methods course for one or two semesters.

Fundamental statistical concepts are introduced in Chapter 1 and the methods used for quantitative data, continuous data following normal and nonnormal distributions, are discussed in Chapters 2 through 4. Regression methodology starting with simple linear regression and discussing logistic regression and PH regression are highlighted in Chapter 5. Chapter 6 briefly sketches miscellaneous topics such as propensity scores, cutoff points of a marker indicating the end point, misclassification errors, interim analysis, conditional power, bootstrap and jackknife, among others.

Lakshmi V. Padgett

1

Introduction

1.1 Types of Data

Data play a crucial part in statistical inference. The type of data one has, determines the type of statistical analysis needed. The methods of analyses performed on one type of data may not necessarily be applicable for other types of data. Further, one needs to have clean data, one without any outliers (observations that do not follow the pattern of the bulk of the data) and holes (chunks of missing observations).

There are *qualitative* and *quantitative* types of data.

Qualitative data include variables such as a persons' eye color, income level (low, middle, high), winning a medal (gold, silver, bronze), an individual having a particular disease or not, and age (<21, 21–35, 36–55, >55). Qualitative data consist of *nominal data* and *ordinal data*. Nominal data have no particular ordering like an individuals' eyecolor, brands of soft drinks, and brands of laptops. Ordinal data can be ranked by category such as income level, winning a medal, movie ratings, and students' letter grades in a course.

Data that can be measured or things that can be counted include age, weight, leaves on a tree, and the number of cars in a household. These types of data are called quantitative data. Quantitative data can be discrete or continuous. Usually all measuring variables are continuous and all counting variables are discrete, with the exception of monetary variable which is treated as continuous. Discrete variables include the number of children in a family, the number of deaths due to a disease at a given time, the number of leaves on a tree, and the number of cars in a household. Age, weight, height, cholesterol level, serum glucose, and blood pressure are examples of continuous variables. Depending on the precision one wants, the continuous variables such as weight can be 125 lbs or 125.1 lbs. The data for the continuous variables may look like discrete variables.

Continuous data can be converted to ordinal data based on the question one is trying to address. Thus, the age of an individual can be given in years, or it can be expressed categorically as a child (<13 years), teenager [13–18], adult [18–55], or senior citizen (≥55 years) depending on whether one is interested in trying to address the average age of people in a community or the proportion of teenagers in a community. The "[" means inclusive of that particular observation and ")" means exclusive of that observation.

1.2 Descriptive Statistics/Data Summaries

Consider the age of 50 people who entered a clinical trial. We want to summarize these age groups by providing quantities that express the nature of the data. These quantities that represent the data are called *descriptive* or *summary statistics*.

All of the summary statistics can be obtained using PROC UNIVARIATE in SAS as follows:

```
Data a;
/***Input data***/
Input Age @@; Cards;
45 55 67 89 78 67 56 43 44 45 57 69 78 76 54 34 23
46 67 65 54 98 78 67 58 49 53 42 74 97 43 45 46 47
48 59 70 89 78 76 65 34 45 36 67 45 47 75 64 61
;
/***end of input data***/
proc univariate; var age;run;
```

The first part of the output which will be used to explain the descriptive statistics is

```
                    The UNIVARIATE Procedure
                        Variable: Age
                          Moments
N                50                Sum weights        50
Mean             59.36 (a1)        Sum observations   2968
Std deviation    16.8713741 (a6)   Variance           284.643265
Skewness         0.32002628        Kurtosis           -0.3227663
Uncorrected SS   190128            Corrected SS       13947.52
Coeff. variation 28.4221262 (a7)   Std error mean     2.38597261


                    Basic Statistical Measures
          Location                         Variability
Mean        59.36000       Std deviation        16.87137
Median      57.50000 (a2)  Variance             284.64327
Mode        45.00000 (a3)  Range                75.00000 (a9)
                           Interquartile range  25.00000 (a8)
```

Note: The mode displayed is the smallest of two modes with a count of 5.

```
                      ***
        Quantile              Estimate
        100% Max              98.0
        99%                   98.0
        95%                   89.0
        90%                   78.0
        75% Q3                70.0 (a5)
        50% Median            57.5
        25% Q1                45.0 (a4)
        10%                   42.5
        5%                    34.0
        1%                    23.0
        0% Min                23.0
```

The commonly used descriptive statistics are mean, median, mode, Q1, Q3, standard deviation, and the coefficient of variation. These statistics are described below:

Mean is the average of the data, and from our output (a1) is 59.36. If the data have two categories, one of them coded as "1" and the other "0," then the mean is the proportion of the category coded as "1."

Approximately 50% of the observations are not more than the *median*, and approximately 50% of the observations are not less than the median. From the output, (a2) represents the median and is 57.5. If the mean and median are close, the mean is used as a central tendency measure of the data. However, if the mean and median are farther apart, then the median is used as the focal point of the data.

Mode is that observation that is repeated the most. From the output, (a3) represents the mode and is 45.0. Sometimes you may have more than one mode. In SAS, the smallest of the modes is reported.

Approximately 25% of the observations are less than or equal to Q1, the *lower quartile*, and approximately 75% of the observations are greater than or equal to Q1. From the output, (a4) represents the lower quartile and is 45.0.

Approximately 75% of the observations are less than or equal to Q3, the *upper quartile*, and approximately 25% of the observations are greater than or equal to Q3. From the output, (a5) represents the upper quartile and is 70.0.

The spread of the data from the mean is indicated by the *standard deviation*. It is 16.87 and is shown by (a6) in our output. The standard deviation is always nonnegative. If the standard deviation is small, the data are clustered near the mean and if the standard deviation is large, the data are widely spread out from the mean. The square of the standard deviation is the variance and is given in the output.

The mean and standard deviation are given in the same units of measurement as the data. If data are collected in different scales or sources, the *coefficient of variation* provides a unit-free measure of the spread of the data. In a group of people with mean annual income of $20,000, a person with an annual income of $21,000 is considered rich, whereas in a group of individuals with an annual income of $100,000, a person making $101,000 is not considered rich, although the squared deviations of the individuals from the group means are the same. Thus, if two groups of data have the same standard deviation with different means, the variability will have practical importance if it is considered in terms of the mean, and the coefficient of variation takes that aspect into consideration and is a better measure to compare the variabilities of groups of data. While comparing the variability of two variables expressed in different units of measurement, the coefficient of variation is also an appropriate measure. From the output, (a7) is the coefficient of variation and is 28.4.

The *interquartile range* for the data from the output at (a8) is 25 and this is Q3–Q1. Approximately 50% of the data is separated by 25 units starting at Q1 = 45 and ending at Q3 = 70. Some researchers indicate the interquartile range as (45, 70).

The *range* for the data from the output at (a9) is 75 and this is the difference between the maximum of all the observations and the minimum of all the observations. Some researchers indicate the range as (23, 98).

For further details, see Raghavarao (1988).

1.3 Graphical and Tabular Representation

Data can either be presented in a tabular form or can be plotted and displayed graphically. Figures sometimes help to get a clearer and a more concise picture of what the data represent. However, one needs to find a balance between figures and tabular forms of data representation.

There are many statistical packages that graph the data, including but not limited to SAS, S-Plus, JMP, and Minitab. Some packages have better graphical qualities, whereas others are more user-friendly. It is not in the scope of this book to evaluate these packages. Some of the common types of graphical displays include stem-and-leaf plots, histograms, bar charts, pie charts, line plots, box plots, scatter plots, and Kaplan–Meier (KM) curves. We will now describe them.

Stem-and-Leaf Plot is similar to the histogram. The advantage of using a stem-and-leaf plot is that we know the individual data points up to the indicated units in the stem-and-leaf plot, whereas in the histogram we only know the class the observation falls into, but not the individual value. Tukey (1977) also provided other graphical representations. Let us consider the age of the 50 people in a clinical trial discussed in Section 1.2.

Figure 1.1 depicts the stem-and-leaf plot.

The leaf is the unit value of the age and the stem is the tens of the age. Leaf 9 at stem 4 corresponds to observation 49. The counts of leaves from the top

Age (Leaf unit = 1)

	Stem	Leaf
1	2	3
4	3	4 4 6
19	4	2 3 3 4 5 5 5 5 5 6 6 7 7 8 9
(8)	5	3 4 4 5 6 7 8 9
23	6	1 4 5 5 7 7 7 7 7 9
13	7	0 4 5 6 6 8 8 8 8
4	8	9 9
2	9	7 8

FIGURE 1.1
Stem-and-leaf plot for age.

and bottom are shown on the left side. The median observation is in the stem where the count is shown within parentheses.

The *histogram* shown in Figure 1.2 is similar to the stem-and-leaf plot except that the information is condensed. The boxes are obtained by dividing the range of a numerically continuous variable, categorizing into several non-overlapping classes with no gaps and the classes may or may not be of equal

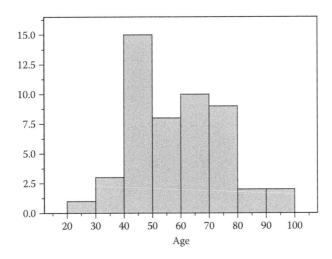

FIGURE 1.2
Histogram for age.

length. The area of the bar indicates the frequency in the corresponding class. In Figure 1.2, we form the classes [20, 30), [30–40), [40–50), [50–60), [60–70), [70–80), [80, 90), and [90, 100).

The *bar chart* is similar to a histogram, where the bars are separated from each other. In a histogram, all the bars are joined together indicating that the data are continuous, whereas in a bar chart, each bar stands separate, indicating that the data are discrete or qualitative. Qualitative or discrete data may be shown by the bars with the frequency indicating the bar height. The average temperature for the 12 months in a year in a city is shown by a bar diagram in Figure 1.3.

Figure 1.3 shows how temperatures in different months fluctuate and indicate the hottest and coldest months in the city.

Suppose one wants to compare the monthly temperatures in four cities for the first 3 months of a year. It can be graphically depicted by multiple bars as shown in Figure 1.4.

A *pie chart* is commonly used to represent frequency type of data on a categorical variable. Classes are mutually exclusive. Figure 1.5 represents a pie diagram of the percentage of hospitals that treated a given number of patients in an emergency room in an average week.

A pie chart can also be used to indicate the percentage of salary spent on housing, food, clothing, entertainment, and savings of a typical American family.

In the longitudinal data graph, the values (*y*-axis) are plotted across time (*x*-axis). A *line plot* is a graph joining all the points by lines. They can be plotted in a single graph for continuous data across time for different groups of

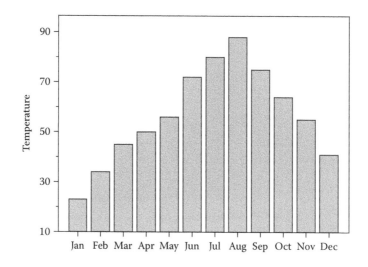

FIGURE 1.3
Bar chart of average temperature for a city.

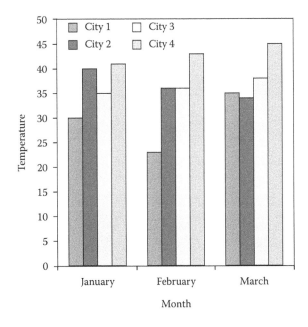

FIGURE 1.4
Bar chart of average temperature in the first 3 months for four cities.

interest. They can also be used to plot the mean or median temperature in a city by month as shown in Figure 1.6.

One can visualize the *box plot* given in Figure 1.7 as an extension of a histogram containing some summary statistics. It is also useful to detect outliers. The line in the middle of the box represents the median value and the dot represents the mean value. The first and third quartiles are the ends of the box. The lines at the end are the whiskers indicating the minimum and maximum observation. Potential outlier points can be indicated on the graph. For this purpose, we form inner fences $Q_1 - 1.5 \, (IQR)$, $Q_3 + 1.5 \, (IQR)$; and outer

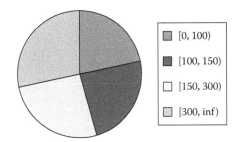

FIGURE 1.5
Pie chart of percentage of hospitals that treated a given number of patients.

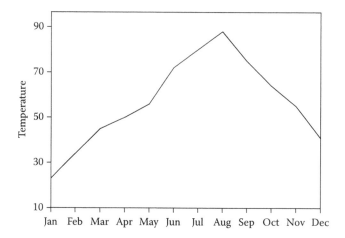

FIGURE 1.6
Line plot of average temperature in a city.

fences $Q_1 - 3$ (IQR), $Q_3 + 3$ (IQR), where IQR is the interquartile range. Observations between inner and outer fences are considered as possible outliers and beyond outer fences are definite outliers.

The *scatter plot* is used to observe an association between two continuous variables such as height and weight (see Figure 1.8). The closer the points are near a straight line, the more correlated are the variables. However, spread-out-points across the plane indicate less correlation of the variables.

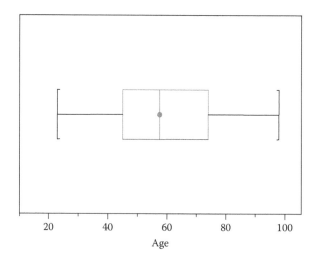

FIGURE 1.7
Box plot for age.

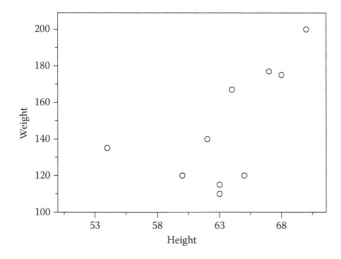

FIGURE 1.8
Scatter plot of height versus weight.

By looking at the scatter plot one detects outliers. It can also help in modeling the dependent variable on the y-axis in terms of the independent variable on the x-axis.

The *KM curve* is a step function indicating the chance of survival at different time points (see Figure 1.9). This is based on the data showing the time of an event like death. This is also used when the exact time of the event is not recorded, but is known that it exceeds some censored value.

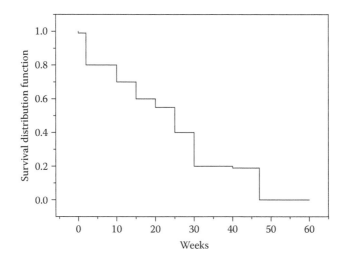

FIGURE 1.9
Survival function.

The histogram is a graphical representation of a frequency table. For the histogram chart displayed in Figure 1.2 one can use PROC FREQ in SAS and get the frequency table as follows:

```
data b;set a;
*Use age data from Sec 1.2; *Categories are defined by the
researcher;
if 20 <= age < 30 then AGECAT = '[20,30)';
else if 30 <= age < 40 then AGECAT = '[30,40)';
else if 40 <= age < 50 then AGECAT = '[40,50)';
else if 50 <= age < 60 then AGECAT = '[50,60)';
else if 60 <= age < 70 then AGECAT = '[60,70)';
else if 70 <= age < 80 then AGECAT = '[70,80)';
else if 80 <= age < 90 then AGECAT = '[80,90)';
else if 90 <= age < 100 then AGECAT = '[90,100)';
proc freq;tables agecat;run;
```

The SAS provides the frequency for the histogram categories in the following output:

```
                        The FREQ Procedure
                                        Cumulative    Cumulative
   AGECAT      Frequency      Percent     Frequency      Percent

   ------------------------------------------------------------------

   [20,30)         1          2.00           1           2.00
   [30,40)         3          6.00           4           8.00
   [40,50)        15         30.00          19          38.00
   [50,60)         8         16.00          27          54.00
   [60,70)        10         20.00          37          74.00
   [70,80)         9         18.00          46          92.00
   [80,90)         2          4.00          48          96.00
   [90,100)        2          4.00          50         100.00
```

From this output we see the range of categories in column 1 and the frequency in column 2. The percentage of observations in each category is shown in column 3. Cumulative frequency given in column 4 is the total frequency upto and including that category. Cumulative percentage given in column 5 is the cumulative frequency expressed as the percentage of the total number of observations. For example, in the [60, 70) age category, 10 in column 2 indicates that 10 individuals are aged 60 and above and less than 70; this number is 20% of the group and is shown by 20 in column 3. The number 37 in column 4 of this row indicates that 37 people are aged less than 70, and this number is 74% of the group and is shown by 74 in column 5.

When two variables are involved, we form a *contingency table* (cross tabulation). If age and systolic blood pressure are measured for 50 people, the following contingency table summarizes the information by using a similar modified command as earlier:

```
Data a;
/***Input data***/
Input age syst @@; cards;
45 100 55 125 67 155 89 145 78 187 67 167
56 163 43 158 44 148 45 157 57 169 69 147
78 178 76 156 54 135 34 167 23 124 46 165
67 147 65 148 54 138 98 144 78 136 67 188
58 168 49 148 53 148 42 158 74 144 97 149
43 137 45 128 46 159 47 157 48 147 59 136
70 135 89 167 78 135 76 164 65 132 34 173
45 145 36 156 67 125 45 156 47 145 75 164
64 183 61 128
;
/***end of input data***/
data b;set a;
if syst < 145 then SYSTD = 'SYST < 145';
else if syst >= 145 then SYSTD = 'SYST >=  145';
if 20 <= age < 30 then AGECAT = '[20,30)';
else if 30 <= age < 40 then AGECAT = '[30,40)';
else if 40 <= age < 50 then AGECAT = '[40,50)';
else if 50 <= age < 60 then AGECAT = '[50,60)';
else if 60 <= age < 70 then AGECAT = '[60,70)';
else if 70 <= age < 80 then AGECAT = '[70,80)';
else if 80 <= age < 90 then AGECAT = '[80,90)';
else if 90 <= age < 100 then AGECAT = '[90,100)';
proc freq;tables systd*agecat;run;
```

This provides the following contingency table:

```
Table of SYSTD by AGECAT

SYSTD AGECAT

Frequency ,
Percent   ,
Row Pct   ,
Col Pct   , [20,30) , [30,40) , [40,50) , [50,60) , [60,70) ,[70,80) , [80,90) , [90,100) , Total
SYST < 145 ,     1,        0,       3,       4,       3,       4,        0,        1,     16
           ,   2.00 ,   0.00 ,   6.00 ,   8.00 ,   6.00 ,   8.00 ,   0.00 ,    2.00 , 32.00
           ,   6.25 ,   0.00 ,  18.75 ,  25.00 ,  18.75 ,  25.00 ,   0.00 ,    6.25 ,
           , 100.00 ,   0.00 ,  20.00 ,  50.00 ,  30.00 ,  44.44 ,   0.00 ,   50.00 ,
SYST >=145 ,     0,        3,      12,       4,       7,       5,        2,        1,     34
           ,   0.00 ,   6.00 ,  24.00 ,   8.00 ,  14.00 ,  10.00 ,   4.00 ,    2.00 , 68.00
           ,   0.00 ,   8.82 ,  35.29 ,  11.76 ,  20.59 ,  14.71 ,   5.88 ,    2.94 ,
           ,   0.00 , 100.00 ,  80.00 ,  50.00 ,  70.00 ,  55.56 , 100.00 ,   50.00 ,
Total            1        3       15        8       10        9        2        2      50
               2.00     6.00    30.00    16.00    20.00    18.00     4.00     4.00 100.00
```

From the output, let us look at [50, 60) age group and syst <145 cell. The first number 4 indicates that four people belong to this category. The number 8 in the second row indicates the percentage of subjects who fall into this cell from all people. The number 25 in the third row is the percentage of people falling into this category out of people with syst <145, row category. The last row is 50 and indicates that 50% of people belong to this category out of people who are in the [50, 60) age group of the column category.

1.4 Population and Sample

Population is the entire group of data on which the experimenter or scientist wants to make a statistical inference. By the entire group we mean all people over 75 years, all households with two cars, all people having a particular disease, and so on. In a population we require measures to describe the characteristics we are interested in. These measures are called parameters. *Parameters* could be the proportion of people above 75 years who had a heart attack, the mean incubation period of a disease, and so forth.

Suppose we are interested in determining the proportion of people over 75 years who had a heart attack. It is very difficult to get all people over 75 years and ask them if they had a heart attack. So we get our information by taking a random *sample* from the population. The sample should represent the people aged over 75 years of different nationalities, different lifestyles, different socioeconomic status, and so forth. The summary measures calculated from the sample are called *statistics*.

Randomization allows one to unbiasedly make an inference on the population parameters based on sample estimates. If we are conducting a survey, then we need to make sure we randomly select our respondents to answer the survey; otherwise, we may be biasing the conclusions. The statistical procedures are only valid if the samples are randomly or probabilistically selected.

In clinical trials, by randomizing subjects to the treatment groups, treatment arms are distributed evenly and unbiasedly among the subjects. The experimental data cannot be used for statistical inferences if the subjects are not randomly assigned to treatments. One may also use stratification based on demographic variables or prognostic factors and randomly assign the treatments to the subjects in each strata. By stratifying one creates homogeneous blocks in order to compare treatment arms unbiasedly without being influenced by other characteristics of the subjects. However, one needs to keep the number of strata to a minimum. Many strata may result in having incomplete blocks (too few subjects in the blocks) and the study at the end may not be balanced for the key factors of interest, like the treatment group.

The easiest form of randomization includes rolling a die or looking at the table of random numbers and assigning treatment A to the odd numbers and treatment B to the even numbers to get the required number of subjects to each of the two treatments. The problem with this method is that it can lead to imbalances in the treatment groups. One advantage is that it is less likely for anyone to guess the treatment assignment. However, when one starts to add stratification variables, this randomization scheme may be inappropriate.

Block randomization is used when subjects are randomized into blocks. If a block has been completed, then the treatment arms will be completely balanced. The smaller the block size, the more likely the balancing among the treatment groups but easier for one to guess the treatment assignment; however, the larger the block size, the more likely the imbalance among the treatment groups but harder for one to guess the treatment assignment. One has to find a balance between these two scenarios.

Suppose a researcher wants to randomly assign three treatments at two sites, using age as a stratum (divided into two groups (>75, ≤75)), with 6 blocks of size 3 in each site and age classification.

From SAS, one can use PROC PLAN with which one can create a simple random list:

```
Data a;
proc plan seed = 1; *test seed for dummy data;
factors site = 2 ordered age = 2 ordered block = 6 ordered
trtgrp = 3;   run;
```

This will provide the following output:

```
              The PLAN Procedure

Factor        Select        Levels        Order

Site            2             2          Ordered
Age             2             2          Ordered
Block           6             6          Ordered
trtgrp          3             3          Random
```

Site	Age	Block		-trtgrp-	
1	1	1	1	3	2
		2	1	3	2
		3	2	3	1
		4	1	3	2
		5	3	2	1
		6	1	2	3
	2	1	3	2	1
		2	2	3	1
		3	2	3	1
		4	2	3	1
		5	3	1	2

		6	3	1	2
2	1	1	2	1	3
		2	1	2	3
		3	1	3	2
		4	2	1	3
		5	2	1	3
		6	2	1	3
	2	1	2	1	3
		2	3	2	1
		3	2	1	3
		4	3	1	2
		5	3	1	2
		6	1	2	3

The above output can be explained as follows. In each site and age group, the subjects are blocked in sets of three people and they are given the indicated treatments. For example, the recruited 10, 11, and 12 subjects at Site 1 age group 1 are assigned treatments 1, 3, and 2, respectively based on block 4.

For a detailed discussion on randomization in clinical trials, refer to Efron (1971), Pocock and Simon (1975), Kalish and Begg (1985), Lachin et al. (1988), and Friedman et al. (1998).

1.5 Estimation and Testing Hypothesis

In scientific or social investigations, the major roles of statistics are as follows:

1. Estimate and test hypotheses about the parameters of interest based on sample data.

2. Find an appropriate model to estimate a dependent variable based on one or several independent variables, test the adequacy of the model, estimate the parameters involved in the model, and test hypotheses about the parameters.

3. Analyze the experimental data using appropriate techniques and determine the efficacy of the treatments.

While estimating parameters, we would like to see some desirable properties in the estimator like *unbiasedness*, *consistency*, and *minimum variance*. An estimator is unbiased if the average of the estimator, in repeated sampling or experimentation, is the parameter. In a single study the unbiased estimator need not be the parameter, but in repeated studies the average value of that estimator is the parameter. A consistent estimator for large samples approaches the parameter. We also want the estimator not to give widely spread-out values in repeated studies. This property is the minimum variance of the estimator. The population mean and proportion are estimated in random sampling by the sample mean and sample proportion. These estimators possess the above properties. Usually, the estimates given by computer packages are based on the estimators with desirable properties. Note that the estimator gives the estimate based on the available data.

The estimate may be given as a single value called *point estimate*. Often, one likes to see an interval of possible values of the parameter, and such an interval is called a *confidence interval* (CI). The CI is associated with *confidence probability* and it can be interpreted as follows. Based on the CI formula, the interval can be calculated from a trial. When many trials are made, out of all those intervals, the actual parameter will be contained in (confidence probability) $\times$ 100% cases.

To test a hypothesis, we form *null* (H_0) and *alternative* (H_A) hypotheses, form a *test statistic* based on the observed data and hypothesis H_0, and find the chance (probability, *p-value*) of getting the present evidence or stronger evidence against H_0. If this chance is small, the evidence is improbable and as we are observing that evidence in the current data, we reject H_0. The test always aims to show that the current data are unlikely to be observed if H_0 is true.

The objective is not to establish H_0 from the data, but to find evidence against H_0 from the data, if possible. In view of this, all claims an investigator wants to make must be taken as alternative hypotheses and their complements are taken as null. If a test rejects (retains) H_0, it is not implied that H_0 is false (true). It is a decision the investigator makes based on the observed data. The truth of H_0 and the decision to reject or retain H_0 can be shown in the following table:

	Actually, H_0	
Decide, H_0	True	False
True	Correct decision	Type II error
False	Type I error	Correct decision

Ideally, the decision should be free of error and it is impossible to make an error-free decision. The decision to reject H_0 is devised controlling the probability of commiting Type I error at a prespecified value and minimizing the probability of committing Type II error. The prespecified probability of committing Type I error is called the *level of significance* and is denoted by α. If a decision to reject a hypothesis H_0 is made, either H_0 is false or the decision is one of those 100α% cases of rejection of H_0 when it is actually true. The *power* of the test is one minus the probability of commiting Type II error (β) and the sample size is usually determined to give a power of at least 80%. The commonly used test statistics are Z, t, χ^2, and F. The normal distribution is specified by its mean and standard deviation, and Z is the standardized normal distribution with mean zero and standard deviation one. The t and χ^2

variables are characterized by their degrees of freedom and when the degrees of freedom are large, they approximate to a normal variable. The F variable is a ratio and is characterized by its numerator and denominator degrees of freedom. The variables Z and t take all possible real values while χ^2 and F take only nonnegative real values.

Since the p-value is the probability of getting evidence against H_0, one decides to reject H_0 if the p-value is less than α. Commonly used α level is 0.05; smaller values like 0.01 or 0.005 are taken when the rejection of H_0 should be cautiously made and larger values like 0.1 is taken when rejection of H_0 has desirable consequences.

When one is interested to establish that two means μ_1, μ_2, or two proportions p_1, p_2 are different without caring for the order, the alternative is taken as $\mu_1 \neq \mu_2$, or $p_1 \neq p_2$, and this setting will give a *two-sided test*. If the alternatives are $\mu_1 > \mu_2$, $\mu_1 < \mu_2$, or $p_1 > p_2$, $p_1 < p_2$, we have *one-sided tests*. In this work we consider one-sided tests with greater than sign in the alternative hypothesis and using the right tail of the test statistic to determine the p-value.

Smallest clinically important effect (SCIE) is the effect size (the treatment difference) meaningful to the clinican or experimenter. In some instances if the p-value is less than 0.05 but the effect size is not large, the test is statistically significant but the result may not be useful to a clinician who does not see enough effect size to change clinical practice. However, in some cases, the p-value is greater than 0.05 and statistically insignificant, but, the effect size is large enough that the clinician may feel the need to change the current practice of treating patients.

The sample size or the number of subjects in a clinical trial plays an important role in estimation and testing hypotheses. In estimation problems, the sample size is determined based on the confidence probability and the maximum error margin the experimenter is willing to take in the study. In hypothesis testing, the sample size is based on the level of significance, expected power for the test for the effect size, and the difference in the treatment effects, indicating a positive outcome of the study. Standard computer packages are available to determine the sample sizes for many types of problems of interest.

1.6 Normal Distribution

If the histogram of a data set is bell shaped with peak at the center and tapering off symmetrically on both sides, the data may be following a normal distribution. This can be tested by the *Shapiro–Wilk test*. For the data on age discussed in Section 1.2, adding the word normal after PROC UNIVARIATE as shown in the programming lines below, we obtain the p-value of the Shapiro–Wilk test.

```
proc univariate normal;var age;run;
```

The output for the Shapiro–Wilk test is shown below.

```
                        Tests for Normality
Test                       Statistic                   p-Value
Shapiro-Wilk         W       0.970878    Pr < W       0.2512  (b1)
Kolmogorov-Smirnov   D       0.110411    Pr > D       0.1297
Cramer-von Mises     W-Sq    0.093805    Pr > W-Sq    0.1356
Anderson-Darling     A-Sq    0.57986     Pr > A-Sq    0.1299
```

The null hypothesis tested here is that the data are normally distributed and hence if the p-value exceeds $\alpha = 0.05$, we retain the null hypothesis that the data are normally distributed. If we look at (b1) the p-value is 0.2512 and we retain the null hypothesis that the data are normally distributed.

By a well-known result known as the *Central Limit Theorem*, most measurement data we come across are normally distributed. For a normally distributed data, if the mean and standard deviation are given, we expect almost all the data to be in the interval, mean ±3 (standard deviation). Many statistical methods are hinged on the assumption of normality of the data. However, some data sets are not normally distributed and we use *nonparametric methods* to analyze such data sets (see Chapter 4).

1.7 Nonparametric Methods

Nonparametric statistical methods are distribution free (they do not need any assumption on distribution), and are thus free of the parameters.

The nonparametric test statistic usually depends on ranks or number of positive or negative differences. The advantages of the underlying nonparametric methods are that they can be used even for parametric tests. There are only mild assumptions to be satisfied for a nonparametric test. However, a disadvantage is that it may be slightly underpowered when the distribution is known and parametric tests are available.

1.8 Some Useful Concepts

If p is the probability of acquiring a disease, then $p/(1-p)$ is defined as the *odds* in favor of acquiring the disease. If p and p^* are the probabilities of getting a disease in two populations, like males and females or smokers and nonsmokers, $\theta = \{p(1-p^*)\}/\{(1-p)p^*\}$ is called the *odds ratio* of the disease in the two populations. When $\theta = 1$, the probabilities of acquiring the disease in the two populations are the same.

Instead of odds ratio, some researchers consider *relative risk, $r = p/p^*$*. The risk of an event is the probability that an event will occur within a stated period of time. Relative risk is the ratio of two risks. Odds ratio and relative risk are estimated by using the sample proportions. Consider the artificial data in Table 1.1 for men and women aged 45 and above for heart disease.

The probability p of men having heart disease is estimated by $15/45 = 0.33$, and the probability p^* of women having heart disease is estimated by $20/55 = 0.36$. Hence, the odds ratio $\theta = ((0.33)(1 - 0.36))/((1 - 0.33)(0.36)) = 0.88$. The relative risk is estimated by $0.33/0.36 = 0.92$. The interpretation of the relative risk is that on an average for 100 women acquiring the disease, 92 men are affected in a population with the same number of men and women. Similarly, the relative risk of women being affected by heart disease over men is $1/(0.92) = 1.09$. The interpretation of the odds ratio is that for every 100 women acquiring heart disease, 88 (100* odds ratio) men are affected. The bases for relative risk and odds ratio are different. The relative risk considers the total population as a base, whereas the odds ratio considers the population of having no event as the base.

While testing the presence or absence of a trait based on laboratory testing, we get *false-positive* or *false-negative* results. A trait actually absent (present) may be determined in a laboratory test as present (absent) and these are known as false-positive (negative) results. The compliment of false-positive (negative) probabilities is known as *sensitivity (specificity)* of the measuring instrument. The statistical tests based on binary responses obtained from laboratory data at α level of significance will actually have a higher α level of significance (Lakshmi, 1995; Lakshmi and Smith, 1993).

Let us consider the example with artificial data given in Table 1.2.

The false-negative error rate is $20/50 = 0.4$ or 40%. The sensitivity = $1 -$ false-negative error rate = $1 - 0.4 = 0.6$ or 60%. The false-positive error rate is $40/100 = 0.4$ or 40%. The specificity = $1 -$ false-positive error rate = $1 - 0.4 = 0.6$ or 60%. Note that although this example shows that the false-positive and false-negative error rates are the same, in reality they may or may not be equal.

TABLE 1.1

Heart Disease for Men and Women Aged above 45 Years

Gender	Heart Disease		Total
	Yes	No	
Men	15	30	45
Women	20	35	55
Total	35	65	100

TABLE 1.2

Trait Detection by Laboratory Test

Presence of a Trait	Laboratory Test		
	Absent	Present	Total
Absent	60	40	100
Present	20	30	50
Total	80	70	150

To see if the laboratory test is a good diagnostic tool, one may plot the false-positive rate (1–specificity) on the *x*-axis and the true positive (sensitivity) of the test on the *y*-axis, and the resulting graph is known as the *relative operative characteristic* (ROC) curve. When the data on the false-positive and true positive rates are available from different laboratories, we can plot the ROC curve as given in Figure 1.10.

Figure 1.10 shows that laboratories corresponding to the two points given in the left top corner produce good diagnostic tests, whereas the point lying on or close to the main diagonal or lower right triangle produces poor results.

ROC is also used in banking to identify the good and bad risk loan applicants based on the credit scores using historic data. The earlier loan applicants are classified as good and bad risk by creating a marker of their credit scores, and by noting the actual loan repayment history, the ROC are

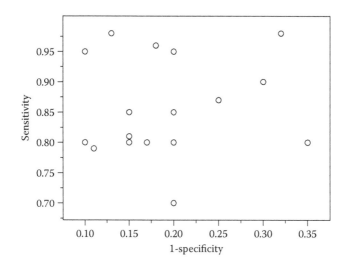

FIGURE 1.10
Relative operative characteristic (ROC) curve.

created. This marker is identified by examining the different ROC curves corresponding to the different markers (see Section 6.2.4).

Clinical trials usually take a long time for completion and hence, one may like to examine the result prior to the completion of the trial, by performing an *interim analysis* (see Section 6.8). The level of significance used at the interim analysis is adjusted so that when the trial is completed the conclusions are drawn at the prechosen α level of significance. At the interim analysis the new drug may be found ineffective and the trial is abandoned, or may be in need of more information to draw a conclusion so that the trial may be continued till the end. At the interim analysis stage, we may determine the *conditional power* (see Section 6.8.2) of the success of the trial based on the observed trend of the results until then or more promising results in the later stage of the trial. It is probable that the study will be successful, given the data observed during the first part of the study, and is discussed by Lan and Wittes (1988).

2

Qualitative Data

2.1 One Sample

2.1.1 Binary Data

Suppose a health scientist is interested in estimating the incidence rate of a particular disease in a large city. One needs to specify the *margin of error* attached to statement, d, and the chance $(1 - \alpha)$ for the validity of the statement. If the scientist estimates the proportion as $\hat{p}$, the real proportion is then in the interval $(\hat{p} - d, \hat{p} + d)$ and in repeated sampling; the statement is true in $(1 - \alpha)$ 100% samples. Usually, $d = 0.03, 0.05,$ or 0.07 and $\alpha = 0.1, 0.05,$ or 0.01. Suppose, the scientist considers $d = 0.03$ and $\alpha = 0.05$, then she needs to have an idea of this proportion and assumes this to the best to her knowledge and experience as $\tilde{p}$. When this information is not available, the scientist considers $\tilde{p} = 0.5$, realizing that the sample size would be larger than required. The number of respondents for the study needs to be determined and the following program will give the necessary sample size, n.

```
data a;
/*** input data***/
d = .03; *margin of error; alpha = .05; * Confidence level = 0.95;
ptilt = .5; *assumed proportion;
/***end of input data ***/
z2side = probit(1 - alpha/2); var = (d/z2side)**2;
N = floor(ptilt*(1 - ptilt)/var) + 1;
keep n;proc print;run;
```

This program will produce the following output:

```
N
1068
```

At least $n = 1068$ individuals from the population need to be selected and each individual is polled and classified based on the presence or absence of the disease. Suppose $n_1 = 500$ individuals and they are found to have the disease. The following program gives in the output, the estimate of the incidence rate at (a2), and a $(1 - \alpha)100\%$ confidence interval (CI) of the incidence rate at [(a1), (a3)]. Choice of the value of α is at the discretion of the investigator.

```
data a;
/***input data**/
n = 1068;*sample size; n1 = 500;*subjects having the disease;
alpha = .05;*Corresponds to 95% CI;
/***end of input data ****/
PHAT = n1/n; z2side = probit(1 - alpha/2);
LOWER_CI = phat-z2side*sqrt(phat*(1 - phat)/n);
UPPER_CI = phat + z2side*sqrt(phat*(1 - phat)/n);
proc print; var lower_ci phat upper_ci; run;
```

The following output is then obtained:

```
LOWER_CI          PHAT                 UPPER_CI
0.43824  (a1)   0.46816  (a2)    0.49809  (a3)
```

The exact CI can be obtained by using the beta distribution as given in Desu and Raghavarao (2004, pp. 45–46).

We can also obtain the exact CI by using the binomial option in PROC FREQ as shown below, when $n = 20$ and $n_1 = 3$ in the example considered earlier.

```
data a;
/***input data***/
n1 = 3;* number of successes; n = 20;* sample size;
/***end of input data***/
n2 = n - n1;
do i = 1 to n1; yes = 1; output; end;
do i = 1 to n2; yes = 2;output; end;
data b;set a; proc freq;;tables yes/binomial;run;
```

The output is as follows:

```
                        ***
              Binomial Proportion for yes = 1
      ---------------------------------------------
                        ***
              Exact Conf Limits
              95% Lower Conf Limit      0.0321  (a4)
              95% Upper Conf Limit      0.3789  (a5)
                        ***
```

The exact CI for the proportion of subjects affected by the disease is given at [(a4), (a5)] and is (0.0321, 0.3789). The exact CI can be used for small or large samples.

Alternatively, let the scientist be interested in testing that the incidence rate is more than (less than, not equal to) a specified value, p_0. Here p_0 is a value prespecified by the investigator. To establish the claim the null hypothesis tested is that the incidence rate is not more than (not less than, equal to) p_0. The level of the test, α needs to be specified. To determine the sample size, the desired power should be specified, usually 80%, 90%, or 95% at an alternative value, p_1, where $p_1 - p_0$ is the smallest clinical effect of interest for detection. The sample size is given by the output of the following program:

```
data a;
/****input data ***/
p0 = .23; p1 = .35; alpha = .05; power = .8;*power of the test;
/**** end of input data ***/
z1side = probit(1 - .05);*if 1 sided;
z2side = probit(1 - .05/2);*if 2 sided; zbeta = probit(power);
N1SIDE = floor((z1side*sqrt(p0*(1-p0)) + zbeta*sqrt(p1*(1-p1)))/
   (p1-p0)**2) +1;
N2SIDE = floor((z2side*sqrt(p0*(1-p0)) + zbeta*sqrt(p1*(1-p1)))/
   (p1-p0)**2) +1;
keep n1side n2side;proc print;run;
```

Output:

```
N1SIDE       N2SIDE
76           86
```

Seventy-six respondents are required in the study in a one-sided test, and 86 respondents for a two-sided test. Suppose $n = 86$ respondents are randomly selected and the presence of the disease among the respondents is determined as $n_1 = 35$. The p-value of the one-sided (two-sided) test is shown to be (b1)[(b2)] of the output of the following program. The claim is statistically supported if the p-value is less than α.

```
data a;
/**input data ***/
n = 86; n1 = 35; p0 = .23; alpha = .05;
/*** end of input data **/
PHAT = n1/n; z = (phat - p0)/sqrt(p0*(1-p0)/n); zabs = abs(z);
PVALUE1 = (1 - probnorm(z)); PVALUE2 = 2*(1 - probnorm(zabs));
keep phat pvalue1 pvalue2; proc print;run;
```

Output:

```
PHAT          PVALUE1                  PVALUE2
0.40698       0.000048111 (b1)         0.000096223 (b2)
```

Note that the variable PVALUE1 is the p-value when the alternative is $p > p_0$. As mentioned in Chapter 1, we will only refer to the right-side alternative for a one-sided test. Since the p-value for a two-sided test at (b2) is 0.000096 we reject the null hypothesis of $p = 0.23$.

Suppose, due to budgetary constraints, one can only get 50 individuals and wants to know what power one can get when $p_1 = 0.35$ while testing

H_0: $p_0 = 0.23$, using 0.05 level of significance. The power can be obtained by the following program:

```
data a;
/***input data ***/
n = 50; p0 = .23; p1 = .35; alpha = .05;
/*** end of input data **/
d = p1 - p0; z2side = probit (1 - alpha/2); z1side = probit (1 - alpha);
sep0 = sqrt (p0* (1 - p0) /n); sep1 = sqrt (p1* (1 - p1) /n);
POWER1 = 1 - probnorm ((z1side*sep0 - d) /sep1);
POWER2 = 1 - probnorm ((z2side*sep0 - abs (d)) /sep1);
keep power1 power2;proc print;run;
```

The output (c1) provides the power for a one-sided alternative and (c2) provides the power for a two-sided alternative.

```
POWER1                    POWER2
0.62844  (c1)             0.51982  (c2)
```

This power implies that by using a sample size of 50 subjects, the probability of rejecting a one-sided (or two-sided) alternative is 0.62844 (or 0.51982). The reduced sample size resulted in obtaining a smaller power than originally planned. One can also use PROC POWER to get these results.

2.1.2 t Categorical Responses

Sometimes an investigator selects a sample of n observations and classifies each observation into t nominal or ordinal categories obtaining the frequencies $n_1, n_2, \ldots, n_t$, in the t categories. Based upon her experience and knowledge of the problem, the scientist wants to test whether the data are in agreement with postulated hypothetical rates of $p_1 = p_{10}, p_2 = p_{20}, \ldots, p_t = p_{t0}$, where $\Sigma_i\ p_{i0} = 1$, and $p_1, p_2, \ldots, p_t$ are the proportions in the t categories. Sometimes $p_{10} = p_{20} = \ldots = p_{t0} = 1/t$ will be a null hypothesis of interest.

For example, the number of people borrowing books from a local library on 5 days of a given week is 200, 180, 170, 150, and 200 and we want to see whether the number of books borrowed is the same on each of the 5 days.

The p-value shown at (d1) of the output of the following program will be used to test the hypothesis and a p-value greater than α indicates that the observed frequencies are in agreement with postulated proportions.

```
data a;
input days freq@@;
cards;
1  200  2  180  3  170  4  150  5  200
;
data a;set a; proc freq order = data; weight freq;
tables days/nocum testp = (20 20 20 20 20);*hypothesized
distribution;run;
```

The output is as follows:

```
                                  ...
                        Chi-Square Test
                   for Specified Proportions
        --------------------------------------------------
        Chi-Square                      10.0000
        DF                              4
        Pr > ChiSq                      0.0404  (d1)
```

From the output, the p-value shown at (d1), 0.04 is less than 0.05 and hence we reject the null hypothesis and conclude that the number of people borrowing books on different days of the week is not the same.

2.2 Two Independent Samples

2.2.1 Two Proportions

In continuation of the binary data considered in Section 2.1.1, let the health scientist be interested in estimating the difference of the incidence rates of the disease for male and female populations. Let p_1 and p_2 be the incidence rates of the disease in male female populations, respectively. The sample sizes taken from the male and the female populations need to be determined to estimate $p_1 - p_2$. The scientist needs to specify the margin of error, d, and the probability that would validate the statement. Let $d = 0.03$ and $1 - \alpha = 0.95$. Usually, the sample sizes n_1 and n_2 are assumed equal. However, one can specify n_1/n_2 to be f. It is considered that $f = 1$, and hence $n_1 = n_2$. This needs to provide the estimated values $\tilde{p}_1$ and $\tilde{p}_2$ and if there is no information to assume, then $\tilde{p}_1 = 0.5$ and $\tilde{p}_2 = 0.5$. In this problem $\tilde{p}_1 = 0.5 = \tilde{p}_2$. The following program provides the sample sizes n_1 and n_2 as output.

```
data a;
/***input data***/
d = .03;*margin of error; alpha = .05; f = 1; ptilt1 = 0.5;
ptilt2 = 0.5;
/***end of input data ***/
z2side = probit(1-alpha/2); var = (d/z2side)**2;
N2 = floor((((ptilt1*(1-ptilt1)/f) + (ptilt2*(1-ptilt2)))/var) + 1;
N1 = n2*f;
proc print; var n1 n2; run;
```

The output is as follows:

```
N1    N2
2135  2135
```

TABLE 2.1

Incidence Rates of the Disease in Females and Males

| Outcome | Gender | | Total |
	Male	Female	
(a)			
No disease	1135 (53.2%)	1123 (52.6%)	2258
Disease	1000 (46.8%)	1012 (47.4%)	2012
Total	2135	2135	4270
(b)			
No disease	1861 (42.7%)	2361 (54.1%)	4222
Disease	2500 (57.3%)	2000 (45.9%)	4500
Total	4361	4361	8722
(c)			
No disease	5 (1.8%)	1 (4.8%)	6
Disease	275 (98.2%)	20 (95.2%)	295
Total	280	21	301

A random sample of $n_1 = 2135$ males and independently a random sample of $n_2 = 2135$ females are taken to determine the number of males and females affected by the disease. The artificial data are given in Table 2.1a.

Point estimate of $p_1 - p_2$ and a $(1 - \alpha)100\%$ CI for $p_1 - p_2$ based on the data of Table 2.1a can be determined using the following program:

```
Data a;
/****input data ****/
n1 = 2135; *sample size for 1st sample;
n2 = 2135; *sample size for 2nd sample; alpha = .05;
P1hat = 1000/n1; *proportion having the disease for 1st
   sample;
P2hat = 1012/n2; *proportion having the disease for 2nd
   sample;
/***end of input data ****/
z2side = probit(1 - alpha/2); DIFFPROP = p1hat - p2hat;
LOWER_CI = diffprop - z2side*(sqrt((p1hat*(1 - p1hat)/n1) +
         (p2hat*(1 - p2hat)/n2)));
UPPER_CI = diffprop + z2side*(sqrt((p1hat*(1 - p1hat)/n1) +
         (p2hat*(1 - p2hat)/n2)));
proc print; var lower_ci diffprop upper_ci; run;
```

The output is as follows:

```
    LOWER_CI            DIFFPROP              UPPER_CI
    -0.035564(e1)      -0.005620609(e2)      0.024323(e3)
```

From the output, the point estimate of $p_1 - p_2$ is -0.006 given at (e2). The 95% CI for $p_1 - p_2$ is $(-0.035, 0.0243)$ given at [(e1), (e3)] in the output. This CI covers zero and hence the null hypothesis, $p_1 = p_2$, will not be rejected with a 0.05 level two-sided test.

Instead of estimating the difference of incidence rates, $p_1 - p_2$, one may sometimes be interested in testing the hypothesis regarding p_1 and p_2. To perform a one-sided test or a two-sided test, we need to determine the sample sizes n_1 and n_2. To this end, we need the smallest clinical effect of interest, $d = p_1 - p_2$, the level of the test α, and the required power to obtain a significant result at d. We assume $n_1 = fn_2$, where f is often 1. Let us take $d = 0.03$, power $= 0.8$, $\alpha = 0.05$, and $f = 1$.

```
Data a;
/**input data ***/
alpha = 0.05; Power = 0.8; d = .03; f = 1;
/**end of input data**/
z2side = probit (1 - alpha/2); z1side = probit (1 - alpha);
zbeta = probit (power);
N21SIDE = floor ((((z1side + zbeta)/d)**2) * ((1/(4*f)) + 1/4)) + 1;
N22SIDE = floor ((((z2side + zbeta)/d)**2) * ((1/(4*f)) + 1/4)) + 1;
N11SIDE = n21side*f; N12SIDE = n22side*f;
proc print; var n11side n21side n12side n22side; run;
```

The sample sizes are on the liberal side because the presumed values $\tilde{p}_1$, $\tilde{p}_2$ are taken to be 0.5. These sample sizes may be more than needed and are given in the following output:

N11SIDE	N21SIDE	N12SIDE	N22SIDE
3435	3435	4361	4361

Now suppose samples of sizes $n_1 = 4361$, $n_2 = 4361$ are taken independently from the two populations for a two-sided test. Let the number of positive responses in the two samples be 2500 and 2000, respectively, as shown in Table 2.1b.

The following program, using normal approximation, provides the p-values at (f1), (f2) of the output. Note that the p-value for the two-sided test here is the same as the p-value at (g2) of the chi-square test given later in this section.

```
data a;
/***input data***/
yes1 = 2500; yes2 = 2000; *number of yes answers for groups 1
  and 2;
n1 = 4361; *sample size for group 1; n2 = 4361; *sample size for
  group 2;
/***end of input data**/
```

```
p1hat = yes1/n1; p2hat = yes2/n2; pcomb = (yes1 + yes2)/(n1 + n2);
z = (p1hat - p2hat)/(sqrt((pcomb*(1 - pcomb)/n1)+ (pcomb*(1 - pcomb)/
   n2))); zabs = abs(z); PVALUE1 = (1 - probnorm(Z));
PVALUE2 = 2*(1 - probnorm(zabs));
keep pvalue1 pvalue2; proc print; run;
```

We obtain the following output:

```
PVALUE1                   PVAUE2
0 (f1)                    0 (f2)
```

From (f2), the p-value is nearly 0, which is less than 0.05. Hence, we conclude that the proportion of males and females affected by the disease are different, based on a 0.05 level for the test.

The two-sided alternative can also be tested based on a chi-square test when the cell frequencies are large, and Fisher's exact test when the cell frequencies are small. The following program executes both tests and if there is a warning indicating that the expected cell frequency is less than 5, the p-value of Fisher's exact test is used to draw conclusions.

```
data a;
/*** input data***/
do OUTCOME = 0 to 1; do GENDER = 0 to 1;
input freq @@; output; end; end; cards;
1861  2361  2500  2000
;
/******end of input data ***/
data a; set a; proc freq; weight freq; tables outcome*gender/
   chisq; run;
```

The required output will appear as follows:

```
                              ***
              Statistics for Table of OUTCOME by GENDER
Statistic                          DF      Value              Prob
-----------------------------------------------------------------------

Chi-Square                          1    114.7692 (g1)     < .0001 (g2)
Likelihood Ratio Chi-Square         1    115.0233          < .0001
Continuity Adj. Chi-Square          1    114.3106          < .0001
Mantel-Haenszel Chi-Square          1    114.7560          < .0001
Phi Coefficient                          - 0.1147
Contingency Coefficient                    0.1140
Cramer's V                               - 0.1147 (g3)
                              ***
```

There is no warning in the output and hence the chi-square test is valid.

From the output, the chi-square value at (g1) has a p-value less than 0.0001 as seen by (g2), and since it is less than 0.05 the disease rate is not the same for males and females. Cramer's V, given at (g3), is −0.1147 and it measures the association between the categorical gender variables and incidence of disease. Larger values of V indicate stronger association. Cramer's V ranges from −1 to 1 for a 2×2 table and ranges from 0 to 1 for other contingency tables.

Suppose in another study, the number of males having the disease is small, say five subjects, and the number of females having the disease is also small, say one subject (see Table 2.1c). Then the chi-square test would be an inappropriate test, since the expected cell frequency is less than five and a warning is given in SAS. In this situation, one may use Fisher's exact test which calculates the exact probabilities.

Running the SAS code given for Table 2.1b on the Table 2.1c, we obtain the following output:

```
                              ***
WARNING: 25% of the cells have expected counts less than 5.
   Chi-Square may not be a valid test.
                      Fisher's Exact Test
   -------------------------------------------------------------
   Cell (1,1) Frequency (F)                 5
   Left-sided Pr <=  F                      0.3545 (h3)
   Right-sided Pr >=  F                     0.9413 (h2)

   Table Probability (P)                    0.2958
   Two-sided Pr <=  P                       0.3545 (h1)
```

By looking at the output, the *p*-value is 0.3545 as shown at (h1) and we retain the hypothesis of equal incidence rates of the disease for male and female subjects. One-sided *p*-values for Fisher's exact test are given in (h2) and (h3).

In the earlier example, if 4361 subjects are not available from each of the two samples and if only 2000 male and 2000 female subjects can be obtained for the study and, with a 0.05 level test, then one would like to know the power of the test when the difference in the incidence rates is $d = 0.03$. The following program provides that power.

```
Data a;
/****input data ****/
d= .03; *difference between the proportions; p1tilt= .5+ (d/2);
p2tilt= .5- (d/2);
n1= 2000; *sample size for 1st sample;
n2= 2000; *sample size for 2nd sample; alpha= .05;
/***end of input data ****/

z1side=probit(1-alpha); z2side=probit(1-alpha/2); n=n1+n2;
POWER1=1-probnorm((z1side*sqrt((1/4)*((1/n1)+(1/n2)))-d)/
       sqrt((p1tilt*(1-p1tilt)/n1)+(p2tilt*(1-p2tilt)/n2)));
POWER2=1-probnorm((z2side*sqrt((1/4)*((1/n1)+
```

```
          (1/n2)))-abs(d))/sqrt((p1tilt*(1-p1tilt)/n1) +
          (p2tilt*(1-p2tilt)/n2))); keep power1 power2;
proc print; run;
```

The output below provides the power for a one-sided test and a two-sided test.

```
     POWER1        POWER2
     0.59972       0.47503
```

PROC POWER can also be used to obtain these results.

2.2.2 Odds Ratio and Relative Risk

Some researchers, instead of considering the problem of two proportions, as discussed in Section 2.2.1, look upon it in terms of odds ratio. The odds ratio ranges from $(0, \infty)$. The odds ratio is equal to 1 when there is no association between the groups and the outcome of the event. If the odds ratio is greater (less) than 1, then the first group is more (less) likely to get the event than the second group. The objective is to compare the odds of a man (woman) contracting the disease to the odds of woman (man) contracting it.

To answer this question one adds "relrisk" after "chisq" as seen in the program below:

```
data a;
/***input data***/
do OUTCOME = 0 to 1;do GENDER = 0 to 1; input freq @@;
    output;end;end;cards;
1861  2361  2500  2000
;
/******end of input data ***/
data a;set a; proc freq; weight freq; tables gender*outcome/
  chisq relrisk;
*the rows are the groups (gender) and the columns are
  the dichotomous response (outcome); run;
```

By doing this on the data given earlier on testing two proportions, one gets the following additional output, in addition to the previous output.

```
                             ***
Statistics for Table of GENDER by OUTCOME
Estimates of the Relative Risk (Row1/Row2)
Type of Study                      Value          95% Confidence
                                                     Limits
-----------------------------------------------------------------
Case-Control (Odds Ratio)  0.6306(i1)     0.5795(i2)   0.6862(i3)
Cohort (Col1 Risk)            0.7882         0.7544       0.8236
Cohort (Col2 Risk)         1.2500(i4)     1.1996(i5)   1.3025(i6)
```

From the output, (i1) provides the odds ratio of not having the disease for a male as 0.6306 times that of a female. This implies that the odds ratio of having the disease for a male was $1/0.6306 = 1.59$ times that of a female. The 95% CI on the odds ratio of 0.6306 is [(i2), (i3)] of the output and is (0.5795, 0.6862). By looking at the 95% CI, we note that it does not include 1; hence, there is a difference between the odds of (not) having the disease for male and female subjects. If the 95% CI had included 1, then we could have concluded that there is no difference in the odds of (not) having the disease for male and female subjects.

Note that if we want to know the odds of (not) having the disease for female over male subjects then we interchange the two columns on the data statement. Also it does not matter which row or column corresponds to the response variable, since it will provide the same odds ratio whether the response variable is a row or a column.

When the dichotomous variable indicates the risk of developing a disease within the two groups, we use the relative risk to indicate the proportions of developing the disease in the two groups. If the condition refers to the prevalence, then we interpret the relative risk as prevalence ratio. This quantity is given in the row corresponding to the positive condition (in the example it is row 2) in the table. In the output, the columns are the rows of Table 2.1b and in (i4) we obtain 1.25 indicating that the ratio of the condition in male and female subjects is 1.25. The 95% CI for this ratio is given at [(i5), (i6)] and is (1.2, 1.3).

2.2.3 Logistic Regression with One Dichotomous Explanatory Variable

To find the relationship between the explanatory variable, like treatment groups or gender and the dichotomous outcome of the response variable, which in this case is having a disease or not having a disease, we may use logistic regression. The outcome variable is coded as "1" for having a disease and "0" for not having a disease. This provides an estimate of the chance of having the disease given the explanatory variable(s). PROC LOGISTIC, PROC CATMOD, or PROC GENMOD can be used to fit a logistic regression equation. We will be discussing PROC LOGISTIC in this chapter and for other procedures, see SAS manual. In this discussion we will assume that the logistic model fits the data and for details of the goodness-of-fit of the model refer to Allison (1999).

For the data given in Table 2.1b, the following program provides the output for the logistic regression.

```
data a;
/***input data***/
do OUTCOME = 0 to 1;do GENDER = 0 to 1;
input freq @@;output;end;end;cards;
1861  2361  2500  2000
;
/******end of input data ***/
```

```
data a;set a;
proc logistic descending; *By using the descending option, the
   model gives the probability of the outcome. If it is not
   used the probability obtained is for the non-occurrence of
   the event;
freq freq; model outcome = gender; run;
```

The required output is as follows:

★★★

The LOGISTIC Procedure
Analysis of Maximum Likelihood Estimates

Parameter	DF	Estimate	Standard Error	Wald Chi-Square	Pr > ChiSq
Intercept	1	0.2952(j6)	0.0306	92.9531	<0.0001
GENDER	1	−0.4611(j7)	0.0431	114.2604	<0.0001(j1)

Odds Ratio Estimates

Effect	Point Estimate	95% Wald Confidence Limits	
GENDER	0.631 (j2)	0.579 (j3)	0.686 (j4)

Association of Predicted Probabilities and Observed Responses

Percent Concordant	31.1	Somers' D	0.115
Percent Discordant	19.6	Gamma	0.227
Percent Tied	49.3	Tau-a	0.057
Pairs	18999000	c	0.557 (j5)

The *p*-value of <0.001 shown in (j1) in the output indicates that the probability of contracting the disease is not the same for the two genders. The probability of the event can be modeled as

$$P = \frac{\exp(0.2952 + (-0.4611)*\text{gender})}{1 + \exp(0.2952 + (-0.4611)*\text{gender})},$$

where 0.2952 and −0.4611 are given at (j6) and (j7), and gender equals 0 or 1 depending on whether the individual is a male or female.

One may also notice the odds ratio estimate given at (j2), in the output is identical to the odds ratio calculated using the chi-square (i1). The CI on the odds ratio is at [(j3), (j4)] is the same as [(i2), (i3)] given earlier. As R^2 indicates the goodness-of-fit of a linear regression model, the *c*-statistic indicated at (j5) in the output, measures the goodness-of-fit (or association) of the logistic regression model and a value more than 0.7 is usually considered to provide a reasonable fit. The c-statistic can be interpreted as the percentage of possible cases in which the model assigns the higher probability to a correct case rather than to an incorrect case and ranges from 0.5 to 1.0. In this case, c-statistic given at (j5) is 0.557 and is not a very good fit. Other measures of association are given in Chapter 5.

If there are other covariates to be considered for the incidence of the disease, the model in the program should be modified to include other variables and the output will have more terms; for further details see Chapter 5.

2.2.4 Cochran–Mantel–Haenszel Test for a 2 × 2 Table

Sometimes the binary data discussed earlier may be available from different strata, such as centers, different age groups, cities, and so on. Then one would like to test the equality of incidence rates adjusted for strata. This is achieved by the Cochran–Mantel–Haenszel (CMH) test as discussed in this section.

This test will also be used in clinical trials when two treatments are compared with a binary endpoint in different centers. Although this test can be used with only one stratum, however, it is more useful to draw conclusions adjusting for more than one stratum. We will motivate the problem in the context of a market research study.

Suppose a marketing researcher wanted to know by collecting data from different cities whether advertising on prime time TV sold more of a product than by not advertising at all. In problems such as this, where one has k strata for a 2 × 2 table and wants to adjust for the strata, the CMH test is used. This test can also be used for an $I \times J$ table (see Section 2.4). In this example, we code 1(0) for sold (not sold) more than expected, and use 1(0) for ad (no ad). Let us consider two cities with the data shown in Table 2.2.

```
data a;
/***input data***/
do city = 0 to 1;do ad = 0 to 1; do soldmore = 0 to 1;
input freq @@;output;end;end;end;cards;
8  10  13  5  6  10  10  10
;
data b;set a; proc sort;by city; proc freq;weight freq;
tables city*ad*soldmore/cmh;run;
```

TABLE 2.2

Effect of Advertisement of Sales in Cities

	City 1		City 2	
	Sold	Not Sold	Sold	Not Sold
Ad	8	10	6	10
No Ad	13	5	10	10

The required output is as follows:

```
                                  ***
                 Summary Statistics for AD by SOLDMORE
                           Controlling for CITY
          Cochran-Mantel-Haenszel Statistics (Based on Table Scores)
      Statistic   Alternative Hypothesis   DF     Value          Prob
      ------------------------------------------------------------------
      1              Nonzero Correlation      1    2.8930(k1)  0.0890(k2)
                                  ***


              Estimates of the Common Relative Risk (Row1/Row2)
      Type of Study       Method         Value    95% Confidence Limits
      ------------------------------------------------------------------
      Case-Control Mantel-Haenszel 0.4348(k3)  0.1669(k4)  1.1329(k5)
      (Odds Ratio) Logit             0.4349      0.1659      1.1402
                                  ***


                          Breslow-Day Test for
                        Homogeneity of the Odds Ratios
                        -----------------------------------
                    Chi-Square                0.4617(k6)
                    DF                        1
                    Pr > ChiSq                0.4968(k7)
```

We first test the homogeneity of the odds ratio in different strata. At the bottom of the output there is a Breslow–Day test, which tests the null hypothesis that the odds ratios for the strata are the same (Breslow and Day, 1980). Breslow–Day test requires a large sample size and is independent of the CMH test. The test statistic is a chi-square with a value of 0.4617 given at (k6) and the associated p-value is 0.4968 given at (k7) of the output, indicating that the odds ratios are the same for the two cities.

When the homogeneity of the odds ratio is not rejected, one can combine the odds ratios adjusted for the strata (cities in the example) based on the CMH statistic. The combined odds ratio is 0.4348 given at (k3) and its 95% CI [(k4), (k5)] is given by (0.1669, 1.1329) from the output. If the homogeneity of the odds ratio is rejected, then the individual stratum odds ratio should be interpreted instead of the combined odds ratio.

The CMH test statistic is 2.893 given at (k1), with a p-value of 0.0890 given at (k2). This test statistic has been adjusted for city differences and compares the sales proportion with and without prime time TV advertisement. Since this p-value is not less than $\alpha = 0.05$, we conclude that sales are similar with and without prime time TV advertisement, after adjusting for cities.

If the responses in the strata are going in opposite directions, then the trend is not as strong as it should be and the conclusions should be drawn cautiously and one should examine the individual tables (see Stokes et al., 1995).

2.2.5 *t* Categorical Responses

With two samples, the response from each individual may be one of the *t* categorical responses. The categorical responses may be ordered or unordered. If they are ordered, we use the Wilcoxon test as discussed in Chapter 4, or Row Mean Score Statistic as discussed in Section 2.6.1, or Cochran–Armitage trend test given in Section 2.6.2, or Ridit Analysis as discussed in Section 2.6.4. If the responses are unordered, one can use the chi-square test as discussed in this section.

One-hundred male and 100 female subjects were asked about their preference on four brands A, B, C, D and no preference (E) of a product and artificial data of the choices are shown in Table 2.3.

With the help of the following program we want to ascertain whether the proportions in each response category are the same for both males and females.

```
data a;
/*** input data***/
do GENDER = 0 to 1;do BRAND = 1 to 5; input count @@;
  output;end;end;cards;
10  15  10  25  40  5  10  10  40  35
;
/******end of input data ***/
data a;set a; proc freq;weight count; tables gender*brand/
  chisq;run;
```

The *p*-value for the test is given at (11) of the following output and is 0.1672 indicating that there is no gender difference. Cramer's *V* at (12) can be interpreted as given in Section 2.2.1.

TABLE 2.3

Artificial Data on Preference of Four Brands by Males and Females

Gender	Brand					Total
	A	B	C	D	E	
Males	10	15	10	25	40	100
Females	5	10	10	40	35	100
Total	15	25	20	65	75	200

```
                                   * * *
                Statistics for Table of GENDER by BRAND
Statistic                           DF       Value              Prob
--------------------------------------------------------------------
Chi-Square                          4        6.4615           0.1672  (11)
Likelihood Ratio Chi-Square         4        6.5323           0.1628
Mantel-Haenszel Chi-Square          1        1.2360           0.2662
Phi Coefficient                              0.1797
Contingency Coefficient                      0.1769
Cramer's V                                   0.1797  (12)
```

One can also use the "cmh" option instead of "chisq" as given below:

```
tables gender*brand/cmh;
```

and interpret the General Association Statistic.

2.3 Paired Two Samples

2.3.1 Binary Responses

Let us consider Instructors A and B passing or failing the same student for two classes. This is the analysis of paired data since we are analyzing the results on the same person by two different instructors. Other examples include analyzing twins for a characteristic, having an assessment of a disease by two different clinicians, determining first and the second place for a pie bake-off by two judges, and especially other case-control studies.

Let $p_1(p_2)$ be the probability that a student passes courses with instructor A(B). The null hypothesis, H_0, of interest here is H_0: $p_1 = p_2$ against the alternative H_A: $p_1 \neq p_2$. Testing this null hypothesis reduces to comparing the two off-diagonal entries (discordant responses) in the 2×2 table, Table 2.4. This test is known as McNemar test and is used for large samples. For the artificial

TABLE 2.4

Paired Data Analyses

	Instructor A		
Instructor B	Passes	Fails	Total
Passes	125	75	200
Fails	275	20	295
Total	400	95	495

data given in Table 2.4, the following program provides the necessary output:

```
data a;
/*****input data**/
do INST2 = 0 to 1;do INST1 = 0 to 1; input freq @@;
  output;end;end;cards;
125  75  275  20
;
/******end of input data ***/
data a;set a;proc freq;weight freq;
tables inst2*inst1/agree; test kappa; run;
```

We obtain the following output:

```
                            ***
                      McNemar's Test
            -----------------------------------
            Statistic (S)            114.2857 (m1)
            DF                           1
            Pr > S                    < 0.0001 (m2)

                  Simple Kappa Coefficient
            -----------------------------------
            Kappa                       -0.2646 (m3)
            ASE                          0.0349
            95% Lower Conf Limit        -0.3331 (m4)
            95% Upper Conf Limit        -0.1961 (m5)

                   Test of H0: Kappa = 0
            ASE under H0                 0.0311
            Z                           -8.5165
            One-sided Pr < Z            <0.0001
            Two-sided Pr > |Z|          <0.0001 (m6)
                            ***
```

The McNemar test is used in these problems and the test statistic (S) is denoted by (m1), 114.2857 and the p-value is <0.0001 given at (m2). Since this p-value is less than $\alpha = 0.05$, we conclude that the passing rates of both instructors are not the same.

To find the CI for $p_1 - p_2$ in the case of paired samples we can use the discordant responses in the following program which provides a CI for the difference in the proportions of passing rates by the two instructors.

```
data b;
/***input data***/
n = 495; alpha = .05;
passa = 275;*instructor a pass and instructor b fail;
passb = 75;*instructor b pass and instructor a fail;
/***end of input data***/
DIFF = (passa - passb)/n; se = (sqrt(passa + passb))/n;
z2side = probit(1 - alpha/2);
UPPER_CI = diff + se*z2side; LOWER_CI = diff - se*z2side;
proc print; var lower_ci diff upper_ci; run;
```

The output is as follows:

```
   LOWER_CI           DIFF            UPPER_CI
   0.32996 (m8)      0.40404 (m7)     0.47812 (m9)
```

The difference in the proportions of passing rates by Instructor A and Instructor B is given by (m7) and is 0.40404. A 95% CI for this difference in the proportions is given at [(m8), (m9)] and in (0.32996, 0.47812).

A measure of agreement of the instructors is given by kappa. Landis and Koch (1977) have provided a table indicating the strength of the agreement to the kappa value. The farther the kappa coefficient is from zero, the larger is the (dis)agreement of the two variables. A kappa value above 0.8 (0.4) is usually considered as an almost perfect (moderate) agreement of the two judges.

In the output of the program (m3) is kappa, and is −0.2646. This tells us that the agreement of the Instructors A and B and rating of the students is less than moderate. The 95% CI on kappa is from (m4) to (m5) of the output and is (−0.3331, −0.1961). Testing for kappa = 0 is based on the *p*-value (m6) for a two-sided test and is less than 0.0001, indicating the conclusion that kappa ≠ 0 at 0.05 significance level. Kappa = 0 implies that the two instructors are independently grading the students.

2.3.2 *t* Categorical Responses

Suppose the head of a hospital wanted to know if both the assisting staff are evaluating the progression of the disease in patients in a similar way. It is decided to create three categories of progression (slow progression, average progression, and fast progression). Clinicians 1 and 2 were asked to evaluate 310 subjects, and the artificial data are given in Table 2.5.

By generalizing the McNemar test, we would like to evaluate whether clinicians 1 and 2 agree on the proportions in the same categories of the disease progression. For this test, a similar code as given in Section 2.3.1 provides the following output.

TABLE 2.5

Evaluations by Two Clinicians

	Clinician 1			
Clinician 2	Slow	Average	Fast	Total
Slow	20	30	40	90
Average	30	40	30	100
Fast	30	50	40	120
Total	80	120	110	310

```
                            ***
       Statistics for Table of CLIN2 by CLIN1
                   Test of Symmetry
       ------------------------------------------

       Statistic (S)                 6.4286
       DF                            3
       Pr > S                        0.0925 (n1)


                  Simple Kappa Coefficient
       ------------------------------------------

       Kappa                         -0.0220 (n2)
       ASE                           0.0394
       95% Lower Conf Limit          -0.0993
       95% Upper Conf Limit          0.0553

                  Test of H0: Kappa = 0
       ASE under H0                     0.0401
       Z                               -0.5478
       One-sided Pr < Z                 0.2919 (n3)
       Two-sided Pr > |Z|               0.5838 (n4)
                            ***
```

The probability 0.0925 given at (n1) is the *p*-value to test the symmetry between the two clinicians (see Bowker, 1948). This symmetry implies that clinicians 1 and 2 classifying the subjects into (i, j) categories is the same as clinician 1 and 2 classifying the subjects as (j, i) categories. This *p*-value is not significant and hence there is symmetry in the clinicians' judgment.

The kappa coefficient −0.022 given at (n2) measures the agreement between the clinicians 1 and 2 is purely coincidence or a real agreement and interpretation can be made as given in Section 2.3.1. In this case, the *p*-values at (n3) and (n4) are not significant and we conclude that the clinicians' agreement is a coincidence.

For ordinal data, weighted kappa will be used to determine the agreement of the two clinicians (judges). It is also useful in certain settings where one clinician's ratings are more important than another clinician's rating. We will return to this topic in Section 2.6.5.

2.4 *k* Independent Samples

2.4.1 *k* Proportions

Suppose we want to know whether the proportions of subjects affected by a disease in three different races are the same. The artificial data are provided in Table 2.6.

By using the same program for chi-square test as shown in Section 2.2.1 we obtain the following output.

```
            Statistics for Table of DISEASE by RACE
Statistic                         DF    Value          Prob
-------------------------------------------------------------
Chi-Square                         2    1.6713         0.4336 (o1)
Likelihood Ratio Chi-Square        2    1.6819         0.4313
Mantel-Haenszel Chi-Square         1    1.5751         0.2095
Phi Coefficient                         0.0641
Contingency Coefficient                 0.0639
Cramer's V                              0.0641 (o2)
```

Looking at (o1) of the output the *p*-value for a chi-square test is 0.4336 and is nonsignificant as it is greater than 0.05. We conclude that there is no evidence to indicate that the incidence rates of the disease are not all same in the three races. The coefficient of association, Cramer's V at (o2), is 0.0641 is very low indicating that there is no association between race and incidence of the disease.

TABLE 2.6

Incidence Rates of Disease for Three Races

Outcome	Race			Total
	White	Black	Other	
No disease	44 (34.6%)	60 (40.0%)	55 (42.3%)	159
Disease	83 (65.4%)	90 (60.0%)	75 (57.7%)	248
Total	127	150	130	407

If the incidence rates were small as described in Section 2.2.1, then SAS puts a warning. However, unlike the 2×2 table, SAS does not display the p-value of Fisher's exact test. One can ask for this test by replacing the "chisq" statement with the "exact" statement as shown below:

```
proc freq;tables variable1*variable2/exact;
```

and obtain the following output for the data in Table 2.6.

```
                            ***
                    Fisher's Exact Test
         ------------------------------------------
         Table Probability (P)      0.0037
         Pr <= P                    0.4330 (p1)
```

The p-value indicated at (p1) will be used to draw the conclusion. Note that for large samples (o1) and (p1) will be nearly equal.

2.4.2 Logistic Regression When the Explanatory Variable Is Not Dichotomous

A clinician was in doubt whether three cities would differ in the outcome of death, of seriously ill patients for a new virus. The data are given in Table 2.7.

For a logistic model when the explanatory variable has t categories, one needs to create $t - 1$ dummy variables, for more details on the use of dummy variables see Section 5.3. Since there are three cities in the example, we use two dummy variables and coded City 1 as 0 0, City 2 as 1 0, and City 3 as 0 1. The following program produces the necessary output.

TABLE 2.7

Incidence of Death for the Three Cities

| Outcome | City | | | Total |
	City 1	City 2	City 3	
No death	15(62.5%)	4(10.8%)	13(56.5%)	32
Death	9(37.5%)	33(89.2%)	10(43.5%)	52
Total	24(28.6%)	37(44.0%)	23(27.4%)	84

```
data a;
/*****input data**/
do dth = 0 to 1; do city = 1 to 3;
input freq @@; output; end; end; cards;
15   4   13   9   33   10
;
/******end of input data ***/

data a1; set a;
if city = 1 then do; Z1 = 0; Z2 = 0; end;
if city = 2 then do; z1 = 1; z2 = 0; end;
if city = 3 then do; z1 = 0; z2 = 1; end;
proc logistic descending; freq freq; model dth = z1 z2; run;
```

The necessary output is

***

The LOGISTIC Procedure
Analysis of Maximum Likelihood Estimates

Parameter	DF	Standard Estimate	Error	Wald Chi-Square	Pr > ChiSq
Intercept	1	-0.5108	0.4216	1.4678	0.2257
Z1	1	2.6210	0.6768	14.9970	0.0001 (q1)
Z2	1	0.2485	0.5956	0.1740	0.6765 (q2)

Odds Ratio Estimates

Effect	Point Estimate	95% Wald Confidence Limits	
Z1	13.750 (q4)	3.649 (q5)	51.809 (q6)
Z2	1.282 (q7)	0.399 (q8)	4.120 (q9)

Association of Predicted Probabilities and Observed Responses

Percent Concordant	64.5	Somers' D	0.529
Percent Discordant	11.6	Gamma	0.695
Percent Tied	23.9	Tau-a	0.253
Pairs	1664	c	0.765 (q3)

In the output, the p-value corresponding to Z1 given at (q1) is the p-value comparing cities 1 and 2, and the p-value corresponding to Z2 given at (q2) is the p-value comparing cities 1 and 3. In this case we conclude that cities 1 and 2 have different death rates, while cities 1 and 3 do not have different death rates, using the 0.05 level test. If the interest is in comparing the death rates of cities 2 and 3, the coding of the dummy variables can be easily modified. The goodness-of-fit is indicated by c at (q3) and this can be used as discussed earlier to determine the model fit. The odds ratio point estimate 13.750 given at (q4) in the line of Z1 is the odds of no death in City 1 versus City 2 and the other estimate (q7) can be similarly interpreted for cities 1 and 3. The CI for the odds ratio with estimate given at (q4) is (3.6, 51.8) given in [(q5), (q6)]. The CI for the odds ratio with estimate given at (q7) is (0.4, 4.1) given at [(q8), (q9)].

2.4.3 CMH Test

Suppose an exercise trainer was wondering which exercising technique works best. The trainer considers three groups. The first group only does aerobic exercises. The second group only lifts weights. The third group does both aerobics and lifts weights. The trainer randomly selected 185 females and 158 males. A person who lost at least 10 pounds in 6 weeks was considered a success and given the value 1; otherwise, the outcome of failure is given the value 0. The following program provides the results needed by the trainer for the artificial data given in Table 2.8.

```
data a;
/***input data***/
do GENDER=0 to 1;do OUTCOME=0 to 1;do EXERCISE =0 to 2;
input freq @@;output;end;end;end;cards;
21  23  34  43  32  32  24  33  20  26  27  28
;
/***end of input data***/
data a;set a; proc freq;weight freq;
  tables gender*outcome*exercise/cmh;run;
```

Output:

```
                              ***
          Summary Statistics for OUTCOME by EXERCISE
                      Controlling for GENDER
  Cochran-Mantel-Haenszel Statistics (Based on Table Scores)
```

TABLE 2.8

Outcome of Exercise Groups Based on Gender

		Exercise			
Gender	**Outcome**	**Group 1**	**Group 2**	**Group 3**	**Total**
Female	Failure	21	23	34	78
	Success	43	32	32	107
	Total	64	55	66	185
Male	Failure	24	33	20	77
	Success	26	27	28	81
	Total	50	60	48	158

```
Statistic  Alternative Hypothesis   DF  Value        Prob
-----------------------------------------------------------------
1          Nonzero Correlation       1   1.4757(r1)  0.2244(r2)
2          Row Mean Scores Differ    1   1.4757      0.2244(r4)
3          General Association (r3)  2   2.1498      0.3413
```

By looking at the output, the CMH statistic given at (r1) is 1.4757 and the associated *p*-value given at (r2) is 0.2244. The statistic is not significant and the trainer concludes that all the three methods are similar for weight reduction, adjusting for gender.

If the two variables of the contingency table are on a nominal scale, the general association measure (r3), is used to draw the inference about the association or independence of the classification variables. The row mean square difference test at (r4) is used when one variable has an ordinal scale and we will discuss this in Section 2.6.

2.4.4 *t* Categorical Responses

The artificial data on the preference of car brands by people of different races are given in Table 2.9. If ordered categories, instead of car brands, are considered then the Kruskal–Wallis test given in Section 4.4 is appropriate. In this problem, the hypothesis of interest is that three races have the same car brand preference proportions. No brand preference is denoted by E.

The necessary program is given below:

```
data a;
/***input data***/
do RACE = 1 to 3;do BRANDS = 1 to 5; input freq @@;
  output;end;end;cards;
5  8  25  7  6  6  6  18  5  5  10  20  16  7  7
;
/***end of input data***/
data a;set a;proc freq;weight freq; tables race*brands/
  chisq;run;
```

TABLE 2.9

Preference of Car Brands by Race

Race	Car Brands					Total
	A	B	C	D	E	
Black	5	8	25	7	6	51
White	6	6	18	5	5	40
Other	10	20	16	7	7	60
Total	21	34	59	19	18	151

The output is as follows:

```
                              ***
                Statistics for Table of RACE by BRANDS
Statistic                          DF     Value          Prob
-----------------------------------------------------------------
Chi-Square                          8     10.2817        0.2458(s1)
Likelihood Ratio Chi-Square         8     10.3734        0.2398
Mantel-Haenszel Chi-Square          1      2.3161        0.1280
Phi Coefficient                            0.2609
Contingency Coefficient                    0.2525
Cramer's V                                 0.1845(s2)
```

In the output, (s1) provides the p-value for the chi-square test and is 0.2458. We conclude that the preference proportions are not different for the three races. An association measure between the categorical variables race and brand preference is given by Cramer's V at (s2) and is 0.1845. These data can be analyzed by using the CMH option as given in Section 2.4 and the general association label given in SAS output provides the chi-square statistic and the p-value. This is the case where both the variables (car brand and race) are on a nominal scale.

2.5 Cochran's Test

When the efficacy of a new treatment has to be evaluated, we match pairs of patients based on demographic variables and randomly assign treatment to one patient and placebo to the other patient in each pair. If the response is binary, the methods of Section 2.4 will be used to draw a conclusion. Sometimes t different treatments including placebo, where $t > 2$, have to be tested for equal effects. In that case we match t patients to form blocks of size t, and in each block patients will be randomly assigned to the treatments using one replication for each treatment in each block. If the response is binary, Cochran's test will be used to test that the effects of the treatments are the same. Alternatively, suppose we take t binary responses on each of the n randomly selected patients, then the equal proportions for the t responses will be tested by Cochran's test.

Suppose a given model car is evaluated by 10 volunteers for roominess (roomy = 1, tight = 0), looks (sharp = 1, dull = 0), gas mileage (good = 1, bad = 0), and reliability (reliable = 1, unreliable = 0). Table 2.10 provides artificial data for the car evaluations. In this example volunteers are blocks and categories for evaluation are the treatments.

To test the hypothesis of equality of the proportions of roomy, good looks, good gas mileage and reliability, we can run the following program and (t1) in the output gives the p-value for the test.

TABLE 2.10

Artificial Evaluation of Four Characteristics of a Car by 10 Volunteers

| Volunteer | Car Evaluation | | | | Total |
	Roominess	Looks	Gas	Reliability	
1	1	0	1	1	3
2	0	1	0	0	1
3	0	1	1	1	3
4	1	1	0	1	3
5	0	1	1	0	2
6	1	1	1	1	4
7	0	0	1	1	2
8	1	1	1	0	3
9	0	0	1	1	2
10	1	1	0	0	2
Total	5	7	7	6	25

```
data a;
input volunteer roominess looks gasmileage reliability @@;
cards;
1 1 0 1 1 2 0 1 0 0 3 0 1 1 1 4 1 1 0 1
5 0 1 1 0 6 1 1 1 1 7 0 0 1 1 8 1 1 1 0
9 0 0 1 1 10 1 1 0 0
;
proc freq;tables roominess*looks*gasmileage*reliability/agree;run;
```

```
                          ***
                  Cochran's Q, for
              roominess by looks, by
                  gas mileage, by
                    reliability
        ----------------------------------------
        Statistic(Q)                 1.0645
        DF                           3
        Pr > Q                       0.7856  (t1)
```

The *p*-value from the output given at (t1) is 0.7856 and we conclude that the proportions of the four characteristics are not different.

2.6 Ordinal Data

2.6.1 Row Mean Score Test

Suppose 230 males and females were recruited to watch the pilot of a new TV show before it aired and rate the show as bad, average, or excellent. Suppose the

TABLE 2.11

Rating of Pilot TV Show based on Gender

Gender		Ratings		Total
	Bad	Average	Excellent	
Female	45(36%)	55(44%)	25(20%)	125
Male	55(52.4%)	35(33.3%)	15(14.3%)	105
Total	100(43.5%)	90(39.1%)	40(17.4%)	230

producer of this show was curious if the males and females judged the show similarly. Since the data follow some ordering, excellent being first, average being second, and bad being third, a regular chi-square test is inappropriate. In this case one can use a row mean score test (see Mantel, 1963) as discussed in this section, or Cochran–Armitage trend test discussed in Section 2.6.2, or Wilcoxon test described in Chapter 4. The artificial data are given in Table 2.11.

The following program gives the output for the row mean score test. This test has the flexibility of attaching equal or unequal scores to the ordinal variable data. If the values are not attached, the default values are assumed equally spaced. The choice of scores is discussed in Stokes et al. (1995).

```
data a;
/***input data***/
do GENDER = 0 to 1;do RATING = 0 to 2;
input freq @@;output;end;end;cards;
45  55  25  55  35  15
;
data a;set a; proc freq;weight freq; tables gender*rating/
   cmh;run;
```

This will then produce the following output:

```
                              ***
              Summary Statistics for GENDER by RATING
      Cochran-Mantel-Haenszel Statistics (Based on Table Scores)

  Statistic  Alternative Hypothesis   DF   Value    Prob
  -------------------------------------------------------------
  1          Nonzero Correlation       1   5.1306   0.0235
  2          Row Mean Scores Differ    1   5.1306   0.0235 (u1)
  3          General Association       2   6.2254   0.0445
```

The *p*-value given at (u1) is 0.0235, and is significant. Thus, the trends in TV ratings are not the same for males and females.

The above row mean scores test statistic and *p*-value obtained in the output can also be obtained by changing the "cmh" option to "chisq" option in the previous programming line. The Mantel–Haenszel test statistic obtained from the chi-square output, is the same as the row mean scores test.

2.6.2 Cochran–Armitage Test

In Cochran–Armitage Test, the ordinal variable is shown across the rows for the two groups thus giving a $t \times 2$ table, where t is the number of ordinal categories. The purpose here is to see whether there is a trend in both the groups. We use the same data of Table 2.11 interchanging the rows and columns to describe this test. This test can be easily obtained from the SAS by adding "trend" at the end of the PROC FREQ programming line.

```
data a;
/***input data***/
do RATING = 0 to 2;do GENDER = 0 to 1;
input freq @@;output;end;end;cards;
45  55  55  35  25  15
;
data a;set a; proc freq;weight freq;
tables rating*gender/trend;run;
```

This will then produce the following output:

```
                              ***
            Statistics for Table of GENDER by RATING
                  Cochran-Armitage Trend Test
      - - - - - - - - - - - - - - - - - - - - - - - - - - - - -
        Statistic (Z)                    2.2700
        One-sided Pr > Z                 0.0116 (v1)
        Two-sided Pr > |Z|               0.0232 (v2)
```

The two-sided p-value given at (v2) is 0.0232, and is significant. Thus, the trends of TV ratings are not the same for males and females. If a one-sided test is of interest then we use the p-value given at (v1). One can also use the CMH option and look at the nonzero correlation to draw this conclusion.

If the ordering of the responses is inconsequential, then the chi-square test of Section 2.2 could have been used.

2.6.3 Measures of Association

Now suppose the producer of the TV wanted to see if the two variables were associated with one another. Since the categories of one variable are ordered, we will not use Cramer's V as before. The commonly used measures of association for ordered variables in this context are Gamma, Kendalls τ, and Spearman's correlation and are obtained if we add "measures" to the PROC FREQ procedure as below:

```
proc freq; weight freq; tables gender*rating/measures;run;
```

The output is as follows:

```
                               ***
         Statistics for Table of GENDER by RATING
    Statistic                    Value            ASE
    -------------------------------------------------------
    Gamma                       -0.2635(w1)      0.1069(w4)
    Kendall's Tau-b             -0.1490(w2)      0.0619(w5)
    Stuart's Tau-c              -0.1664          0.0691
    Somers' D C|R               -0.1676          0.0696
    Somers' D R|C               -0.1325          0.0551
    Pearson Correlation         -0.1497          0.0649
    Spearman Correlation        -0.1566(w3)      0.0650(w6)
                               ***
```

The gamma ranges from –1 to 1. When both the variables are ordinals and follow the same sort of agreement then we say that both the variables follow a linear relationship. The closer the gamma value is to ±1, the more linear are the data. In this setting, tied pairs are ignored.

Kendalls Tau given at (w2) is –0.1490. It is based on the concordant and discordant responses of every pair of variables. The concordant responses go in the same direction and the discordant responses go in different directions. In the example, a female rating a show bad and a man rating a show excellent is a concordant pair; whereas a woman rating a show excellent and a man rating a show average is a discordant pair. A positive Tau indicates more concordant pairs of responses, whereas a negative Tau indicates more discordant pairs. Tau considers these concordant and discordant responses and provides a measure of association between the variables and is between –1 and 1. This is similar to the gamma; however, it uses a correction for ties. The gamma given at (w1) of the output has a value of –0.2635, indicating a weak tendency that male subjects score the TV show lower than the female subjects.

The Spearman correlation can also be used to measure the association. The Spearman correlation like the gamma is between –1 and 1, with correlation of 0 being no association. If the variables increase or decrease together, then there is a positive correlation. If the variables go in opposite directions, there is a negative correlation. This correlation coefficient is computed using ranks. The Spearman correlation given at (w3) of the output is –0.1566.

The ASE for testing Gamma, Kendall's Tau, and Spearman correlation to be zero is given at (w4), (w5), and (w6). The statistics are significant if their values are more than 2*ASE of the statistic, or smaller than (–2)*ASE.

2.6.4 Ridit Analysis

When ordinal data are available from two samples, the equality of the distributions of the two samples can be tested nonparametrically by using the

Wilcoxon test as discussed in Chapter 4 or by a ridit analysis (Bross, 1958) as discussed here. One of the samples can be taken as a reference sample and another sample can be taken as the test sample. Both the samples should have the same number of categories for the ordinal data. The ridits are calculated from the reference sample. The ridit for a category is the proportion of half the observations belonging to that category and the sum of the observations belonging to the lower categories. The test sample is tested against the ridits. Consider the data given in Table 2.11. The following program provides the *p*-value at (x1) for testing the equality of the distributions for the two samples. From the output, the required *p*-value is less than $\alpha = 0.05$. Hence, the distribution of ratings by male and female subjects is not the same.

```
data a;
/***input data***/
*reference sample;
input refsamp@@; cards;
45  55  25
;
/***end of input data***/
data a1;set a; count = _n_;refhalf = refsamp/2; proc sort; run;
data a2;set a1; if count = 1 then refcum = refsamp; else
  refcum + refsamp;
reflag = lag(refcum); if reflag = . then reflag = 0;
refsum = reflag + refhalf;a = 1;
keep refsamp refsum a;proc sort;by a;
data b;
/***input data***/
*Test sample;
input testsamp@@; cards;
55  35  15
;
data b1;set b; a = 1;proc sort;by a;
data final;merge a2 b1;by a;drop a;
prod1 = testsamp*refsum;prod2 = (refsamp + testsamp)**3;
proc univariate noprint;var refsamp testsamp prod1 prod2;
output out = sum sum = m n o p;
data sum;set sum;RBAR = o/(m*n);
serbar = (1/(2*sqrt(3*n)))*sqrt(1 + ((n + 1)/m) +
        (1/(m*(m + n-1)))-(p/(m*(m + n)*(m + n - 1))));
z = abs((rbar -.5)/serbar); PVALUE = 1 - probnorm(z);
keep rbar pvalue; proc print;run;
```

The output is as follows:

```
  RBAR        PVALUE
  0.41619     0.008894851(x1)
```

2.6.5 Weighted Kappa

When data on t ordered categorical responses are given for two independent samples, where $t > 2$, weighted kappa measures the agreement between the two samples. Usually this situation arises, when each of the two judges or raters classify the items on an ordinal scale and one judge's rating may be more important. The weights commonly used to measure the agreement are

$$w_{ij} = 1 - \frac{|i - j|}{(t - 1)} \quad \text{or} \quad w_{ij} = 1 - \frac{(i - j)^2}{(t - 1)^2},$$

where w_{ij} is the weight given when one judge classifies the item in the ith category and the other judge classifies the same item in the jth category (also see SAS manual, Cicchetti and Allison, 1971; Fleiss and Cohen, 1973). The w_{ij} range from 0 to 1.

This implies that larger weights are given when the classification of the judges are close, with full weight for complete agreement and zero weight for complete disagreement. For $t = 2$, weighted kappa is the same as ordinary kappa.

In SAS, the coding given in Section 2.3.2 provides the test for the weighted kappa by adding *wtkappa* to the test statement as shown below:

```
test kappa wtkappa;
```

The Cicchetti–Allison weight is used by default and Fleiss–Cohen weight can be used with the AGREE option as follows:

```
tables outcome*gender/agree (wt = fc);run;
```

For the data discussed in Section 2.3.2, for the weighted kappa using Cincchetti–Allison weight, the output is

```
                        ***
                Weighted Kappa Coefficient
    ------------------------------------------------
    Weighted Kappa                      -0.0433 (y1)
    ASE                                  0.0438
    95% Lower Conf Limit                -0.1291
    95% Upper Conf Limit                 0.0426
              Test of H0: Weighted Kappa = 0
    ASE under H0                         0.0444
    Z                                   -0.9753
    One-sided Pr < Z                     0.1647
    Two-sided Pr > |Z|                   0.3294 (y2)
```

In this example, as we are discussing the progression of the disease which is in ordinal scale, weighted Kappa is the appropriate measure of the agreement between the two clinicians and from the output at (y1) it is −0.0433. To test the independence of evaluation of the two clinicians we use the test for weighted kappa = 0 given in the output. The *p*-value for this test is given in (y2) and is 0.3294 which is not significant. Hence, the two clinicians are independently rating the progression of the disease in the patients.

2.6.6 Ordinal Logistic Regression

2.6.6.1 Two Samples

Suppose a magazine was ranking two cities in terms of their cleanliness as clean, moderate, and dirty. Simulated data are given in Table 2.12.

The data here are ordinal data for the explanatory variable with three categories and we need to perform ordinal logistic regression. The procedure is based upon proportional odds assumption. The following program gives the necessary output.

City 1 is coded as 0, and city 2 is coded as 1. Further, dirty is coded as 0, moderate is coded as 1, and clean is coded as 2. The program and output are shown below:

```
data a;
/***input data***/
input CLEAN CITY freq @@;cards;
0  0  17  0  1  9  1  0  19  1  1  11  2  0  8  2  1  5
;
/***end of data***/
data a;set a; proc logistic descending; model clean = city;
  freq freq;run;
```

TABLE 2.12

Cleanliness Analysis of Two Cities

Cleanliness	City 1	City 2	Total
		City	
Dirty	17	9	26
Moderate	19	11	30
Clean	8	5	13
Total	44	25	69

***

Score Test for the Proportional Odds Assumption

Chi-Square	DF	Pr > ChiSq
0.0001	1	0.9938 (z1)

***

```
           Analysis of Maximum Likelihood Estimates
                   Standard              Wald
Parameter      DF  Estimate   Error   Chi-Square    Pr > ChiSq
..................................................................
Intercept 2     1  -1.5028    0.3544    17.9839     < 0.0001
Intercept 1     1   0.4620    0.2997     2.3760       0.1232
CITY            1   0.1145    0.4683     0.0597       0.8069 (z2)
                                ***
```

Our first test of the proportional odds assumption (see Section 5.6) is based on the *p*-value at (z1) of the output. Since this *p*-value is 0.9938 and is not significant, the proportional odds assumption is valid. One should note that if the number of categories of the response variable is large, then ordinary least-squares regression is appropriate. In addition, we also need a large sample size. When the proportional odds assumption is valid, we test that the two cities are similar for cleanliness by looking at the *p*-value given in (z2). Since this *p*-value is not significant, we conclude that the two cities are similar for their cleanliness.

2.6.6.2 k Samples

Suppose now instead of two cities as in Section 2.6.6.1, the magazine wants to rank four cities in terms of their cleanliness as dirty, moderate, and clean as shown in Table 2.13.

Using dummy variables as discussed in Chapter 5, we need to introduce three dummy variables to represent the four cities. City 1 is coded as 0 0 0, city 2 is coded as 1 0 0, city 3 is coded as 0 1 0, and city 4 is coded as 0 0 1. The program and output are shown below:

TABLE 2.13

Cleanliness Analyses of Four Cities

Cleanliness	City				
	City 1	City 2	City 3	City 4	Total
Dirty	17	9	13	6	45
Moderate	19	11	20	8	58
Clean	8	5	10	6	29
Total	44	25	43	20	132

```
data a;
/***input data***/
input clean city @@;cards;
0 1 0 2 0 3 0 4 1 1 1 3 1 3 1 4 1 1 1 2 1 3 1 2 1 1 1 2 1 3 1
4 0 1 0 2 0 3 0 1 1 1 1 2 1 3 1 3 0 1 0 2 0 3 0 4 1 1 1 3 1
```

```
3 1 4 0 1 1 1 0 1 1 1 1 1 0 2 0 3 0 4 1 2 1 2 1 3 1 1 0 1 0 2
0 3 0 1 1 1 1 2 1 3 1 4 0 1 0 3 0 3 0 1 1 1 1 2 1 3 1 1 0 1 0
2 0 3 0 4 1 4 1 2 1 3 1 4 0 1 1 1 0 1 1 1 0 1 0 2 0 3 0 4 1 1
1 3 1 3 1 1 0 1 0 2 0 3 2 4 2 1 2 2 2 3 2 4 2 2 0 2 0 3 0 4 1
1 1 2 1 3 2 4 2 1 2 2 2 3 2 4 2 2 1 2 1 3 1 4 0 1 1 1 0 1 1 1
2 3 2 3 2 3 2 4 2 3 1 3 1 3 1 4 0 3 1 3 0 3 1 3 2 3 2 3 2 3 2
3 2 1 2 1 2 1 2 2 2 1 2 4 2 1 2 1
;
/***end of input data**/
data a;set a;
if city = 1 then do; Z1 = 0; Z2 = 0;Z3 = 0; end;
if city = 2 then do; z1 = 1; z2 = 0; z3 = 0; end;
if city = 3 then do; z1 = 0; z2 = 1; z3 = 0; end;
if city = 4 then do; z1 = 0; z2 = 0; z3 = 1; end;
proc logistic descending; model clean = z1 z2 z3; run;
```

***

Score Test for the Proportional Odds Assumption

Chi-Square	DF	Pr > ChiSq
0.2805	3	0.9636 (aa1)

***

Analysis of Maximum Likelihood Estimates

Parameter	DF	Estimate	Standard Error	Wald Chi-Square	Pr > ChiSq
Intercept 2	1	-1.4877	0.3198	21.6367	< 0.0001
Intercept 1	1	0.4549	0.2910	2.4437	0.1180
Z1	1	0.1137	0.4679	0.0590	0.8081 (aa2)
Z2	1	0.3431	0.4010	0.7324	0.3921 (aa3)
Z3	1	0.5160	0.5041	1.0478	0.3060 (aa4)

Odds Ratio Estimates

Effect	Point Estimate (aa5)	95% Wald Confidence Limits (aa6)	(aa7)
Z1	1.120	0.448	2.803
Z2	1.409	0.642	3.093
Z3	1.675	0.624	4.500

Association of Predicted Probabilities and Observed Responses

Percent Concordant	41.0	Somers' D	0.093
Percent Discordant	31.7	Gamma	0.128
Percent Tied	27.4	Tau-a	0.060
Pairs	5597	c	0.547

The *p*-value given at (aa1) for the proportional odds assumption is not sig-nificant, and the proportional odds assumption is valid. Based on the coding for the cities used (aa2) is the p-value for comparing cities 1 and 2 for cleanliness and this p-value is not significant. Similarly, the p-value comparing cities 3 and 1 is given in (aa3) and cities 4 and 1 is given at (aa4). None of these three p-values are significant and each of the three cities 2, 3, and 4 are similar to city 1 in terms of cleanliness.

In the column (aa5) we have the point estimates of three odds ratios. For example, 1.120 is the odds for increased cleanliness of City 2 to City 1. Its CI is (0.448, 2.803) given in [(aa6), (aa7)]. The CIs for all the three explanatory variables covers 1 showing that the odds ratio of 1 for all the three variables is not rejected, similar to the conclusions drawn from the p-values given at (aa2), (aa3), and (aa4).

3

Continuous Normal Data

3.1 One Sample

In most of the standard textbooks, the inferences on one- and two-sample means are discussed when population variance(s) is (are) known or unknown, using standard normal and *t*-distributions. In practice, the population variance(s) is (are) unknown and as such we will discuss the results using only the *t*-distribution in this book. The *t*-distribution assumes normal distribution for the underlying data. When the sample size(s) is (are) small, the normal distribution of the data has to be ascertained using the Shapiro–Wilk test or other tests, as discussed in Chapter 1. When the sample size(s) is (are) large, the sample mean(s) is (are) approximately normally distributed based on the central limit theorem, and as the *t*-distribution also approximates normal distribution with increased degrees of freedom, the methods discussed in this and the next section are valid without testing the normality assumption of the data. With ordinal data, sometimes we associate numerical values to the categories and analyze the data using the quantitative methods. If the point scale is seven or more, it may be reasonable to use methods of this chapter, but if the scale is two or three points, these methods are inappropriate and one should use methods for discrete data as discussed in Chapter 2.

For the sample size and power calculations, we use the standard normal distribution as an approximation. When the population variance(s) is (are) unknown, the sample size(s) can be more accurately determined by using Stein's two-stage procedures, and the interested reader is referred to Desu and Raghavarao (1990, pp. 4–5, 25) for further details.

Let us now consider an example where a market researcher is interested in estimating the mean age of customers in a mall. The researcher needs to know the margin of error to be attached to the statement, d, and the chance $(1 - \alpha)$ for the statement to be true. If the mean age is estimated to be $\bar{x}$, the real mean then is in the interval $(\bar{x} - d, \bar{x} + d)$ and in repeated sampling, the statement is true in $(1 - \alpha)$ 100% samples. Usually $\alpha = 0.1$, 0.05, or 0.01. Suppose, the researcher takes $\alpha = 0.05$ and wants a margin of error, $d = 3$. The researcher needs to determine the number of respondents for the survey and for this purpose the researcher needs to know the standard deviation of the response variable. Since there is no idea about the standard deviation, an approximate value for the standard deviation as range/6 is presumed. If the ages of the customers in the mall being surveyed are approximately between 12 and 72 years, then the standard deviation can be approximately taken as $(72 - 12)/6 = 10$. The following program will give the necessary sample size, n.

```
data a;
/*** input data***/
sd = 10; *guessed standard deviation;  alpha = .05; *alpha level;
  d = 3; *assumed error margin;
/***end of input data ***/
z2side = probit(1 - alpha/2);  N = floor((sd*z2side/d)**2) +1;
keep n; proc print; run;
```

This program will produce the following output:

```
    N
    43
```

The researcher needs to randomly select $n = 43$ individuals from the population and each individual is asked his (her) age.

The following program gives the $(1 - \alpha)100\%$ confidence interval (CI) of the mean, at [(a2), (a3)] of the output for the age data in the input statement. The mean is given at (a1). Selection of α is at the researcher's discretion.

```
data a;
/***input data***/
input AGE @@; cards;
34 15 45 45 56 41 72 14 16 34 46 23 15 28 28 30 39 23 70 28 10
60 32 24 16 17 18 36 22 24 43 72 45 47 28 49 12 11 57 23 35
37 14
;
/***end of input data***/
proc ttest alpha = .05;*if alpha is not specified it is assumed
  to be .05;
var age; run;
```

The necessary output is as follows:

```
                        The TTEST Procedure
                            Statistics
                   Lower CL                    Upper CL
Variable    N       Mean          Mean          Mean
AGE        43     28.125 (a2)   33.349 (a1)   38.572 (a3)     ***
                                 ***
```

Alternatively, the researcher should be interested in testing that the mean is more than (less than, not equal to) a specified value, μ_0. Here μ_0 is a value prespecified by the researcher. To establish the claim, the null hypothesis tested is that the mean is not more than (not less than, equal to) μ_0. The researcher has to specify the level of the test, α. To determine the sample size, the desired power, usually 80%, 90%, or 95%, at an alternative value, μ_1 should be specified, where $\mu_1 - \mu_0$ is the smallest meaningful effect of interest required to detect. The approximate value of the standard deviation is needed to determine the sample size for the estimation discussed earlier in this section. The following program produces approximate sample sizes for one-sided or two-sided tests.

```
data a;
/***input data***/
sd = 10; * standard deviation guess;
mu0 = 35;  *hypothesized mean;
mu1 = 40;  *alternative mean needed to detect;
alpha = .05;*alpha level; power = .8;  *power of the test at mu1;
/***end of input data***/
delta = mu1-mu0 ;  z2side = probit(1-alpha/2);  *2 sided;
z1side = probit(1-alpha);*1 sided;  zbeta = probit(power);
N1SIDE = floor((sd*(z1side+zbeta)/delta)**2) +1;
N2SIDE = floor((sd*(z2side+zbeta)/delta)**2) +1;
keep n1side n2side; proc print;run;
```

The output is

N1SIDE	N2SIDE
25	32

The researcher randomly selects 32 subjects (25 for a one-sided test) and collects the data.

If the null hypothesis is $\mu = 0$, the following program provides the necessary tests and output for the age data in the input statement. If the null hypothesis is $\mu = \mu_0$ ($\neq 0$), the subsequent program provides the necessary output.

```
data a;
/***input data***/
input AGE @@; cards;
55 45 49 16 21 62 14 66 34 23 15 39 23 41 28 20
40 32 24 46 37 18 42 25 17 28 49 12 57 23 24 72
;
/***end of input data***/
proc univariate normal;run;
```

The following output is provided:

```
                                  ***
                    Tests for Location:  Mu0 = 0
Test                   ---Statistic---          ----p Value----
Student's t            T     11.83976   Pr > |t|      <0.0001 (b2)
Sign                   M     16         Pr >= |M|     <0.0001 (b3)
Signed Rank            S     264        Pr >= |S|     <0.0001 (b4)


                    Tests for Normality
Test                   ----Statistic---         ----p Value----
Shapiro-Wilk           W      0.936202   Pr < W       0.0585 (b1)
Kolmogorov-Smirnov     D      0.152025   Pr > D       0.0590
Cramer-von Mises       W-Sq   0.109082   Pr > W-Sq    0.0846
Anderson-Darling       A-Sq   0.67099    Pr > A-Sq    0.0764
                                  ***
```

The normality assumption is first checked using the *p*-value at (b1). If this *p*-value exceeds α, the level of significance, the *p*-value at (b2) based on *t*-distribution is used for inference of the null hypothesis μ = 0. If (b1) is less than α, then the data are not normal, then the sign test or the signed-rank test with the corresponding *p*-values given at (b3) and (b4) is used. These tests will be discussed in Chapter 4.

In the example, the *p*-value from the Shapiro–Wilk test given at (b1) is 0.0585 which is >0.05 and it can be concluded that the data are normally distributed. Hence, we proceed with testing the hypothesis H_0: μ = 0 by the *t*-test with a two-sided *p*-value <0.0001 given at (b2). Obviously, this *p*-value implies the rejection of μ = 0 in favor of the alternative, μ ≠ 0 at the 0.05 level of significance. The one-sided *p*-value is half the two-sided *p*-value in the positive or negative direction based on the sign of the *t*-statistic.

Suppose the researcher wanted to test the null hypothesis that H_0: μ = 35. Thus, the null hypothesis of interest is H_0: $μ = μ_0 = 35$, and the following program provides the *p*-value for a one-sided or two-sided test. Note that "h0" in the PROC TTEST is the hypothesis of interest. The default value of "h0" is zero.

```
data a;
/***input data***/
input AGE @@;cards;
55 45 49 16 21 62 14 66 34 23 15 39 23 41 28 20
40 32 24 46 37 18 42 25 17 28 49 12 57 23 24 72
;
/***end of input data***/
proc ttest alpha = .05 h0 = 35; var age;  run;
```

The output is as follows:

```
                          ***
                       T-Tests
       Variable   DF    t Value        Pr > |t|
       Age        31    -0.25        0.8056 (c1)
```

The p-value is 0.8056 as shown by (c1) for a two-sided test, and is not significant. Thus, the researcher retains the null hypothesis and concludes that the mean age is 35 years. The p-value for a one-sided test with alternative hypothesis $\mu > 35$ years is $1 - 0.8056/2 = 0.5972$, because the t-value is negative. The p-value for a one-sided test with alternative $\mu < 35$ is $0.8056/2 = 0.4028$.

The researcher presumes that there may be more variability in the data than he would like to see. He would like to test the hypothesis $H_0: \sigma^2 = \sigma_0^2$ against $H_A: \sigma^2 > \sigma_0^2$, where $\sigma_0^2 = 100$. The following program gives the necessary test.

```
data a;
/***input data***/
input AGE @@; cards;
55 45 49 16 21 62 14 66 34 23 15 39 23 41 28 20
40 32 24 46 37 18 42 25 17 28 49 12 57 23 24 72
;
/***end of input data***/
proc univariate noprint; output out = stats n = n var = S2;
Data a; set stats;
/***input data***/
Var = 100;  *null hypothesis of the variance;
/***end of input data***/
CHISQ = ((n - 1) * s2/var);  PVALUE = 1 - probchi (chisq, n - 1);
proc print; var s2 chisq pvalue;  run;
```

The output is as follows:

```
        S2            CHISQ              PVALUE
   268.273 (d1)    83.1647     0.000001172 (d2)
```

The value 268.273 at (d1) is the sample variance, s^2. The p-value for testing the null hypothesis $\sigma_0^2 = 100$ is 0.000001172 given at (d2). The p-value is significant and the null hypothesis that the variance is 100 against the one-sided alternative is rejected.

Suppose the researcher's budget can only support a sample of 20 people. In testing $H_0: \mu = 35$ at α-level test, the power for one-sided (or two-sided) test at the alternative $\mu = \mu_1 = 40$ can be determined from the following program:

```
data a;
/***input data***/
n = 20;*sample size;   sd = 10;*standard deviation guess;
alpha = .05;*alpha level;
```

```
mu0 = 35;*hypothesized mean;   mu1 = 40;*alternative mean needed to
  detect;
/***end of input data***/
delta = mu1-mu0;
z2side = probit(1-alpha/2);*2 sided;
z1side = probit(1-alpha);*1 sided;   a = (delta*sqrt(n))/sd;
POWER1 = 1-probnorm(z1side-a);   POWER2 = 1-probnorm(z2side-abs(a));
keep power1 power2; proc print;run;
```

Output:

```
POWER1                POWER2
0.72281(e1)    0.60877(e2)
```

Based on the above output, (e1) and (e2) are the powers for the one-sided and two-sided tests and are 72.3% and 60.9%, respectively. Power can also be calculated in SAS by PROC POWER procedure.

3.2 Two Samples

3.2.1 Independent Samples

3.2.1.1 Means

Continuing the situation considered in Section 3.1, suppose the researcher is interested in estimating the difference in the mean ages of males and females. The researcher needs to specify the margin of error in the estimate, d, and the confidence $1-\alpha$, in the truth of the statement. Furthermore, the researcher needs to provide an approximation for the standard deviations $\tilde{\sigma}_1$ and $\tilde{\sigma}_2$ of the male and female age, respectively. Usually, the sample sizes n_1 and n_2 are assumed to be equal. However, one can specify n_1/n_2 as f. The researcher assumes $f = 1$, and hence $n_1 = n_2$. The following program provides the required sample sizes n_1 and n_2 as the output.

```
Data a;
/**input data**/
sd1 = 10;* assumed sd for sample 1;   sd2 = 9;* assumed sd for
  sample 2;
alpha = .05;   d = 2.5;   f = 1;
/**end of input data**/
z2side = probnorm(1-alpha/2);
N2 = floor(((z2side/d)**2)*(((sd1**2)/f) + (sd2**2))) + 1;
  N1 = n2*f;
proc print; var n1 n2; run;
```

The output is

```
N1                    N2
21                    21
```

A random sample of $n_1 = 21$ males and independently another random sample of $n_2 = 21$ females is taken and the age of the sampled males and females is obtained.

Point estimate of $\mu_1 - \mu_2$ and a $(1 - \alpha)100\%$ CI for $\mu_1 - \mu_2$ based on the input data can be determined using the following program. The output also gives the p-value for testing the null hypothesis H_0: $\mu_1 = \mu_2$.

```
Data group1;* input data for group 1, in our example the
  males;
/***input data***/
input AGE @@; cards;
30 54 34 48 23 46 16 49 24 36 23 35 45 28 49 35 28 48 56 45 56
;
/***end of input data***/
proc univariate noprint;var age;output out = stats1
  std = sdgroup1;run;
data group1;set group1; group = 1;
data group2; * input data for group 2, in our example
  the females;
/***input data***/
input AGE @@;  cards;
35 50 24 30 24 39 35 20 34 29 34 65 30 50 25 46 34 74 36 54 49
;
/***end of input data***/
proc univariate noprint;var age;output out = stats2
  std = sdgroup2;run;
data group2;set group2;  group = 2;
data stats1;set stats1;  proc print;run;
data stats2;set stats2;proc print;run;  data final;set group1
  group2;
proc ttest h0 = 0;*if the null hypothesis is mu1 - mu2 = d0
  replace h0 = 0 by h0 = d0;
var age;class group;  run;
```

The necessary output is as follows:

sdgroup1

12.1145 (f8)

sdgroup2

13.9675 (f9)

The TTEST Procedure

Statistics

Variable	GROUP	***	Lower CL Mean	Mean	Upper CL Mean	***
			***			
AGE	Diff (1-2)		−8.583 (f4)	−0.429 (f5)	7.7258 (f6)	

```
                                  T-Tests
Variable Method               Variances     DF      t Value      Pr > |t|
AGE       Pooled              Equal         40      -0.11     0.9159(f2)
AGE       Satterthwaite       Unequal    39.2(f7)   -0.11     0.9159(f3)
                        Equality of Variances
Variable Method               Num DF      Den DF    F Value      Pr > F
AGE       Folded F              20          20       1.33     0.5303 (f1)
```

The difference in the two mean values is given at (f5) and is −0.429. The researcher first tests that the two population variances are equal by looking at the p-value given at (f1). If this p-value exceeds $\alpha = 0.05$, the equal variance assumption is tenable and the pooled variance for testing $\mu_1 = \mu_2$ is used, giving p-value at (f2) and CI for $\mu_1 - \mu_2$, at [(f4), (f6)]. If the p-value at (f1) is less than $\alpha = 0.05$, the two populations have different variances and then the t tests are used with approximate degrees of freedom given by Satterthwaite at (f7). The p-value for testing $\mu_1 = \mu_2$ is then given at (f3) and the CI for $\mu_1 - \mu_2$ at [(f10), (f11)] can be obtained by using the program as shown below:

```
data stats;
/***input data***/
MEAN = -.43;* mean for the difference (f5);
df = 39.2;* degrees of freedom for Satterthwaite (f7);
  alpha = .05;
n1 = 21; *sample size for group 1;   n2 = 21; *sample size for
  group 2;
sd1 = 12.11;* obtain the standard deviation for group 1(f8);
sd2 = 13.97;* obtain the standard deviation for group 2(f9);
/***end of input data***/
t = tinv((1 - alpha/2),df);
UPPER_CI = mean + t*(sqrt(((sd1**2)/n1) + ((sd2**2)/n2)));
LOWER_CI = mean - t*(sqrt(((sd1**2)/n1) + ((sd2**2)/n2)));
proc print; var lower_ci mean upper_ci;   run;
```

Output is:

```
     LOWER_CI             MEAN             UPPER_CI
    -8.58912 (f10)      - 0.43           7.72912 (f11)
```

In the example (f1) is 0.5303 and is >0.05, implying that the two population variances are equal. Looking at (f2) p-value 0.9159 which is >0.05 it is concluded that the mean age for male and female subjects are not different. The CI for the differences in the mean age for male and female subjects based on [(f4), (f6)] is (−8.583, 7.726).

If (f1) was less than 0.05, then the variances would not be equal, then (f3) will be looked at, for the p-value of the test, which is 0.9159. The CI for the difference in the mean age for male and female subjects based on [(f10), (f11)] is (−8.589, 7.729).

It may be noted that in this example, the p-values for testing the two means and the CIs for the difference of the two means are almost the same with Satterthwaite degrees of freedom and pooled variance. This is because the null hypothesis of equality of the two variances is retained based on the p-value at (f1).

Note that the sample sizes used in the above program are not necessarily the required sample sizes for the testing problem. The required sample sizes for testing will now be given.

Let the researcher be interested in testing the null hypothesis that the difference in the means μ_1 and μ_2 is not more than (not less than, equal to) d_0. Clearly, $d_0 = \mu_1 - \mu_2$. Let d_1 be the smallest clinical difference that is prespecified by the researcher, who will also need to specify the level of the test α, the desired power 80%, 90%, or 95% of detecting a difference $d_1 = \mu_1 - \mu_2$, and the approximate standard deviations, $\tilde{\sigma}_1$, $\tilde{\sigma}_2$ of the two populations. To perform a one-sided or two-sided test, the sample sizes n_1 and n_2 need to be determined. Assume $n_1 = f n_2$, where f is often 1.

```
data a;
/**input data ***/
alpha = 0.05;  Power = 0.8;  f = 1;  d0 = 2.5;  d1 = 5;
sd1 = 10;*assumed sd from sample 1;  sd2 = 9;*assumed sd from
  sample 2;
/**end of input data**/
d = d1 - d0;  z2side = probit (1 - alpha/2);
z1side = probit (1 - alpha);  zbeta = probit (power);
N21SIDE = floor ((((z1side + zbeta)/d)**2)
  *(((sd1**2)/f) + (sd2**2))) + 1;
N22SIDE = floor ((((z2side + zbeta)/d)**2)
  *(((sd1**2)/f) + (sd2**2))) + 1;
N11SIDE = n21side*f;  N12SIDE = n22side*f;
keep n11side n12side n21side n22side;  Proc print;
var n11side n21side n12side n22side;  run;
```

The output is as follows:

N11SIDE	N21SIDE	N12SIDE	N22SIDE
180 (g1)	180 (g2)	228 (g3)	228 (g4)

Thus, a sample size of 228 for both genders is needed to test H_0: $\mu_1 - \mu_2 = 2.5$ against the alternative H_A: $\mu_1 - \mu_2 \neq 2.5$ for a two-sided test as shown in (g3) and (g4). One-hundred-and-eighty subjects are required if it is a one-sided test shown in (g1) and (g2). This sample size for the two samples enable the researcher to reject H_0 with a probability of 0.8, when $\mu_1 - \mu_2 = 5$.

For a two-sided test, the researcher needs to take independent random samples of $n_1 = 228$ males and $n_2 = 228$ females and get the data on all $n_1 + n_2$

individuals. The previous program(s) can be used to draw the necessary inferences as described earlier.

Suppose the researcher only obtains 100 subjects in each group. Then he would like to know the power of the test. The following program provides the necessary output at (h1) and (h2).

```
data a;
/***input data***/
n1 = 100;*sample size for n1;   n2 = 100;*sample size for n2;
sd1 = 10;*standard deviation guess sample 1;
sd2 = 9;*standard deviation guess sample 2;
alpha = .05;*alpha level;   d0 = 2.5;*hypothesized mean
   difference;
d1 = 5;*alternative mean difference needed to detect;
/***end of input data***/
d = d1 - d0;
z2side = probit(1 - alpha/2);*2 sided;   z1side = probit(1 - alpha);*1
   sided;
se = sqrt(((sd1**2)/n1) + ((sd2**2)/n2));
POWER1 = 1 - probnorm(z1side - (d/se));
POWER2 = 1 - probnorm(z2side - (abs(d)/se));
keep power1 power2;   proc print;run;
```

| POWER1 | POWER2 |
| 0.58449 (h1) | 0.45949 (h2) |

The power is 58.4% at (h1) for the one-sided test and 45.9% at (h2) for the two-sided test as displayed by the output.

3.2.1.2 Variances

The equality of population variances can be tested by using the PROC TTEST procedure of the previous section obtaining the necessary *p*-value at (f1).

3.2.2 Paired Samples

Suppose a pediatrician was interested in estimating the difference in mean birth weight of first- and second-born twins. This is the case of paired samples, the twins forming the pairs of observations. The pediatrician needs to specify the margin of error attached to the statement, d, and the chance $(1 - \alpha)$ taken for the truth of the statement. If the pediatrician estimates the mean birth-weight difference to be $\bar{\delta}$, the real mean is then in the interval $(\bar{\delta} - d, \bar{\delta} + d)$ and in repeated sampling, the statement is true in $(1 - \alpha)$ 100% samples. Usually, $\alpha = 0.1, 0.05$, or 0.01. Let $d = 0.25$ and $\alpha = 0.05$. To find the variance of the differences in weights, the variances of the birth weights of first- and second-born twins and the correlation between the two birth weights should be known. Usually, this correlation, ρ, is high, like 0.8. Let the standard

deviation, taken as range/6, be 0.5 for both variables, since no approximations can be taken for the two groups' standard deviations. The pediatrician
needs to determine the number of respondent pairs needed to address this
question. The following program will give the necessary number of pairs, n,
needed in this investigation.

```
data a;
/***input data***/
sd1 = .5; *standard deviation of the group 1 data;
sd2 = .5; *standard deviation of the group 2 data;
rho = 0.8;* correlation between the two groups; alpha = .05; *
  alpha level;
d = .25; *error margin in estimating difference;
/***end of input data ***/
var = (sd1**2) + (sd2**2) - 2*rho*sd1*sd2;  z2side = probit (1-alpha/2);
  sd = sqrt(var);  N = floor((z2side*sd/d)**2) +1;  keep n;
proc print;  run;
```

This program will produce the following output:

```
N
7
```

He needs to randomly select $n = 7$ sets of twins from the population and
each twins' mean birth-weight difference is measured. The following program gives the required CI for the difference in mean δ and a test for the
hypothesis H_0: $\delta = 0$ for data given in the input of the program.

```
data pairs;
/***input data***/
input group1 group2 @@;  cards;
6.0 6.5 3.3 3.7 4.6 4.3 5.6 6.3 3.9 3.2 5.5 5.9 5.2 5.3
;
/***end of input data***/
data pairs;set pairs;  DIFF = group2 - group1;  proc ttest;
  var diff;  run;
```

The following output is obtained:

```
                    The TTEST Procedure
                       Statistics
                  Lower CL                           Upper CL
Variable    N       Mean            Mean               Mean
DIFF        7    -0.302 (i2)     0.1571 (i1)       0.616 (i3)    ***
                            T-Tests
                Variable    DF    t Value     Pr > |t|
                DIFF         6      0.84      0.4342 (i4)
```

The estimated mean difference of birth weights for second- and first-born twins is 0.16 lbs given at (i1) and the lower and upper bounds of CI of the twin difference in birth weights is (–0.302, 0.616) given at [(i2), (i3)]. This is the mean and CI of the mean for the differences in weights whereas the expressions considered in Section 3.2.1.1 are the differences in the overall means and its CI. The *p*-value for a two-sided test of H_0: $\delta = 0$ is given at (i4) and is 0.4342, which is not significant.

Suppose the pediatrician was interested in testing H_0: $\delta = \delta_0$, where δ_0 is a prespecified value. Then "h0" should be specified as δ_0 in the PROC TTEST statement as given below using $\delta_0 = 0.25$ and the output can be interpreted as before:

```
proc ttest h0 = .25; var diff; run;
```

The sample size needed for testing the differences of means will now be discussed. Let the pediatrician be interested in concluding that the difference in mean birth weight, be more than (less than, not equal to) a specified value, δ_0. Here δ_0 is a value prespecified by the researcher. To establish the claim, the null hypothesis tested is that the mean is not more than (not less than, equal to) δ_0. The pediatrician has to specify the level of the test, α. To determine the sample size, the desired power should be specified, which is usually 80%, 90%, or 95% at an alternative value, δ_1, where $\delta_1 - \delta_0$ is the smallest weight difference of interest the pediatrician wants to detect.

Suppose the interest is to test H_0: $\delta = \delta_0 = 0.25$ against the one-sided or two-sided alternative. Assume the variances and correlations as discussed earlier. The pediatrician has to determine the sample size of twins that would be needed to test the null hypothesis for a 0.05 level test with power of rejecting "h0" as 0.8 when $\delta_1 = 0.50$. The following program would give the necessary sample size, *n*.

```
data a;
/***input data***/
d0 = .25;   d1 = 0.5;   sd1 = .5;  *standard deviation of the group 1
    data;
sd2 = .5;  *standard deviation of the group 2 data;
rho = 0.8;*  correlation between the two groups;  alpha = .05;
  *  alpha level;  power = .8;*power of the test;
/***end of input data***/
var = (sd1**2) + (sd2**2) - 2*rho*sd1*sd2;   sd = sqrt(var);
d = d1 - d0;  *effect of interest;
z2side = probit(1-alpha/2);*2 sided;   z1side = probit(1-alpha);
  *1 sided;   zbeta = probit(power);
N2SIDE = round(((sd*(z2side + zbeta))/d)**2);
N1SIDE = round(((sd*(z1side + zbeta))/d)**2);
keep n1side n2side; proc print; run;
```

The output is:

```
 N1SIDE          N2SIDE
 10               13
```

Thus, a sample size of 13 twins will be needed to test H_0: $\delta = 0.25$ against the two-sided alternative, with 80% power when $\delta = 0.5$.

For testing a hypothesis H_0: $\delta = \delta_0$, where $\delta_0 \neq 0$, the PROC TTEST is used, where H_0 is δ_0 and interpret the output as described above.

The pediatrician has limited funds for the research and decides to go with only four sets of twins and wants to know the power for testing the hypothesis. The following program provides the power of the test.

```
data a;
/***input data***/
n = 4;*sample size; d0 = .25; d1 = 0.5;
sd1 = .5; *standard deviation of the group 1 data;
sd2 = .5; *standard deviation of the group 2 data;
rho = 0.8;* correlation between the two groups; alpha = .05;
  * alpha level;
/***end of input data***/
var = (sd1**2) + (sd2**2) - 2*rho*sd1*sd2; sd = sqrt(var);
d = d1 - d0;  z2side = probit(1-alpha/2);*2 sided;
 z1side = probit(1-alpha);*1 sided;
 a1 = z1side - (d*sqrt(n)/sd);  a2 = z2side - (d*sqrt(n)/sd);
POWER1 = 1-probnorm(a1);  POWER2 = 1-probnorm(abs(a2));
keep power1 power2; proc print;run;
```

The output is as follows:

```
        POWER1          POWER2
      0.47460(j1)    0.35241(j2)
```

The power is 47.5% at (j1) for the one-sided test and 35.2% at (j2) for the two-sided test as displayed in the output.

3.3 *k* Independent Samples

3.3.1 One-Way Analysis of Variance

One uses the *t*-distribution to draw inferences on one or two population means as in Sections 3.1 and 3.2. However, to draw inferences on more than two population means, the *F* test based on the analysis of variance (ANOVA) is used. This reduces to the methods discussed in Section 3.2 for the two-sample case. The analysis presented in this section is required in two different scenarios. Random samples will be independently drawn from k populations and the researcher would be interested in drawing inferences on the k population means $\mu_1, \mu_2, \ldots, \mu_k$. The other setting is where k treatments are given to n identical experimental units by randomly dividing the units into k groups of $n_1, n_2, \ldots, n_k$ units and applying k treatments to the k groups randomly. The interest is to draw inferences on the effects of the k treatments. Although the symbols $\tau_1, \tau_2, \ldots, \tau_k$ are normally used to represent the treatment effects, in this work μ_i is used to denote treatment effects also.

The global null hypothesis of primary interest is that all means (effects) are equal against the alternative that at least one pair of means (effects) is different. The test is based on comparing the variability between the groups to the variability within the groups of data. To this end, the total variability in the data will be partitioned into the variability between groups and within groups and this division is shown by the ANOVA table in the computer output of this section and the p-value given at (k1) of the output is used to test $H_0: \mu_1 = \mu_2 = \cdots = \mu_k$. If this p-value is less than the significance level, say 0.05, then H_0 will be rejected.

If $H_0: \mu_1 = \mu_2 = \cdots = \mu_k$ is rejected, the interest will then be to compare a set of means to another set of means. An expression of the type $\sum_{i=1}^{k} a_i \mu_i$, where $\sum_{i=1}^{k} a_i = 0$ is called a *contrast* of the means and inferences are drawn on contrasts in this context. For example, if $k = 5$, a contrast $\mu_1 - 2\mu_3 + \mu_4$ will be written in the contrast statement of the program as

```
1   0   -2   1   0,
```

where "0" represents the mean that is not included in the contrast statement.

The contrasts $\sum_{i=1}^{k} a_i \mu_i$ and $\sum_{i=1}^{k} b_i \mu_i$ are said to be *orthogonal* if $\sum_{i=1}^{k} a_i b_i = 0$, where a_i and b_i are the coefficients of the means. For example, the contrasts $\mu_1 - \mu_2$, and $\mu_1 + \mu_2 - 2\mu_3$ are orthogonal because $(1)(1) + (-1)(1) + (0)(-2) = 0$.

With k means, $k - 1$ contrasts can be formed, which are pair-wise orthogonal, and thus usually at most $k - 1$ contrast statements of orthogonal contrasts are included in the program. When these $k - 1$ pair-wise orthogonal contrasts are considered, it is interesting to note that the global hypothesis may be rejected while none of the contrasts are significant, or vice versa.

As mentioned earlier, when the global hypothesis is rejected, the experimenter may be interested in identifying which pairs of means (effects) are different. If k is large and if all pair-wise comparisons are made each at α level, by chance, concluding that some pairs of means are significant, when all the k means are same. This is so because $(k(k - 1)/2)\alpha$ contrasts are concluded significant, when the null hypothesis is true. To remedy this situation, family-wise error rate is used in multiple comparisons. In $100\alpha\%$ experiments, with all k means the same, we are willing to find at least one significant pair of means.

The commonly used multiple comparison methods are *Tukey, least-significant difference (LSD), Scheffe, Bonferroni, Duncan, Student–Newman–Keuls (SNK)*, and *Sidak. Dunnett's* procedure is used when comparing $k - 1$ active treatment means against a control mean. Each of these tests has its pros and cons and they will briefly be described here.

The LSD test should be used only for testing the significance of preplanned contrasts. A very common mistake among researchers is to use this method when the comparisons were formulated after looking at the data. This method can be thought of as a *t*-test using the pooled error variance. The LSD should not be used when making all pair-wise comparisons of the means for the reason stated earlier. Usually, the number of comparisons made, is at most the model degrees of freedom ((k10), of the output). For this method the overall alpha is not controlled, no adjustments are made for any of the comparisons. When k is large, some pairs of means are declared significant, when they are actually not. This test uses the smallest difference between the means that would result in concluding significantly different means.

Tukey's method is known as honestly significant difference (HSD). It declares fewer significant differences compared to LSD, Duncan, and SNK.

Duncan's multiple range test first ranks the means and then tests the means accounting for the distance between the means. This method may provide more significant results compared to Tukey.

The SNK method is similar to Duncan. It gives fewer significant differences than Duncan but more than Tukey. This method also takes into account the number of group means between the tested means.

The Bonferroni method performs multiple *t*-tests for the difference between the means. It is a very conservative method and provides few significant results. It makes adjustments based on the number of comparisons made. The α level for each comparison is α/m, where m is the number of planned comparisons.

The Sidak test is not as conservative as the Bonferroni method. Like the Bonferroni method, it makes adjustments based on the number of comparisons tested.

The conclusions of the Scheffe test for the comparisons are similar to the overall *F*-test conclusions. If the F test produces significant results, then this method will also provide significant means. If the F test does not produce significant results, then this method will also not provide significant results.

The Dunnett procedure is used when comparing active treatments against a control treatment or placebo. It does not include all possible comparisons. Note that the LSD method can also be used for this purpose. However, the criteria for the critical difference used between the Dunnett's procedure and LSD are different.

In the program in the model line Tukey's test is used to obtain the inferences based on this method. One can replace this method in the model line of the program, by any other method of interest or can use all methods to see whether the inferences based on all methods provide similar conclusions.

Consider an example where a physician is interested in finding the most effective way for the patients to lose weight using four different methods. The physician would want to put the patients on four different regimens, one group would not exercise or take any diet pills, one group would only exercise, one would only take diet pills, and the last group would exercise and take diet pills. The physician would want to observe the weight lost in 12 weeks by the four methods and compare the methods.

All the methods discussed here assume normal distribution for the data and assume equal variability within each of the k groups. The determination of the sample size needed in each group is first discussed.

To begin the study the physician needs to know the number of subjects to be assigned to each group. Usually, equal number of subjects are assigned to each group. If n_i is the number of subjects assigned to the ith group, taking $n_1 = n_2 = n_3 = n_4$. The physician must specify the largest difference Δ in weight loss in the groups to be detected with probability $1 - \beta$, which is the power of the test. If Δ is specified, and if the maximum difference in the mean weight losses is less than Δ, then the four regimens will be considered not significant. The physician should also have an idea of the standard deviation σ, of the weight losses between subjects. Let α be the level of the test. When k, Δ, σ, α, and $1 - \beta$, are specified the required $n_1 = n_2 = n_3 = n_4$ can be determined by the following program based on the approximation given in Desu and Raghavarao (1990, p. 49).

```
Data a;
/**input data**/
alpha = .05;  power = .8;  k = 4;  delta = 7;
sigma = 5;*assuming range of weight loss of the programs is
  30 lbs (range) and taking sigma as range over 6;
/**end of input data **/
Chisq = cinv(1 - alpha, k - 1); Zbeta = probit(power);
N = floor(2*((sqrt(chisq - (k - 2)) + zbeta)**2)*((sigma/
  delta)**2)) + 1;
keep n; proc print; run;
```

Output:

```
N
11
```

The physician selects 11 subjects for each of the four groups and records the weight lost in pounds in 12 weeks and the daily caloric intake on an average. Initially, 44 subjects are randomly placed into four groups and assigned the four regimens to the four groups. Artificial data are displayed in Table 3.1 indicating the weight loss. Data are also provided for baseline body weight and the diet caloric intake and this information will be used in the next section.

The physicians' primary interest is to see whether the four regimen effects are not the same, and if they are different, to identify which of the regimens are different. The program below provides the overall F test, contrasts and

TABLE 3.1

Weight Loss at 12 Weeks by Various Weight-Loss Strategies

No Exercise and Diet Pills			Diet Pills			Exercise			Exercise and Diet Pills		
Weight Loss	Calories/ Day	Initial Body Weight	Weight Loss	Calories/ Day	Initial Body Weight	Weight Loss	Calories/ Day	Initial Body Weight	Weight Loss	Calories/ Day	Initial Body Weight
5	2100	150	5	1200	145	7	1300	165	8	1250	167
2	1500	165	5	1300	164	5	1200	170	7	1200	235
2	2300	132	4	1250	137	6	1100	215	9	800	210
3	2425	165	5	2000	211	8	1450	213	10	1500	184
3	2000	147	3	1300	189	5	1200	189	9	1200	175
2	1900	214	6	1000	157	7	1300	159	7	1300	149
5	2500	210	5	1400	189	5	1500	150	9	1250	195
3	1750	178	7	1350	174	6	1600	190	10	1300	204
2	2000	176	5	1800	203	5	1500	197	12	1200	174
2	1250	186	7	1250	134	6	1400	186	9	1350	196
1	2100	155	4	1350	176	6	1600	168	10	1200	179

the code for the commonly used multiple comparisons. Note that SAS provides other methods which will not be discussed here, but they can be interpreted in a similar manner. Interested readers may review the SAS manual for further details. The various multiple comparison procedures of interest are stated in the MEANS option in the program.

Suppose the physician is interested in drawing inferences on the following three comparisons before beginning the study.

```
No exercise or diet pill vs others
Diet pill vs exercise
Exercise or diet pill vs (diet pill + exercise)
```

Starting with the first comparison of no exercise or diet pill versus others (diet pill alone, exercise alone, and both exercise and diet pill) results in drawing inference on

$$\mu_1 - \frac{\mu_2 + \mu_3 + \mu_4}{3} \quad \text{or} \quad 3\mu_1 - \mu_2 - \mu_3 - \mu_4.$$

This corresponds to the contrast statement

$$3 - 1 - 1 - 1.$$

The second comparison of interest corresponds to the contrast statement:

$$\mu_2 - \mu_3$$

written as

$$0 \quad 1 \quad -1 \quad 0.$$

The third contrast statement of interest corresponds to

$$\frac{\mu_2 + \mu_3}{2} - \mu_4$$

written as

$$0 \quad 1 \quad 1 \quad -2.$$

The above 3 contrasts are pair-wise orthogonal.

The program is as follows.

```
Data a;
/***input data ***/
Input GROUP WGTLOSS  @@;
cards;
1 5 1 2 1 2 1 3 1 3 1 2 1 5 1 3 1 2 1 2 1 1 2 5 2 5 2 4 2 5 2
3 2 6 2 5 2 7 2 5 2 7 2 4 3 7 3 5 3 6 3 8 3 5 3 7 3 5 3 6 3 5
3 6 3 6 4 8 4 7 4 9 4 10 4 9 4 7 4 9 4 10 4 12 4 9 4 10
;
/***end of input data***/
```

```
proc glm; class group; model wgtloss = group;run;
* Update the contrast statements based on hypothesis of
  interest;
contrast 'no exercise or diet vs others' group  -3 1 1 1;
contrast 'diet vs exercise' group 0 1  -1 0;
contrast 'diet or exercise vs exercise and diet'
  group 0 1 1  -2;
run; means group/TUKEY;
*means group/ TUKEY CLDIFF alpha = .05;  *Use if you would like
  the 95% CL difference of the means; run;
```

The necessary output is as follows:

The GLM Procedure
Dependent Variable: WGTLOSS

Source	DF	Sum of Squares	Mean Square	F Value	Pr > F
Model	3 (k10)	228.7272727	76.2424242	49.19	<0.0001 (k1)
Error	40	62.0000000	1.5500000		
Corrected Total	43	290.7272727			

R-Square	Coeff Var	Root MSE	WGTLOSS Mean
0.786742	21.73792	1.244990	5.727273

Source	DF	Type I SS	Mean Square	F Value	Pr > F
GROUP	3	228.7272727	76.2424242	49.19	<0.0001

Source	DF	Type III SS	Mean Square	F Value	Pr > F
GROUP	3	228.7272727	76.2424242	49.19	<0.0001

The GLM Procedure
Dependent Variable: WGTLOSS

Contrast	DF	Contrast SS	Mean Square	F Value	Pr > F
No exercise or diet vs others	1	132.0000000	132.0000000	85.16	<0.0001 (k2)
Diet vs exercise	1	4.5454545	4.5454545	2.93	0.0946 (k3)
Diet or exercise vs exercise and diet	1	92.1818182	92.1818182	59.47	<0.0001 (k4)

The GLM Procedure
Tukey's Studentized Range (HSD) Test for WGTLOSS

Note: This test controls the Type I experiment wise error rate, but it generally has a higher Type II error rate than REGWQ.

```
Alpha                                        0.05
Error Degrees of Freedom                     40
Error Mean Square                            1.55
Critical Value of Studentized Range          3.79069
Minimum Significant Difference               1.4229(k5)
```

```
Means with the same letter are not significantly different.
Tukey Grouping        Mean(k6)            N              GROUP
        A              9.0909             11               4
        B              6.0000             11               3
        B
        B              5.0909             11               2
        C              2.7273             11               1
```

The following output is based on the additional programming line commented above.

means group/ TUKEY CLDIFF alpha = .05;

                     The GLM Procedure
       Tukey's Studentized Range (HSD) Test for WGTLOSS

Note: This test controls the Type I experiment wise error rate.

```
Alpha                                        0.05
Error Degrees of Freedom                     40
Error Mean Square                            1.55
Critical Value of Studentized Range          3.79069
Minimum Significant Difference               1.4229
```

Comparisons significant at the 0.05 level are indicated by ***.

GROUP Comparison (k7)	Difference Between Means (k8)	Simultaneous 95% Confidence Limits (k9)		
4 −3	3.0909	1.6680	4.5139	***
4 −2	4.0000	2.5771	5.4229	***
4 −1	6.3636	4.9407	7.7866	***
3 −4	−3.0909	−4.5139	−1.6680	***
3 −2	0.9091	−0.5139	2.3320	
3 −1	3.2727	1.8498	4.6957	***
2 −4	−4.0000	−5.4229	−2.5771	***
2 −3	−0.9091	−2.3320	0.5139	
2 −1	2.3636	0.9407	3.7866	***
1 −4	−6.3636	−7.7866	−4.9407	***
1 −3	−3.2727	−4.6957	−1.8498	***
1 −2	−2.3636	−3.7866	−0.9407	***

The *p*-value for the *F* test, given in (k1), is used to test the equality of all the means and is <0.0001. The *p*-value is significant and leads to a conclusion that the four regimen groups do not have same mean weight loss levels.

The first contrast statement for regimen groups 1 versus 2, 3, and 4 has highly significant *p*-value <0.0001 given at (k2). The second contrast statement of 2 versus 3 is not significant and the last contrast statement of 2, 3 versus 4 is highly significant as the *p*-value is <0.0001, as indicated by the *p*-values given at (k3) and (k4).

The critical difference to compare any two means by Tukey's method is given by (k5) and is 1.4. The means for the four regimens are provided in the (k6) column. The last column indicates the Group label. The letters in the left-most column under Tukey grouping are used to compare the treatment means using Tukey's method. The regimens with the means given by the same letter are not significantly different and the means given by different letters are significant. The means corresponding to regimens 3 and 2 are 6.0 and 5.1, respectively, and have the same letter B next to the means and hence regimens 3 and 2 are not significantly different. The mean of the fourth regimen 9.1 and the mean of the first regimen 2.7 do not have the same symbol next to the means and hence are significantly different. The significance of the means is determined by comparing the difference of the means against the critical value given at (k5).

Table 3.2 provides the critical values for adjacent means based on all of the selected multiple comparisons. The higher the critical value, the stringent the test, implying that it will be difficult to detect significant differences between the means.

Tukey's critical value is 1.4, whereas Duncan and SNK critical values are both 1.1, and thus Tukey's test gives less significant differences than Duncan and SNK methods.

The $(1 - \alpha)$ 100% CIs for the difference in the means can also be requested by the CLDIFF option by selecting α of your choice of the multiple comparison method as shown in the above program. Comparisons that are

TABLE 3.2

Critical Values for Adjacent Means Based on Selected Multiple Comparisons

Test	Critical Value for Two Adjacent Means
Scheffe	1.5
LSD	1.1
Sidak	1.5
Bonferroni	1.5
Dunnett	1.3
Duncan	1.1
Student–Newman–Keuls	1.1
Tukey	1.4

significantly different at the 0.05 levels are indicated by ***. In the output the first line in the (k7) column is the comparisons between the third and fourth age group. The difference between the means given in the column (k8) is 3.1 and the CI for this difference given in the column (k9) is (1.67, 4.51). The other lines can be similarly interpreted.

3.3.1.1 Variance

One can check the equality of the variances of the k populations by using homogeneity of variance test (HOVTEST) option in PROC MEANS as shown below, using Levene's and/or Bartlett's test. Levene's test is less sensitive to normality of the underlying data whereas Bartlett's test is sensitive. The null hypothesis is that all the variances are equal against the alternative that the variances are not all equal. In our output below at (l1) the p-value for Levene's test (1960) is 0.7044, and the p-value for Bartlett's test (Bartlett, 1937b) at (l2) is 0.7307 and both p-values are greater than the 0.05 level and conclude that the variances are equal. If the p-value is <0.05, then one would conclude that the variances are not equal and in that case would use Welch's ANOVA (1951) by using the option WELCH along with the MEANS option in PROC GLM to draw conclusions on the equality of means by using the p-value at (l3) of Welch's ANOVA. The p-value of the Welch ANOVA is significant indicating the four group means are not all the same. The following programming lines provide the necessary output:

```
Data a;
/***input data ***/
Input GROUP WGTLOSS  @@;  cards;
1 5 1 2 1 2 1 3 1 3 1 2 1 5 1 3 1 2 1 2 1 1 2 5 2 5 2 4 2 5 2
3 2 6 2 5 2 7 2 5 2 7 2 4 3 7 3 5 3 6 3 8 3 5 3 7 3 5 3 6 3 5
3 6 3 6 4 8 4 7 4 9 4 10 4 9 4 7 4 9 4 10 4 12 4 9 4 10
;
/***end of input data***/
proc glm; class group;  model wgtloss = group ; run;
means group/hovtest = levene welch hovtest = bartlett; run;
```

***

The GLM Procedure
Levene's Test for Homogeneity of WGTLOSS Variance
ANOVA of Squared Deviations from Group Means

Source	DF	Sum of Squares	Mean Square	F Value	Pr > F
GROUP	3	5.4838	1.8279	0.47	0.7044 (l1)
Error	40	155.3	3.8834		

Bartlett's Test for Homogeneity of wgtloss Variance

Source	DF	Chi-Square	Pr > ChiSq
GROUP	3	1.2934	0.7307 (l2)

```
                 Welch's ANOVA for WGTLOSS
    Source        DF        F Value        Pr > F
    GROUP        3.0000       38.94      < 0.0001(13)
    Error       22.0349
```

3.3.2 Covariance Analysis

Null hypothesis related to the means will have a greater chance of rejection when the variability within groups is reduced. One way to reduce the variability is to adjust the responses to a common level by regressing it on a variable called a covariate that is unrelated to the treatment. This type of analysis is known as analysis of covariance (ANCOVA). This method is a combination of an ANOVA and regression analysis.

If the covariate measure is available before randomizing the experimental units to the treatment groups, it is reasonable to assume that there is a common slope between the response variable and the covariate. However, if the covariate is measured after the assignment of the treatment and during the course of the experiment, it is likely that there may be different slopes between the response variable and covariate, and there is a need to consider an interaction term between the covariate and treatment groups. The significance of treatment effects is considered after adjusting for different slopes.

These ideas are illustrated with examples below.

Assume that a network was wondering whether the number of hours of TV watched by white, African-American, and other race groups are the same. Race can be considered as the treatment. The network considered the number of years in school, since it may affect TV watching habit. The number of years of schooling is a covariate, which may interact with race and in the analysis of watching TV, an interaction term for groups and covariate is considered.

Returning to the weight loss problem discussed in the previous section, two covariates were listed along with the response variable in Table 3.1. Initial body weight can be considered as a covariate with no interaction on the regimen groups, as the treatments are randomly assigned and the initial body weight is measured before the randomization of the patients into four groups. The randomization justifies equal slope assumption for the loss of weight to the baseline body weight for the four groups. The diet caloric intake may depend on the treatment regimen and it is possible that the slopes of the response variable on caloric intake may be different for the treatment groups. Hence, the covariate caloric intake with an interaction term with the treatment groups needs to be considered.

While one covariate is usually included in the analysis, it is possible to include any number of covariates and interactions of covariates with treatment groups, if needed. The following program provides the required ANCOVA.

The weight loss data are analyzed using diet calorie intake as a covariate. If the *p*-value of the interaction given at (m1) is more than 0.05, some researchers reanalyze the data excluding the interaction term. However, the author prefers to draw conclusions with the original model and the interaction term.

The output will show Type I and Type III sum of squares. Type I sum of squares are the unadjusted treatment, SS in the one-way ANCOVA, if the treatment is followed by another variable in the model statement. The TYPE III sum of squares is the adjusted treatment sum of squares and enables us to test the treatment effects adjusted for all other factors included in the model. One should look at the Type III sum of squares in the analysis.

```
Data a;
/***input data***/
Input GROUP WGTLOSS CALORIES INITIALBW @@; cards;
1 5 2100 150 1 2 1500 165 1 2 2300 132
1 3 2425 165 1 3 2000 147 1 2 1900 214
1 5 2500 210 1 3 1750 178 1 2 2000 176
1 2 1250 186 1 1 2100 155 2 5 1200 145
2 5 1300 164 2 4 1250 137 2 5 2000 211
2 3 1300 189 2 6 1000 157 2 5 1400 189
2 7 1350 174 2 5 1800 203 2 7 1250 134
2 4 1350 176 3 7 1300 165 3 5 1200 170
3 6 1100 215 3 8 1450 213 3 5 1200 189
3 7 1300 159 3 5 1500 150 3 6 1600 190
3 5 1500 197 3 6 1400 186 3 6 1600 168
4 8 1250 167 4 7 1200 235 4 9 800 210
4 10 1500 184 4 9 1200 175 4 7 1300 149
4 9 1250 195 4 10 1300 204 4 12 1200 174
4 9 1350 196 4 10 1200 179
;
/***end of input data***/
proc glm;class group;
model wgtloss = group calories initialbw group*calories;run;
```

The following is the necessary output:

```
                        The GLM Procedure
                  Dependent Variable: WGTLOSS
                          Sum of         Mean          F
Source            DF     Squares        Square       Value      Pr > F
Model              8   231.8424201   28.9803025     17.23      <0.0001
Error             35    58.8848526    1.6824244
Corrected Total   43   290.7272727
```

```
        R-Square    Coeff Var    Root MSE    WGTLOSS Mean
        0.797457    22.64748     1.297083      5.727273
```

Source	DF	Type I SS	Mean Square	F Value	Pr > F
GROUP	3	228.7272727	76.2424242	45.32	< 0.0001
CALORIES	1	1.2149943	1.2149943	0.72	0.4012
INITIALBW	1	0.0944567	0.0944567	0.06	0.8141
CALORIES*GROUP	3	1.8056963	0.6018988	0.36	0.7838

Source	DF	Type III SS	Mean Square	F Value	Pr > F
GROUP	3	11.16762713	3.72254238	2.21	0.1040 (m4)
CALORIES	1	0.31632389	0.31632389	0.19	0.6672 (m2)
INITIALBW	1	0.02844717	0.02844717	0.02	0.8973 (m3)
CALORIES*GROUP	3	1.80569635	0.60189878	0.36	0.7838 (m1)

On the basis of the p-value 0.7838 given in (m1) for the interaction, we conclude that the slopes for caloric intake are the same for the four different diet regimens. The caloric intake p-value of 0.6672 given in (m2) indicates that there is no effect due to the covariate. The initial body weight with p-value of 0.8973 given in (m3) indicates that the initial body weight has no impact on the loss of weight. There are no group differences as indicated by the p-value 0.1040 given in (m4). Note the groups are significant without covariates indicated by Type I sum of squares and our previous analysis.

3.4 Multivariate Methods

Sometimes multiple responses will be taken from each experimental unit and in that case we stack all the responses in a column to get a response vector. Let us consider p responses. Although it is possible to analyze each response by using univariate methods as discussed earlier, it is appropriate to analyze all these responses together by using multivariate methods. By using multivariate methods, one can consider the joint probability and the relationship between the responses. Examples of multivariate problems include components of midterm and final grades for students, city and highway miles for a car, MAYO score components (stool frequency, rectal bleeding, endoscopy, physician global assessment), different lab tests (e.g., glucose, cholesterol), and so on.

Let us start by first discussing some basic concepts of multivariate analysis.

The vector of population means is the stacked array of the population means and will be denoted by

$$\mu = \begin{bmatrix} \mu_1 \\ \vdots \\ \mu_k \end{bmatrix}.$$

The sample mean vector

$$\bar{X} = \begin{bmatrix} \bar{x}_1 \\ \vdots \\ \bar{x}_k \end{bmatrix}.$$

The joint variability between two variables is known as the covariance between them, and will be denoted by σ_{ij}. If there is no linear relationship between the two variables, then the covariance is 0. The covariances and the variances are put together to form a variance and covariance matrix. The variances are all placed in a diagonal and the covariances are placed in off-diagonal positions to form the variance and covariance matrix, and denote them by

$$\Sigma = \begin{bmatrix} \sigma_{11} & \cdots & \sigma_{k1} \\ \vdots & \cdots & \vdots \\ \sigma_{1k} & \cdots & \sigma_{kk} \end{bmatrix}$$

for the population, and

$$\mathbf{S} = \begin{bmatrix} s_{11} & \cdots & s_{k1} \\ \vdots & \cdots & \vdots \\ s_{1k} & \cdots & s_{kk} \end{bmatrix}$$

for the sample.

All the variances and covariances in the matrix may not necessarily be in the same unit of measurement. To make the matrix unit free a correlation matrix is constructed. The correlation ρ_{ij} is $\sigma_{ij}/(\sqrt{\sigma_{ii}}\sqrt{\sigma_{jj}})$ and is always between –1 and 1. The population correlation matrix will be denoted by

$$\mathbf{P} = \begin{bmatrix} 1 & \cdots & \rho_{1k} \\ . & \cdots & . \\ \rho_{k1} & \cdots & 1 \end{bmatrix}$$

and the sample correlation matrix is denoted by

$$\mathbf{R} = \begin{bmatrix} 1 & \cdots & r_{1k} \\ . & \cdots & . \\ r_{k1} & \cdots & 1 \end{bmatrix}.$$

if the correlation between two variables is positive (negative), then the covariance between the two variables is also positive (negative), and vice versa.

Almost all methods considered in this section assume that the data are distributed as multivariate normal and the variance–covariance matrix for different groups are equal. Testing these assumptions is beyond the scope of this book and the interested reader is referred to Johnson and Wichern (1998). Readers interested in matrix manipulation are referred to Graybill (1969).

TABLE 3.3

Artificial Data on City and Highway Gas Mileage, Weight-to-Power Ratio, and Front Headroom of Cars

Car	City	Highway	Weight-to-Power Ratio (lb/hp)	Front Headroom (in)	Car	City	Highway	Weight-to-Power Ratio (lb/hp)	Front Headroom (in)
1	26	32	18	40	11	34	37	17	39
2	30	33	17	43	12	24	37	16	36
3	28	31	16	39	13	28	32	14	37
4	29	32	17	36	14	30	36	15	36
5	31	34	19	38	15	29	35	16	39
6	25	34	20	39	16	27	34	15	40
7	35	37	13	37	17	26	31	16	42
8	32	35	14	36	18	23	36	15	41
9	28	31	15	39	19	27	32	15	42
10	27	31	16	36	20	23	33	18	39

Let us consider city and highway gas mileage, weight-to-power ratio (lb/hp), and front headroom (in) for 20 cars. The artificial data are given in Table 3.3.

The necessary descriptive statistics can be obtained by using PROC CORR. The COV option produces the variance–covariance matrix structure.

```
data a
/***input data***/;
input CITY HWAY WGTTOPOW HEADROOM @@; cards;
26 32 18 40 30 33 17 43 28 31 16 39 29 32 17 36 31 34 19 38 25
34 20 39 35 37 13 37 32 35 14 36 28 31 15 39 27 31 16 36 34
37 17 39 24 37 16 36 28 32 14 37 30 36 15 36 29 35 16 39 27 34
15 40 26 31 16 42 23 36 15 41 27 32 15 42 23 33 18 39
;
/***end of input data***/
proc corr cov;run;
```

This produces the following output:

```
The CORR Procedure 4 Variables: CITY HWAY WGTTOPOW HEADROOM

                  Covariance Matrix (n1), DF = 19
                CITY            HWAY            WGTTOPOW        HEADROOM
CITY       10.83157895      2.24736842      -1.69473684     -1.91578947
HWAY        2.24736842      4.66052632      -0.59473684     -1.26842105
WGTTOPOW   -1.69473684     -0.59473684       3.04210526      0.71578947
HEADROOM   -1.91578947     -1.26842105       0.71578947      4.85263158
```

```
                        Simple Statistics
                    Mean
Variable    N      (n2)      Std Dev      Sum       Minimum    Maximum
CITY        20   28.10000    3.29114   562.00000   23.00000   35.00000
HWAY        20   33.65000    2.15883   673.00000   31.00000   37.00000
WGTTOPOW    20   16.10000    1.74416   322.00000   13.00000   20.00000
HEADROOM    20   38.70000    2.20287   774.00000   36.00000   43.00000
```

```
           Pearson Correlation Coefficients (n3),  N = 20
                     Prob > |r| under H0: Rho = 0
                 CITY          HWAY          WGTTOPOW       HEADROOM
CITY          1.00000       0.31631        -0.29524       -0.26425
                            0.1742 (n4)      0.2063         0.2602
HWAY          0.31631       1.00000        -0.15795       -0.26672
              0.1742                         0.5060         0.2556
WGTTOPOW     -0.29524      -0.15795          1.00000        0.18630
              0.2063        0.5060                          0.4316
HEADROOM     -0.26425      -0.26672          0.18630        1.00000
              0.2602        0.2556           0.4316
```

All the four means are given in the column (n2) and the variance–covariance matrix for the four variables is given in the matrix (n1). The correlation matrix is given in (n3). These are the sample values and we express this output in the following matrix form:

$$\bar{X} = \begin{bmatrix} 28.1 \\ 33.7 \\ 16.1 \\ 38.7 \end{bmatrix}, \quad S = \begin{bmatrix} 10.8 & 2.2 & -1.7 & -1.9 \\ 2.2 & 4.7 & -0.6 & -1.3 \\ -1.7 & -0.6 & 3.0 & 0.7 \\ -1.9 & -1.3 & 0.7 & 4.9 \end{bmatrix},$$

$$R = \begin{bmatrix} 1 & 0.3 & -0.3 & -0.3 \\ 0.3 & 1 & -0.2 & -0.3 \\ -0.3 & -0.2 & 1 & 0.2 \\ -0.3 & -0.3 & 0.2 & 1 \end{bmatrix}.$$

The first entry 28.1 in $\bar{X}$ represents the mean city mileage of the 20 cars and similar interpretations for other entries in $\bar{X}$.

The variance for city mileage is 10.8 given in the first row and first column of S. The value 2.2 given in the first row and the second column of S is the covariance between the city and highway gas mileage for the 20 cars. The other entries in **S** can be similarly interpreted. The entry 0.3 given in the first row and the second column of **R** is the correlation between the city and highway gas mileage. The entry −0.3 given in the first row and the fourth column of **R** is the correlation between the city gas mileage and head room of the 20 cars. The 0.3 correlation implies that higher the city gas mileage, the highway gas mileage is also higher. The −0.3 correlation means that the higher the head room, the lower the city gas mileage. The other correlations in **R** can be similarly interpreted.

When the correlation is 0 the variables are independent. For testing the population correlation 0, the *p*-values are given in the Pearson correlation coefficients output, at the bottom of the correlations. The *p*-value 0.1742 given at (n4) is used to test the null hypothesis that the correlation between the city and highway gas mileages is 0 against a two-sided alternative and as this *p*-value is >0.05, concluding that the 0 population correlation is not rejected at 0.05 level of significance for a two-sided test. The remaining *p*-values can be interpreted similarly.

The data can be plotted. We will not go into details about the various plotting techniques. Johnson and Wichern (1998) describe various graphical procedures including linked scatter plots and brushing techniques.

3.4.1 Correlation, Partial, and Intraclass Correlation

Let the car manufacturer be interested in testing that the correlation of weight-to-power ratio and front headroom is more than (less than, not equal to) a specified value, ρ_0. Here ρ_0 is a value prespecified by the investigator. To establish the claim, the null hypothesis tested is that the correlation is not more than (not less than, equal to) ρ_0. The level of the test α has to be specified. To determine the sample size, the desired power, usually 80%, 90%, or 95% has to be specified at an alternative value, ρ_1. The distribution of the correlation coefficient is complicated. When the variables for which the correlation is calculated have a normal distribution, and the population correlation is zero, a transformation of ρ has a *t*-distribution. However, with any population correlation, Fisher's Z-transformed variable is approximately normally distributed with variance $1/(n-3)$, where n is the sample size and this variance does not involve the population correlation. The following program produces sample sizes for one-sided or two-sided tests assuming $\rho_0 = 0$ and $\rho_1 = 0.59$.

```
proc power;
    onecorr dist = fisherz nullc = 0  corr = 0.59 ntotal =.
        sides = 1 sides = 2 alpha = .05 power = .80;
*nullc is the correlation for the null hypothesis;
*corr is the correlation for the alternative hypotheis; run;
```

This produces the following output:

```
                        The POWER Procedure
                Fisher's z Test for Pearson Correlation
                     Fixed Scenario Elements
        Distribution                  Fisher's z transformation of r
        Method                        Normal approximation
        Null Correlation              0
        Nominal Alpha                 0.05
        Correlation                   0.59
        Nominal Power                 0.8
        Number of Variables           0
          Partialled Out


        Index    Actual Sides    Actual Alpha    Power    N Total
          1           1             0.0497        0.811      16
          2           2             0.0498        0.818      20
```

In all, 16 subjects are needed for a one-sided test, and 20 subjects for a two-sided test.

Suppose the manufacturer was interested in testing $H_0: \rho = 0$ against $H_A: \rho \neq 0$ for the weight-to-power ratio and front headroom. He selects 20 cars based on the above-determined sample size. The data collected are given in Table 3.3. The FISHER option in PROC CORR, provides a Fisher's Z transformation. The sample correlation in column (o1) is the correlation between the indicated variables in the line of the correlation. The Fisher's Z transformation of (o1) can be found in column (o2). The 95% CI is given at [(o3), (o4)] and the p-value for testing 0 correlation is given in column (o5).

```
proc corr nosimple fisher (biasadj = no); var city hway
    wgttopow headroom; run;
```

```
                Pearson Correlation Statistics (Fisher's z Transformation)
With        Sample                                                           p Value for
Variable    variable   N Correlation   Fisher's z   95% Confidence Limits    H0:Rho=0
                            (o1)          (o2)          (o3)        (o4)        (o5)
city        hway       20   0.31631      0.32754      0.146754    0.665655    0.1769
city        wgttopow   20  -0.29524     -0.30429     -0.652508    0.169419    0.2096
city        headroom   20  -0.26425     -0.27067     -0.632776    0.201879    0.2644
hway        wgttopow   20  -0.15795     -0.15928     -0.561242    0.305956    0.5113
hway        headroom   20  -0.26672     -0.27333     -0.634368    0.199326    0.2598
wgttopow    headroom   20   0.18630      0.18850     -0.279243    0.580927    0.4370
                            (o6)          (o7)          (o8)        (o9)       (o10)
```

The correlation between weight-to-power ratio and front headroom is 0.18630 given at (o6). The Fisher's Z transformation of the correlation 0.18630 is 0.18850 given at (o7). The 95% CI of this population correlation is (−0.28, 0.58) given at [(o8), (o9)]. The *p*-value for testing zero correlation for these variables is 0.4370 given at (o10) and as this *p*-value is >0.05 the null hypothesis of zero correlation is not rejected.

Suppose the manufacturer was interested in testing H_0: $\rho = \rho_0$ (0.5) against H_A: $\rho \neq \rho_0$ (0.5) for the weight-to-power ratio and front headroom. The necessary program and output follow:

```
proc corr nosimple nocorr fisher(rho0 = .5 biasadj = no);
var wgttopow headroom;run;
```

```
                    The CORR Procedure
              2 Variables: WGTTOPOW HEADROOM
     Pearson Correlation Statistics (Fisher's z Transformation)
               With           Sample                    95% Confidence
Variable Variable   N   Correlation Fisher's z           Limits
WGTTOPOW HEADROOM  20     0.18630      0.18850   -0.279243 0.580927


     Pearson Correlation Statistics (Fisher's z Transformation)
                                   --H0:Rho = Rho0--
    Variable      With Variable      Rho0            p Value
    WGTTOPOW      HEADROOM           0.50000         0.1231 (o11)
```

The *p*-value is 0.1231 given at (o11) for testing $\rho = 0.5$ against the two-sided alternative and this *p*-value indicates that the null hypothesis of the correlation between weight-to-power ratio and front head room is 0.5 is not rejected.

Suppose due to budgetary constraints, the car manufacturer can only get 10 cars, and wants to know what power one can get when $\rho_1 = 0.59$ while testing H_0: $\rho_0 = 0$, using 0.05 level of significance. The power can be obtained by the following program:

```
proc power;
   onecorr dist = fisherz  nullc = 0 corr = 0.59 ntotal = 10
          sides = 1 sides = 2 alpha = .05 power = .; run;
```

```
                    The POWER Procedure
            Fisher's z Test for Pearson Correlation
                  Fixed Scenario Elements
    Distribution                    Fisher's z transformation of r
    Method                          Normal approximation
    Null Correlation                0
    Nominal Alpha                   0.05
    Correlation                     0.59
    Total Sample Size               10
    Number of Variables             0
      Partialled Out
```

```
                  Computed Power
                      Actual
     Index    Sides    Alpha        Power
       1        1      0.0488    0.600 (o12)
       2        2      0.0484    0.473 (o13)
```

The power of the one-sided test is 60.0% given at (o12) and is 47.3% for a two-sided test given at (o13).

Partial correlations are those between variables while controlling (adjusting) the effect for the other variables. Suppose instead of the standard correlation between city and highway gas mileages, the manufacturer wanted to know the correlation of city and highway gas mileages while controlling the effect of the weight-to-power ratio. The following program is used. The PARTIAL option is used for the variables that need to be controlled.

```
proc corr nosimple nocorr fisher(biasadj = no);
var city hway; partial wgttopow; run;
```

```
                  The CORR Procedure
          1   Partial Variables:    WGTTOPOW
          2   Variables:            CITY HWAY
```

```
  Pearson Partial Correlation Statistics (Fisher's z Transformation)
              With            N          Sample    Fisher's    95% Confidence
Variable  Variable  N partialled  Correlation      z            Limits
CITY        HWAY    20       1       0.28585     0.29404  -0.193484 0.655012
                                      (p1)                   (p2)      (p3)
```

```
       Pearson Partial Correlation Statistics (Fisher's z
                         Transformation)
Variable          With Variable        p Value for H0: Rho = 0
CITY                  HWAY                     0.2395 (p4)
```

The partial correlation for city and highway gas mileages adjusted for weight-to-power ratio is 0.28585 given at (p1). The 95% CI for this partial correlation is (−0.19, 0.66) given at [(p2), (p3)]. The p-value for testing this partial correlation is 0 against the two-sided alternative is 0.2395 given at (p4) and the partial correlation is not significant.

Inference on the partial correlations similar to the ordinary correlations can be drawn by using the effective sample size for sample size, which is the sample size minus the number of variables adjusted to obtain the partial correlation.

Often times, one is interested in testing whether the correlations are the same among the k groups. The null hypothesis $H_0: \rho_1 = \rho_2 = \cdots = \rho_k$ is tested against the alternative that at least one pair is not the same. Consider the correlations between the mid-term and final exam test scores in three subjects: Math, English, and Biology and let the correlations be 0.80, 0.85, and 0.70, respectively. Let the number of students considered in the three subjects be 45, 55, and 50. The following is the necessary program to test this null hypothesis and estimate the correlation coefficient by combining the k sample correlation coefficients when the null hypothesis is retained.

```
data a;
/***input data***/
numgrps = 3;*input the number of groups;
alpha = .05;counter = 0;zsum = 0;  nsum = 0;  zsumsq = 0;
/***end of input data ***/
%macro calc(ssize,group,rho);
counter = counter + 1;  n&group = &ssize;  nsum = (n&group - 3) + nsum;
r&group = &rho;  Rho&group = .5*(log((1 + r&group)/(1 - r&group)));
z&group = ((n&group - 3)*rho&group);
zsum = z&group + zsum;
zsumsq = zsumsq + ((n&group - 3)*rho&group**2);
if counter = numgrps then zbar = zsum/nsum;
if counter = numgrps then CHISQ = zsumsq - ((zsum**2)/nsum);
%mend calc;
/***input data***/
*input sample size, group number, rho;
%calc(45,1,.8);
%calc(55,2,.85);
%calc(50,3,.7);
/*** end of input data ***/
data b;set a;
PVALUE = 1 - probchi(chisq,numgrps - 1);
RCOMB = (((exp(2*zbar)) - 1)/((exp(2*zbar)) + 1));
keep chisq pvalue rcomb; proc print; run;
```

CHISQ	PVALUE	RCOMB
3.75441	0.15302 (q1)	0.79305 (q2)

The p-value for testing the null hypothesis that the three correlations are the same is 0.153 given at (q1) of the output and we conclude that the three correlations are the same. The estimated common correlation is 0.793 given at (q2) of the output.

Let us consider k randomly selected treatments experimented with r replications of each treatment. The correlation between observations in each of these k groups is intraclass correlation. This is obtained from the one-way ANOVA table as given in Section 3.3.1. Consider the weight loss for the four regimens given in that section resulting in the following ANOVA table:

Source	DF	Sum of Squares	Mean Square	F Value	Pr > F
Model	3	228.7272727	76.2424242	49.19	<0.0001
Error	40	62.0000000	1.5500000		

The intraclass correlation is obtained by the following program:

```
data a;
/***input data***/
betwnms = 76.24;*mean square model; withinms = 1.55;*mean square
  error;  df = 3;*model degrees of freedom;
/***end of input data***/
ICORR = (betwnms − withinms) / (betwnms + df*withinms);
keep icorr; proc print;run;

  ICORR
  0.92335
```

The intraclass correlation between the weight loss for the four regimens is 0.923. Testing the significance of this correlation is the same as testing for the equality of effects of the k groups and the p-value for this test is <0.001 given in the ANOVA table.

3.4.2 Hotelling's T^2

Hotelling's T^2 is an extension of the univariate t-test to a multivariate setting. Its application will be discussed in one- and two-sample problems.

3.4.2.1 One Sample

Manufacturer of Model A cars claims that the city and highway mileage delivered by that model car is 25 and 30 mpg, respectively. A consumer protection agency wants to disprove that claim. They randomly select $n = 10$ cars from that population of cars and test the mileage. The data obtained by them are displayed in Table 3.4.

The following program gives a test for the multivariate hypothesis that the city and highway gas mileages are, respectively, 25 and 30 mpg. The $(1 − \alpha)100\%$ simultaneous CIs of the means and differences of means are also given in the program. For convenience, the operations will be performed in steps.

TABLE 3.4

Artificial Data on the City and Highway Mileage of Model A Cars

Car Number	City Mileage	Highway Mileage	Car Number	City Mileage	Highway Mileage
1	26	32	6	25	34
2	30	33	7	35	37
3	28	31	8	32	35
4	29	32	9	28	31
5	31	34	10	27	31

Step 1

```
data in;
/***input data***/
input CITY HWAY @@;  cards;
26 32 30 33 28 31 29 32 31 34 25 34 35 37 32 35 28 31 27 31
;
/***end of input data***/
proc corr cov; run;
```

Output from Step 1

```
                   The CORR Procedure
          2 Variables: CITY HWAY
                 Covariance Matrix (r1), DF = 9
                          CITY                 HWAY
          CITY         8.988888889         4.333333333
          HWAY         4.333333333         4.000000000
                       Simple Statistics
Variable   N   Mean (r2)   Std Dev    Sum      Minimum   Maximum
CITY      10   29.10000    2.99815  291.00000  25.00000  35.00000
HWAY      10   33.00000    2.00000  330.00000  31.00000  37.00000
                             ***
```

Step 2: Calculation of T² and p-value

```
data a; proc iml;
/***input data***/
p = 2;*number of items;  alpha = .05;  n = 10;*sample size;
mu = {25, 30}; *hypothesized means;
xbar = {29.1, 33};*from (r2) of Step 1;
s = {8.99 4.33,4.33 4.0};* from (r1) of Step 1. Each row is
  separated by comma;
/***end of input data***/
nminusp = n - p;  sinv = inv(s);
xbarmmu = xbar - mu;  xbarmmut = xbarmmu`;
T2 = n*xbarmmut*sinv*xbarmmu;
F = (nminusp/(p*(n - 1)))*T2;  PVALUE = 1 - probf(f,p,nminusp);
print t2 pvalue;  quit;
```

Output from Step 2

```
  T2                PVALUE
  24.189041      0.0054074 (r3)
```

Step 3: Calculation for the CI for the Means

```
data ci;
%macro ci(var,varname);
```

```
data &var;set in;*Data from step 1;
proc univariate noprint;var &var;output out = stats n=n
  var = var mean = MEAN;run;
data &var;set stats;
/***input data***/
p = 2;*number of components; alpha = .05;
/***end of input data***/
nminusp = n - p; f = finv(1 - alpha, p,nminusp);
LOWER_CI = mean - (sqrt(p*(n-1)*f/(nminusp))*sqrt(var/n));
UPPER_CI = mean + (sqrt(p*(n-1)*f/(nminusp))*sqrt(var/n));
VARNAME = &varname;  keep varname mean lower_ci upper_ci;
%mend ci;
data b;
/*** input data***/
*Call macro for the number of components of interest;;
%ci(city,'City';);
%ci(hway,'Hway');
/*** end of input data***/
data final;set city hway; proc print;
var varname lower_ci mean upper_ci; run;
```

Output from Step 3

VARNAME	LOWER_CI	MEAN	UPPER_CI
city	26.0970 (r4)	29.1	32.1030 (r5)
hway	30.9967 (r6)	33.0	35.0033 (r7)

Step 4: Confidence Interval for the Difference of the Means

```
data a;  proc iml;
/***input data***/
p = 2;*number of items;  alpha = .05;  n = 10;
xbar = {29.1, 33};*These are the means from (r1) for the
  components of the required difference;
s = {8.99 4.33,4.33 4.0};* The 1st and 4th are the 2 variance
  for the variables of interest and the 2nd/3rd component is
  the covariance for the two variables from (r2) of the output;
/***end of input data***/
onet = {1 - 1};  one = {1,-1};  nminusp = n - p;  vardiff = onet*s*one;
sterdiff = sqrt(vardiff/n);  diff = onet*xbar;
f = finv(1 - alpha,p,nminusp);
LOWER_CI = diff - (sqrt(p*(n-1)*f/nminusp))*sterdiff;
UPPER_CI = diff + (sqrt(p*(n-1)*f/nminusp))*sterdiff;
print lower_ci diff upper_ci;  quit;
```

Output from Step 4

LOWER_CI	DIFF	UPPER_CI
−5.984263 (r8)	− 3.9	− 1.815737 (r9)

TABLE 3.5

Artificial Data of City and Highway Mileage for Model A and B Cars

Car Number	City Mileage	Highway Mileage	Car Number	City Mileage	Highway Mileage
1	26	32	11	23	29
2	30	33	12	31	33
3	28	31	13	29	35
4	29	32	14	22	32
5	31	34	15	21	31
6	25	34	16	25	36
7	35	37	17	27	34
8	32	35	18	32	35
9	28	31	19	24	32
10	27	31	20	22	33

Based on the above output the null hypothesis H_0: $\mu = \begin{bmatrix} 25 \\ 30 \end{bmatrix}$ is tested by using the p-value at (r3). Since this p-value is 0.005, the null hypothesis is rejected and hence the manufacturer's claim is rejected. The 95% CI for the city mileage based on these cars is (26.1, 32.1) given at [(r4), (r5)]. The 95% CI for the highway mileage based on these cars is (31.0, 35.0) given at [(r6), (r7)]. The 95% CI for the difference between city and highway mileages is (−6.0, −1.8) given at [(r8), (r9)].

To test whether the means of the variables are the same one can use the CI [(r8), (r9)]. If zero is contained in this interval, then it is concluded that the means of the component variables are the same, otherwise different.

3.4.2.2 Two Samples

We would like to test whether the mean gas mileage for city and highway driving for car Models A and B are the same. This is the two-sample version of Hotelling T^2 statistic. Let us take $n_1 = 10$ Model A cars and $n_2 = 10$ Model B cars and the gas mileage data are given in Table 3.5. The first 10 cars are Model A cars given in Table 3.4 and the additional cars are Model B cars. We assume that the variance–covariance matrices of the variables are the same for both models.

The following program provides the necessary output. For convenience, the program is shown in three steps.

Step 1

```
data group1;*Model A cars;
/***input data***/
input city hway @@; cards;
```

```
26 32 30 33 28 31 29 32 31 34 25 34 35 37 32 35 28 31 27 31
;
/***end of input data***/
proc corr cov;run; data group1;set group1;  group=1;
data group2;*Model B cars;
/***input data***/
input city hway @@; cards;
23 29 31 33 29 35 22 32 21 31 25 36 27 34 32 35 24 32 22 33
;
/***end of input data***/
proc corr cov; run; data group2;set group2;  group=2;
```

Output from Step 1

```
                         The CORR Procedure
               2 Variables: CITY HWAY
                    Covariance Matrix (s1), DF=9
                                 CITY              HWAY
              CITY            8.988888889      4.333333333
              HWAY            4.333333333      4.000000000

                         Simple Statistics
                     Mean
Variable    N      (s2)     Std Dev     Sum      Minimum    Maximum
CITY        10   29.10000   2.99815   291.00000  25.00000   35.00000
HWAY        10   33.00000   2.00000   330.00000  31.00000   37.00000
                            ***

                    Covariance Matrix (s3), DF=9
                                 CITY              HWAY
              CITY           15.60000000      4.88888889
              HWAY            4.88888889      4.44444444

                         Simple Statistics
                     Mean
Variable    N      (s4)     Std Dev     Sum      Minimum    Maximum
CITY        10   25.60000   3.94968   256.00000  21.00000   32.00000
HWAY        10   33.00000   2.10819   330.00000  29.00000   36.00000
                            ***
```

Step 2: Calculation of T2 and p-value

```
data a; proc iml;
/***input data***/
p=2;*number of items; alpha=.05;
n1=10;*sample size for group 1; n2=10;* sample size for
  group 2;
x1bar={29.1, 33};*means from (s2) of Step 1 for Model A cars;
x2bar={25.6, 33};*means from (s4) of Step 1 for Model B cars;
```

```
s1 = {8.99 4.33,4.33 4.0};* from (s1) of Step 1. Each row is
  separated by comma for Model A cars;
s2 = {15.6 4.9,4.9 4.4};* from (s3) of Step 1. Each row is
  separated by comma for Model B cars;
/***end of input data***/
nminusp = n1 + n2 - p - 1;  spooled = ((n1-1)*s1+(n2-1)*s2)/(n1+n2-2);
sinvp = inv(spooled);  diff = x1bar-x2bar;  difft = diff`;
T2 = (n1*n2/(n1+n2))*difft*sinvp*diff;  F = (nminusp/
    (p*(n1+n2-2)))*T2;
PVALUE = 1 - probf(f,p,nminusp);  print t2 pvalue;  quit;
```

Output from Step 2

T2	PVALUE
8.4786892	0.0376007 (s5)

Step 3: Calculation for the CI for the Means

```
data ci;set a;
%macro ci(var,varname);
data &var;set group1 group2;* Data from step 1;
proc sort;by group;
proc univariate noprint;var &var;
output out = stats n = n var = var mean = MEAN;by group;run;
data group11;set stats;  if group = 1;
mean11 = mean;var11 = var;  n11 = n;
a = 1;drop group mean n var;  proc sort;by a;
data group12;set stats;if group = 2;
mean12 = mean;var12 = var;n12 = n;
a = 1;drop group mean n var;
proc sort;by a;
data &var;merge group11 group12;  by a;
/***input data***/
p = 2;*number of components; alpha = .05;
/***end of input data***/
MEANDIFF = mean11 - mean12;
s1pooled = (((n11-1)/(n11+n12-2))*var11 + ((n12-1)/
          (n11+n12-2))*var12);
n = n11 + n12;  f = finv(1-alpha,p,n-p-1);
LOWER_CI = meandiff - (sqrt(p*(n-2)*f/(n-p-1)))
  *sqrt(s1pooled*(n/(n11*n12)));
UPPER_CI = meandiff + (sqrt(p*(n-2)*f/(n-p-1)))
  *sqrt(s1pooled*(n/(n11*n12)));
VARNAME = &varname;  keep varname meandiff lower_ci upper_ci;
%mend ci;
data b;
/*** input data***/
*Call macro for the number of components of interest;;
%ci(city,'City';);
```

```
%ci(hway,'Hway');
/*** end of input data***/
data a;set city hway;
proc print;  var varname lower_ci meandiff upper_ci;  run;
```

Output from Step 3

***

VARNAME	LOWERCI	MEANDIFF	UPPERCI
city	− 0.82450 (s6)	3.5	7.82450 (s7)
hway	− 2.53427 (s8)	0.0	2.53427 (s9)

The null hypothesis that the mean vectors are the same for both populations is tested using the p-value at (s5). Since the p-value of 0.038 at (s5)
is <0.05, we conclude that the two mean vectors are different for models
A and B. The 95% CI for the differences in the city gas mileage means for
Models A and B is (–0.8, 7.8) given at [(s6), (s7)]. The 95% CI for the differences in the highway gas mileage means for Models A and B is (–2.5, 2.5)
given at [(s8), (s9)].

3.4.3 One-Way Multivariate Analysis of Variance

One uses the ANOVA to draw inferences on more than two univariate population means, using the F test. The extension is a multivariate analysis of
variance (MANOVA). In this situation, the responses are more than one continuous variables. With two populations, the problems discussed here reduce
to the two sample Hotelling's T^2 problem discussed in Section 3.4.2.

The global null hypothesis of primary interest is that all mean (effect) vectors are equal for all the populations (treatments) against the alternative that
mean (effect) vectors for at least one pair of populations (treatments) are
different.

If the null hypothesis for the global test is rejected, then tests are performed
to see which population (treatment) mean vectors are different. If the global
null hypothesis is not rejected, then these tests are not usually performed.
Note that in some cases even if the global test is rejected, the pair-wise tests
may not show any pairs that are significantly different or vice versa.

Contrast statements are used to draw inferences about which populations
(treatments) are different from each other. An expression of the type $\sum_{i=1}^{k} a_i \mu_i$,
where $\sum_{i=1}^{k} a_i = 0$ is called a contrast of the mean vectors.

Post hoc comparisons can also be made using the Hotelling's T^2 or using
Bonferroni intervals for all pairs of groups.

An instructor examines the scores for test 1, test 2, and test 3 between
whites, African-Americans, and other races. The test scores are correlated
since they are obtained from the same individual. These scores for each
of the races are given in the programming lines. If the responses were not

correlated, then a univariate analysis would have been more appropriate. The MANOVA is provided below:

```
Data group1;
/***input data***/
Input test1 test2 test3 @@; cards;
40 30 45 50 55 70 73 67 46 55 50 40 42 46 57 35 58 78
;
/***end of input data***/
data group1;set group1; group = 'White';
Data group2;
/***input data***/
Input test1 test2 test3 @@; cards;
60 40 55 44 55 60 72 77 60 65 73 60 72 45 35
;
/***end of input data***/
data group2;set group2; group = 'Black';
Data group3;
/***input data***/
Input test1 test2 test3 @@; cards;
80 50 55 60 58 70 80 65 20 50 45 75 72 62 45
;
/***end of input data***/
data group3;set group3; group = 'Other';
data group;set group1 group2 group3;
proc glm; class group; model test1 test2 test3 = group;
  manova h = group / printe printh;
contrast 'black vs white' group 1 0 -1;*Note SAS groups
  alphabetically;
  manova h = group; run;
```

The necessary output is as follows:

***

MANOVA Test Criteria and F Approximations for the Hypothesis
of No Overall GROUP Effect

H = Type III SSCP Matrix for GROUP

E = Error SSCP Matrix

$S = 2$ $M = 0$ $N = 4.5$

Statistic	Value	F Value	Num DF	Den DF	Pr > F
Wilks' Lambda	0.54095182	1.32	6	22	0.2905 (t1)
Pillai's Trace	0.46951500	1.23	6	24	0.3273
Hotelling-Lawley Trace	0.82924455	1.47	6	13.032	0.2627
Roy's Greatest Root	0.80521506	3.22	3	12	0.0613 (t2)

Note: F Statistic for Roy's Greatest Root is an upper bound.
Note: F Statistic for Wilks' Lambda is exact.

***

```
                          The GLM Procedure
                   Multivariate Analysis of Variance
          MANOVA Test Criteria and Exact F Statistics for the
             Hypothesis of No Overall black vs white Effect
                 H = Contrast SSCP Matrix for black vs white
                        E = Error SSCP Matrix
                      S = 1  M = 0.5  N = 4.5
Statistic                Value      F Value   Num DF   Den DF      Pr > F
Wilks' Lambda      0.75419329       1.20        3        11      0.3567 (t3)
Pillai's Trace     0.24580671       1.20        3        11      0.3567
Hotelling-         0.32592004       1.20        3        11      0.3567
  Lawley Trace
Roy's Greatest     0.32592004       1.20        3        11      0.3567
  Root
                                  * * *
```

The four commonly used statistics are provided in the output. Wilks' Lambda is based on the likelihood ratio test and Roy's Greatest Root is based on the union–intersection principle. These are widely used in drawing inferences. The p-value for Wilk's Lambda statistic is 0.2905 given in (t1). The p-value for Roy's Greatest Root is 0.0613 given in (t2). Both these tests indicate nonsignificant results between the races. The p-value for testing the African-American race against the white race excluding others based on the test scores is 0.3567 given in (t3) and is not significant. Note that in SAS nonnumerically represented groups are ordered alphabetically.

3.4.4 Profile Analysis

Sometimes the data on tests administered are collected on the same experimental unit at the same (different) time point(s) and if the data are plotted on the y-axis and time points on the x-axis, the profile of the responses on that unit is obtained. Some statistical problems related to such profiles are considered.

Let the interest be to test the effectiveness of three drugs A, B, and C on controlling the sugar levels of Type II diabetic patients. A sample of say, 15 patients, with similar demographics and disease conditions is taken. Randomly, the 15 patients are divided into three groups of five each and randomly the patients are assigned to the three treatments A, B, and C. For each patient the A1C test data are obtained at three-month intervals for one year getting four observations on each of the 15 patients and artificial data are given in Table 3.6.

The means for the three drugs at each of the four time points can be plotted. The first test is that the profiles are parallel, which means that the drugs are not interacting with the time periods and nonparallel profiles indicate the interaction between drugs and time periods.

TABLE 3.6

Artificial Data of A1C for Three Drugs in Four Periods

A				B				C			
3 mo	6 mo	9 mo	12 mo	3 mo	6 mo	9 mo	12 mo	3 mo	6 mo	9 mo	12 mo
7.1	7.2	6.9	6.8	7.5	8.0	7.7	7.4	8.1	8.2	7.9	8.1
7.0	6.9	7.3	7.1	8.0	7.6	7.7	7.4	8.0	7.9	8.1	7.8
6.8	7.0	6.9	7.0	7.9	7.7	7.6	7.3	7.9	8.0	8.2	8.0
7.5	7.2	7.3	7.4	7.4	7.6	7.5	7.2	8.3	8.1	7.8	7.9
7.7	7.5	7.4	7.6	7.4	7.4	7.2	7.1	8.2	8.0	7.9	7.9

Abbreviation: mo, month.

If the profiles are parallel, then the effectiveness of the drugs is tested and the equality of responses over the time periods. Note that the data on each unit over time periods are correlated and hence multivariate methods can be used (see Morrison, 1976). If the profiles are nonparallel, we can test the treatment effects at each period by using univariate ANOVA, and test the equality of responses at different time points for each treatment by taking the vectors of differences in responses for successive periods and testing the population mean vector to be zero by using Hotellings T^2, as discussed earlier.

However, one can use univariate ANOVA and conservatively test the required hypothesis and we use the univariate ANOVA method in this section.

The necessary program and output are given below.

```
Data group1;
/***input data***/
Input PERIOD SUBJECT RESPONSE @@; cards;
3 1 7.1 3 2 7.0 3 3 6.8 3 4 7.5 3 5 7.7 6 1 7.2 6 2 6.9 6 3
7.0 6 4 7.2 6 5 7.5 9 1 6.9 9 2 7.3 9 3 6.9 9 4 7.3 9 5 7.4 12
1 6.8 12 2 7.1 12 3 7.0 12 4 7.4 12 5 7.6
;
/***end of input data***/
data group1; set group1; DRUG = 'A';
Data group2;
/***input data***/
Input PERIOD SUBJECT RESPONSE @@; cards;
3 6 7.5 3 7 8.0 3 8 7.9 3 9 7.4 3 10 7.4 6 6 8.0 6 7 7.6 6 8
7.7 6 9 7.6 6 10 7.4 9 6 7.7 9 7 7.7 9 8 7.6 9 9 7.5 9 10 7.2
12 6 7.4 12 7 7.4 12 8 7.3 12 9 7.2 12 10 7.1
;
/***end of input data***/
data group2; set group2; DRUG = 'B';
Data group3;
/***input data***/
```

```
Input PERIOD SUBJECT RESPONSE @@;cards;
3 11 8.1 3 12 8.0 3 13 7.9 3 14 8.3 3 15 8.2 6 11 8.2 6 12
7.9 6 13 8.0 6 14 8.1 6 15 8.0 9 11 7.9 9 12 8.1 9 13 8.2 9
14 7.8 9 15 7.9 12 11 8.1 12 12 7.8 12 13 8.0 12 14 7.9 12 15
7.9
;
/***end of input data***/
data group3; set group3; DRUG = 'C';
data final;set group1 group2 group3;
proc glm outstat = a1 noprint; class drug period subject;
model response = period drug subject(drug) period*drug; run;
data drug;set a1; if _type_ = 'SS3'; meansq = ss/df;
if _source_ = 'DRUG' or _source_ = 'SUBJECT(DRUG)';
lagmnsq = lag(meansq); keep meansq _source_ lagmnsq;
data drug1;set drug; f = lagmnsq/meansq; source = 'DRUG'; a = 1;
if f = . then delete; keep source f a; proc sort; by a;
data df;
/***input data***/
k = 3;*number of drugs; n = 15;*number of subjects; a = 1;
/***end of input data***/
proc sort; by a; data drug1;merge drug1 df;by a;
data a;set a1; a = 1; proc sort; by a; data a;merge a df;by a;
if _type_ = 'SS3'; if _source_ = 'PERIOD' then do;
pvalue = 1 - probf(f,1,n - k); source = 'Period   '; end;
if _source_ = 'DRUG*PERIOD' then do;
  pvalue = 1 - probf(f,k - 1,n - k);
source = 'Drug*Period'; end; if source = ' ' then delete;
  keep source pvalue;
data final;set a drug1;
if source = 'DRUG' then do; pvalue = 1 - probf(f,k - 1,n - k);
  source = 'Drug';
end; keep pvalue source; proc print; var source pvalue; title
  'p-value with adjusted df'; run;
```

The output is

```
           p-value with adjusted df
             source             pvalue
             Period          0.06315 (u1)
             Drug*Period     0.22769 (u2)
             Drug            0.00004 (u3)
```

The p-value given at (u2) is more than 0.05 level and hence there is no interaction between the drugs and period indicating the parallelism of the profiles for the three drugs across the periods. The p-value given at (u1) is more than 0.05 and hence there is no difference between the periods of the responses. The p-value for the drug given at (u3) is highly significant indicating the difference in the effects for the three drugs controlling the sugar levels of diabetic patients.

3.4.5 Discriminant Functions

While considering multivariable responses in k groups, one can come across the statistical tools of discriminant analysis and cluster analysis. These two methods serve different roles. We distinguish the methods and discuss discriminant analysis in this section. Cluster analysis will be discussed in the next section.

When there is a p-dimensional response vector $(X_1, X_2, ..., X_p)$ it should be classified into one of the k known populations (groups). To this end, we have training samples of p-dimensional responses available from each of the k populations (groups). Using the available sample data from all the k populations a criterion of classifying a new observation into one of the k populations is developed. Knowing the family income, family size, and assets and liabilities a lender wants to classify the individual as a credit liability or asset. Based on the GRE score, undergraduate GPA, and interests of the student, a graduate school decides to give admission or deny admission to a student. Based on the skull measurements, an anthropologist classifies the skull.

In a sample of multivariable responses and one does not have any predetermined classes, the sample data are clustered into groups, where the units within a group are homogeneous and between the groups are different, in "some sense." Using the data and clustering algorithms the groups are formed. It is emphasized that in this case there are no predetermined groups and the data indicate the newly formed groups. Although instructors give grades with predetermined test scores cutoff points, a statistical way of giving grades is to cluster the midterm and final examination scores. Families can be classified as wealthy, middle class, and poor based on family income, home price, and assets and liabilities.

In discriminant analysis, if the responses follow a multivariate normal distribution with the same dispersion matrix for all k populations, the linear discriminant function coefficients $l_{i0}, l_{i1}, ..., l_{ip}$ for the ith group, $i = 1, 2, ..., k$ are estimated. The new observation $x_1, x_2, ..., x_p$ will have a score of

$$l_{i0} + l_{i1}x_1 + \cdots + l_{ip}x_p$$

for the ith group and will be classified to the group in which it has a maximum score. When the population dispersion matrices are different, the quadratic discriminant function is formed and when the data are nonnormal a nonparametric discriminant function is formed and these are beyond the scope of this work.

A credit card company classified its customers into three categories based on their payment pattern for a calendar year of 12 months, as follows:

```
A: Made full payment each month;
B: Made full payment some months and
   minimum payment some months; and
C: Made minimum payment all 12 months.
```

TABLE 3.7

Artificial Data on Three Variables in
Three Groups of Credit Card Holders

Group	X_1	X_2	X_3
A	100	40	700
	80	38	625
	125	45	750
	150	50	800
	75	45	675
B	80	35	635
	100	40	725
	90	30	575
	120	35	650
	75	40	600
C	70	30	450
	80	40	550
	60	25	625
	100	50	675
	60	35	425

The company is interested in classifying new applicants into these three categories based on their annual income in thousand dollar (X_1), age (X_2), and credit score (X_3). The artificial data are given in Table 3.7 for a sample of five customers in each group.

To classify an individual into one of the three groups based on X_1, X_2, X_3, a linear discriminant function is developed assuming the X values to follow a normal distribution with equal dispersion matrices in the three groups. The program is as follows:

```
data group1;
/***input data***/
input INCOME AGE CSCORE @@;cards;
100 40 700 80 38 625 125 45 750 150 50 800 75 45 675
;
/***end of input data***/
data group1;set group1;group = 1;
data group2;
/***input data***/
input INCOME AGE CSCORE @@;cards;
80 35 635 100 40 725 90 30 575 120 35 650 75 40 600
;
/***end of input data***/
data group2;set group2;group = 2;
data group3;
/***input data***/
```

```
input INCOME AGE CSCORE @@;cards;
70 30 450 80 40 550 60 25 625 100 50 675 60 35 425
;
/***end of input data***/
data group3;set group3;group = 3; data group;set group1 group2
   group3;
proc discrim ; class group; var income age cscore ; run;
```

The required output is

```
                               ***
           Linear Discriminant Function for GROUP
   Variable            1(v1)            2(v2)            3(v3)
   Constant         -43.86550        -34.19671        -27.88233
   INCOME            -0.12802         -0.11190         -0.13255
   AGE                0.53806          0.38377          0.52352
   CSCORE             0.10964          0.10202          0.08574
                               ***
```

```
Number of Observations and Percent Classified into group (v4)
From GROUP          1              2              3            Total
   1               4              1              0              5
                  80.00          20.00          0.00         100.00
   2               1              3              1              5
                  20.00          60.00          20.00        100.00
   3               1              1              3              5
                  20.00          20.00          60.00        100.00
   Total           6              5              4              15
                  40.00          33.33          26.67        100.00
                               ***
```

In the output the columns (v1), (v2), and (v3) provide the linear discriminant function coefficients. Limiting the interest to classify an individual with $X_1 = 90$, $X_2 = 40$, and $X_3 = 750$, the discriminant scores for the individual to be in groups A, B, and C are formed. Using (v1), (v2), and (v3) the discriminant scores are obtained by plugging in 90 for income, 40 for age, and 750 for cscore and the results are

Group A = $-43.86550 + (-0.12802)(90) + (0.53806)(40)$
$+ (0.10964)(750) = 48.3651$
Group B = $-34.19671 + (-0.11190)(90) + (0.38377)(40)$
$+ (0.10202)(750) = 47.5981$
Group C = $-27.88233 + (-0.13255)(90) + (0.52352)(40)$
$+ (0.08574)(750) = 45.4340.$

The maximum discriminant for Group A's score is 48.3651 and hence this individual is classified into Group A.

In the output at (v4) the misclassification error rates are given. It is observed that from Group A, 20% observations are misclassified into group B and 80% are correctly classified into Group A. From Group B 20% observations are misclassified into each of Group A and C, and 60% are correctly classified. From Group C 20% observations are misclassified into each of Group A and B, and 60% are correctly classified.

These overestimate the superiority of the procedure because the data provide the classification function. One can form the criteria deleting one observation at a time and classifying it using the function obtained by deleting it and determine the misclassification error rate which will not be discussed here.

One can test the significance of the coefficients of the linear discriminant function and also test whether a particular discriminant function can be used replacing the actual discriminant function obtained in the program. The interested reader can refer to multivariate analysis textbooks like Johnson and Wichern (1998), to obtain further details.

3.4.6 Cluster Analysis

Given multivariable data, one can form clusters based on the similarity between the observations and the procedure of aggregating these observations into clusters by using an appropriate measure. There are several similarity measures and methods of aggregating the observations. In this section, the simplest, Euclidean distance similarity measure, and aggregating the observations by the centroid procedure will be discussed.

Once the distances are determined, various clustering algorithms are used to form the clusters. There is no set number of clusters. These clustering algorithms are formed using hierarchical and nonhierarchical algorithms. Each step of clustering can be displayed in diagrams known as dendogram.

As mentioned above, there are various clustering methods (Punj and Stewart, 1983). SAS has several clustering algorithms. The centroid method for illustration is used. In this method one can start with $n-1$ clusters and go on to obtain one cluster, where n is the number of observations.

Consider the data on two midterm and final tests in a class of 15 students in Table 3.8 and divide them into groups to give grades.

The program and output are as follows:

```
data group;
/***input data***/
input midterm1 midterm2 final @@; cards;
80 85 87 75 77 72 60 65 70 90 86 85 97 90 92 65 80 75 89 84 80
69 75 65 68 76 70 46 50 45 60 55 50 70 72 71 55 55 50 40 45 50
60 62 65
;
/***end of input data***/
data group1;set group;  subjid=_n_;
proc cluster noeigen method=centroid
out=tree nonorm; *specify method of interest;
```

```
id subjid; var midterm1 midterm2 final;  run;
proc tree horizontal spaces = 2;  id subjid; copy midterm1
  midterm2 final; run;
```

TABLE 3.8

Test Scores of Students for Midterms 1 and 2 and Finals

Student	Midterm 1	Midterm 2	Final
1	80	85	87
2	75	77	72
3	60	65	70
4	90	86	85
5	97	90	92
6	65	80	75
7	89	84	80
8	69	75	65
9	68	76	70
10	46	50	45
11	60	55	50
12	70	72	71
13	55	55	50
14	40	45	50
15	60	62	65

```
                     The CLUSTER Procedure
               Centroid Hierarchical Cluster Analysis
    Root Mean Square Total - Sample Standard Deviation = 14.97649
                        Cluster History
NCL       -----Clusters Joined-----       FREQ   Cent Dist  Tie
14              9               12          2      4.5826
13             11               13          2      5
12              4                7          2      5.4772
11              8     CL14                  3      5.5902
10              3               15          2      5.831
 9              2     CL11                  4      7.3636
 8      CL9                      6          5      9.2466
 7             10               14          2      9.2736
 6              1     CL12                  3     10.512
 5      CL6                      5          4     14.24
 4      CL8          CL10                   7     15.944
 3      CL7          CL13                   4     16.515
 2      CL5          CL4                   11     30.869
 1      CL2          CL3                   15     44.868
```

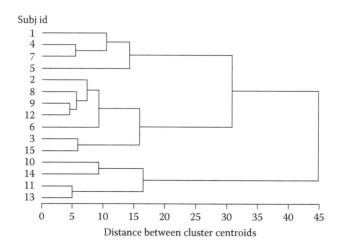

The optimal number of clusters can be determined as given in Sharma (1996, p. 198). However, one may decide the number of clusters to be formed based on the problem, and in that case the required number of clusters can be formed by visual inspection of the dendogram or by the cluster history.

Suppose the instructor wants to give four grades A, B, C, and D. Four clusters can be found as {1,4,7,5}, {2,8,9,12,6}, {3,15}, {10,14,11,13}. Suppose instead the instructor wants to give three grades A, B, and C then these three clusters are {1,4,7,5}, {2,8,9,6,12,3,15}, {10,14,11,13}. The grades are assigned by examining the scores for the students in the clusters.

3.4.7 Principal Components

When data are available where the responses are p-dimensional and p is large, it is difficult to express the phenomenon in terms of all response variables. It is desirable to reduce the dimensionality into a maximum of three or four latent factors in terms of original p variables. The new factors may be a linear combination of original variables or more complicated functions of original variables. Principal components and factor analyses provide new latent factors as linear combinations of the original variables. In principal components, the new factors are uncorrelated and explain the total variance of the p original variables in terms of the new factors. Thus, these can be used instead of the original variables without the loss of information. The variance of the ith principal component is not less than the $(i + 1)$th principal component for $i = 1, 2, \ldots$. In other words, the first principal component has the maximum explained variance, the second principal component has the second largest variance, and so on. In factor analysis, the original variables are expressed as linear combinations of uncorrelated two or three latent factors to explain the correlation structure of the original p variables. The principal components will be discussed in this section and factor analysis in the next section.

Principal components can be formed using the dispersion matrix or correlation matrix of the p original variables. The eigenvectors are principal components. We will discuss them in terms of the correlation matrix in this section. Theoretically, p principal components can be formed; but in practice the first two or three components explain most of the total variance of the original p variables. It is preferable to have at least five observations for every variable.

The eigenvalues of the dispersion matrix are the amount of variance explained by the principal component using the corresponding eigenvector. Usually, the components are selected where the eigenvalues are greater than 1. When the difference between two consecutive eigenvalues is very small the principal components corresponding to those eigenvalues will not be considered. The principal components are uniquely defined by making the sum of squares of coefficients of each principal component, as 1.

Consider the patients who have stroke and a clinician is interested to identify the latent factors which is more variable in causing the stroke. In Table 3.9, the artificial data on 20 patients on the variables such as age, weight,

TABLE 3.9

Artificial Data on Age, Weight, Systolic and Diastolic Blood Pressure, Job Stress, and Pay for the Stroke Patients

Patient	Age	Weight (lbs)	Systolic BP	Diastolic BP	Job Stress	Pay
1	27	130	140	85	1	40
2	50	180	160	100	7	125
3	60	160	150	90	4	55
4	35	200	155	90	8	32
5	42	195	120	80	4	140
6	22	110	100	75	2	30
7	45	125	120	85	7	40
8	50	100	100	80	5	80
9	60	175	130	90	4	65
10	33	160	140	90	3	45
11	43	105	125	85	4	75
12	67	171	130	85	1	40
13	37	130	120	85	1	35
14	48	155	103	75	10	80
15	62	193	120	85	4	100
16	65	150	90	65	3	55
17	39	140	140	91	9	70
18	29	182	130	85	2	40
19	62	185	120	80	4	35
20	28	110	100	70	5	130

systolic blood pressure, diastolic blood pressure, job stress on a point scale of 1–10, and the pay in thousand dollars are provided.

The program is as follows:

```
data a;
/***input data***/
input age weight sysbp diasbp jobstres pay @@; cards;
27 130 140 85 1 40 50 180 160 100 7 125 60 160 150 90 4 55
35 200 155 90 8 32 42 195 120 80 4 140 22 110 100 75 2 30
45 125 120 85 7 40 50 100 100 80 5 80 60 175 130 90 4 65
33 160 140 90 3 45 43 105 125 85 4 75 67 171 130 85 1 40
37 130 120 85 1 35 48 155 103 75 10 80 62 193 120 85 4 100
65 150 90 65 3 55 39 140 140 91 9 70 29 182 130 85 2 40
62 185 120 80 4 35 28 110 100 70 5 130
;
/***end of input data***/
proc princomp; var age weight sysbp diasbp jobstres pay ; run;
```

The output is as follows:

```
                                  ***
                     Eigenvalues of the Correlation Matrix
                 Eigenvalue(w2)    Difference    Proportion    Cumulative
        1           2.25682521     0.88236076      0.3761        0.3761
        2           1.37446445     0.21688457      0.2291        0.6052
        3           1.15757988     0.50241486      0.1929        0.7981
        4           0.65516501     0.16738959      0.1092        0.9073
        5           0.48777542     0.41958540      0.0813        0.9886
        6           0.06819002                     0.0114        1.0000

                                Eigenvectors
             PRIN1(w1)     PRIN2       PRIN3       PRIN4       PRIN5       PRIN6
AGE          0.134556    0.420559    0.687180  -0.267343    0.499684    0.107945
WEIGHT       0.455439    0.216819    0.403731   0.199742  -0.716557  -0.170928
SYSBP        0.618875   -0.225668   -0.138259   0.067506    0.091675    0.730747
DIASBP       0.600359   -0.189827   -0.172988   0.020759    0.387598  -0.650344
JOBSTRES     0.175711    0.512505   -0.472888  -0.669082  -0.187461    0.005316
PAY          0.012611    0.653068   -0.303516   0.660281    0.207567    0.046537
```

From the output the eigenvectors provide the new linear combinations of the six variables. As mentioned there are six new eigenvectors (six latent factors) corresponding to the six variables. The first principal component (eigenvector) given by (w1) is 0.13*age + 0.46*weight + 0.62*systbp + 0.60*diasbp + 0.18*jobstress + 0.01*pay. For this factor, the coefficients of the variables systolic and diastolic blood pressure are high. Hence, the first principal component is representing the blood pressure of the patients. On the second principal component the coefficients for job stress and pay are high and hence it is work related. In the third principal component, the coefficients for age and weight are high and they represent the physical attributes of the patient. Since the fourth eigenvalue of 0.655 given in column w2 is <1, we will not consider the principal component 4 and subsequent ones.

The principal components are also helpful in fitting multiple regression equations. When the independent variables in a multiple regression are correlated, we get *multicollinearity* and the regression coefficients cannot be accurately determined. In such cases, by using principal components as independent variables, we remove the difficulty of multicollinearity in fitting and interpreting multiple regression equations.

Principal components are also useful in stock markets to form portfolios which are highly volatile.

3.4.8 Factor Analysis

Factor analysis is commonly used in social sciences and psychology. We explain the correlations between the response variables in terms of latent factors.

The two common factoring techniques used are principal components factoring and principal axis factoring. In this section the principal components factoring will be discussed. The latent factors (eigenvectors) determined may be difficult to interpret and the axis is rotated to simplify the task of interpretation. *Varimax rotation* is a widely used rotation of the factors. It is an orthogonal rotation focusing on making as many values in each column of the factor loading coefficient table to be as close as possible to zero. This attempts to provide a simple explanation of the latent factors.

The data given in Table 3.9 of the previous section are considered and the principal component factoring using the following program is carried out. In this program varimax rotation provides a unique solution of the latent factors. The program automatically picks up the required number of latent factors based on the criteria that the eigenvalue is greater than 1.

```
data a;
/***input data***/
input age weight sysbp diasbp jobstres pay @@; cards;
27 130 140 85 1 40 50 180 160 100 7 125 60 160 150 90 4 55
35 200 155 90 8 32 42 195 120 80 4 140 22 110 100 75 2 30
45 125 120 85 7 40 50 100 100 80 5 80 60 175 130 90 4 65
33 160 140 90 3 45 43 105 125 85 4 75 67 171 130 85 1 40
37 130 120 85 1 35 48 155 103 75 10 80 62 193 120 85 4 100
65 150 90 65 3 55 39 140 140 91 9 70 29 182 130 85 2 40
62 185 120 80 4 35 28 110 100 70 5 130
;
/***end of input data***/
proc factor rotate=v;  var age weight sysbp diasbp jobstres
  pay ; run;
```

```
                           The FACTOR Procedure
                 Initial Factor Method: Principal Components
                       Prior Communality Estimates: ONE
         Eigenvalues of the Correlation Matrix: Total = 6  Average = 1
                  Eigenvalue    Difference    Proportion    Cumulative
           1      2.25682521    0.88236076      0.3761        0.3761
           2      1.37446445    0.21688457      0.2291        0.6052
           3      1.15757988    0.50241486      0.1929        0.7981
           4      0.65516501    0.16738959      0.1092        0.9073
           5      0.48777542    0.41958540      0.0813        0.9886
           6      0.06819002                    0.0114        1.0000
         3 factors will be retained by the MINEIGEN criterion.
                                     ***

                       Rotated Factor Pattern (aa1)
                         FACTOR1        FACTOR2        FACTOR3
            AGE          -0.10962       0.90425        0.03015
            WEIGHT        0.47367       0.70194        0.06586

            SYSBP         0.97608       0.06060       -0.00970
            DIASBP        0.94560       0.04133        0.04164
            JOBSTRES      0.17633      -0.03502        0.81070
            PAY          -0.13851       0.11080        0.81348

                 Variance Explained by Each Factor (aa2)
                    FACTOR1          FACTOR2          FACTOR3
                   2.1335528        1.3292624        1.3260543

           Final Communality Estimates: Total = 4.788870 (aa3)
        AGE        WEIGHT        SYSBP        DIASBP      JOBSTRES        PAY
     0.83058922 0.72141881 0.95650209 0.89759725 0.68955829 0.69320388
```

On the basis of the output at (aa1) we represent the response factors using three latent factors. The first latent factor has a high score for the response factors of the systolic and diastolic blood pressures. This latent factor represents blood pressure. The second latent factor represents the age and weight, which represents the baseline characteristics. The third latent factor represents job stress and pay and is related to job. The three latent factors are l_1, l_2, and l_3. We then have

$$\text{Age} = -0.11 * l_1 + 0.90 * l_2 + 0.03 * l_3$$

and similarly for the other response factors. The coefficients −0.11, 0.90, and 0.03 are called *factor loadings*. The variance explained by each of the three latent factors is given in (aa2). These are the sums of squares for the columns in (aa1). The communalities in (aa3) are the sums of squares of the rows (variables) in (aa1) and these should be close to 1 in order that the latent factors explain the response factors closely in terms of correlations. The communality is an index of the portion of the variance of the variable accounted by the latent factors.

Explanatory factor analysis is used to determine the factors whereas confirmatory factor analysis allows the researcher to see how well that model explains the responses. For further details see Sharma (1996).

3.4.9 Canonical Correlation

Principal components provide ordered latent factors maximizing the variance of the original variables. When the original variables form two sets of variables we would like to determine the linear combinations of the first set of variables with the second set of variables, maximizing the correlations between them.

In the example of the variables listed in stroke patients in Section 3.4.7, the variables age, weight, and systolic and diastolic blood pressure, are the physical characteristics of the patient and job stress and pay are work-related variables. One may like to form linear combinations of the physical variables and linear combinations of the work-related variables maximizing the correlation between those two. The factors obtained in this way for the first and second set are called canonical factors giving the canonical correlations.

The first linear combination has the highest correlation and the second has the next highest correlation not accounted for by the first pair of variables. The correlations from the last linear combination may be small and so one may be able to drop this variable, thus reducing the number of variables in the analysis. Usually two or three sets of canonical variables explain the correlations between the two sets of variables. The number of sets of canonical variables formed is the minimum of the number of variables in the two sets of variables.

The program for forming the canonical factors for the physical and work-related variables for stroke patients of Table 3.9 is

```
data a;
/***input data***/
input age weight sysbp diasbp jobstres pay @@; cards;
27 130 140 85 1 40 50 180 160 100 7 125 60 160 150 90 4 55
35 200 155 90 8 32 42 195 120 80 4 140 22 110 100 75 2 30
45 125 120 85 7 40 50 100 100 80 5 80 60 175 130 90 4 65
33 160 140 90 3 45 43 105 125 85 4 75 67 171 130 85 1 40
37 130 120 85 1 35 48 155 103 75 10 80 62 193 120 85 4 100
65 150 90 65 3 55 39 140 140 91 9 70 29 182 130 85 2 40
62 185 120 80 4 35 28 110 100 70 5 130
;
/***end of input data***/
proc cancorr; var age weight sysbp diasbp; with jobstres pay;
  run;
```

The output is as follows:

<pre>
                    The CANCORR Procedure
               Canonical Correlation Analysis
                     Adjusted   Approximate   Squared
     Canonical   Canonical   Standard   Canonical
     Correlation   Correlation   Error   Correlation
1 0.224860 (bb3) -0.487042   0.217816   0.050562
2 0.168887 (bb6)   .   0.222872   0.028523
</pre>

***

<pre>
                    The CANCORR Procedure
               Canonical Correlation Analysis
       Standardized Canonical Coefficients for the VAR Variables
                         V1(bb1)   V2(bb4)
        AGE   -0.1533   0.0481
        WEIGHT   0.8505   0.4751
        SYSBP   -2.0769   -1.1385
        DIASBP   1.0746   1.7155
           Standardized Canonical Coefficients for the
                         WITH Variables
                         W1(bb2)   W2(bb5)
        JOBSTRES   -0.4406   0.9603
        PAY   1.0511   0.1071
</pre>

***

The first set of canonical factors given at (bb1) and (bb2) are

$$V_1 = -0.153\text{*age} + 0.85\text{*weight} + (-2.077)\text{*sysb} + 1.07\text{*diasbp}$$
$$W_1 = -0.44\text{*jobstres} + 1.05\text{*pay}$$

with a canonical correlation given at (bb3) of 0.225. Looking at the coefficients in V_1 and W_1 it is noted that the blood pressure measurements constitute the variables V_1 and pay W_1 as they got high coefficients in the variables.

The second set of canonical factors given at (bb4) and (bb5) are

$$V_2 = 0.048\text{*age} + 0.475\text{*weight} + (-1.139)\text{*sysbp} + 1.716\text{*diasbp}$$
$$W_2 = 0.9603\text{*jobstres} + 0.1071\text{*pay}$$

with a canonical correlation given at (bb6) of 0.169. Here V_2 is the difference between the two blood pressure measurements and W_2 is the job stress.

One can test the significance of the canonical correlations before interpreting them from the deleted output and we have not considered the testing in this discussion.

3.5 Multifactor ANOVA

3.5.1 Crossed Factors

Consider a study involving two factors A at "a" levels and B at "b" levels. If we form all "ab" treatment combinations associating each level of A with each level of B, we say that factors A and B are crossed in the experiment. If $b > a$ and we divide the b levels of factor B into "a" groups of disjoint levels b_1, b_2, ..., b_a and associate the b_i levels of B to the ith level of factor A, we have the experiment where factor B is nested in factor A. Similarly if $a > b$, one can nest factor A in factor B. If A and B are crossed, one will be able to study the interaction effect for factors A and B. If there is no interaction between factors A and B, then the differential response between any two levels of one factor remains the same at each level of the other factor. If this differential response between any two levels of one factor is different for any two levels of the other factor, then factors A and B are said to be interacting. With nested factors, inferences cannot be drawn on the interaction effect of the factors.

Consider an experiment where the effect of the number of cylinders in a car and the horse power of car engines on the gas mileage delivered by the car has to be determined. Cars with three levels for cylinders 4, 6, and 8 are considered. If we take horse power 140, 160, and 180 and consider nine types of cars with i cylinders and j horse power, where $i = 4$, 6, and 8 and $j = 140$, 160, and 180 and record the gas mileages, we get data of an experiment with crossed factors.

Instead, if we take 4-, 6-, and 8-cylinder engines and consider five horse powers, 140, 150, 160, 170, and 180 and consider 4-cylinder engine with horse powers 140, 150; 6-cylinder engine with horse power 160; and 8-cylinder engine with horse powers 170 and 180 we get an experiment where horse power is nested in the number of cylinders. The concept of crossed and nested factors can be extended to any number of factors. The experiment on crossed factors is discussed in this Section and that of nested factors in Section 3.5.3.

In crossed factors to draw inference on interaction, we need multiple observations. If only one observation is taken with two crossed factors, inferences can be drawn on interaction using Tukey's 1 df nonadditivity term (see Section 3.5.2 for more detail).

Sometimes the experimenter will be interested to study only the effect of the levels of the factor used in the experiment then in that case they are considered as fixed effects of the factor. When the interest is to study the effects on population levels, a random sample of effects will be experimented which is a random effect factor. For a random effects factor, the interest is in seeing whether the variability of the responses for the factor levels is different. This is done by performing variance components analysis (see Section 3.6).

TABLE 3.10

City and Highway Gas Mileages of Cars

Horse Power	Cylinders					
	4		6		8	
	Weight (lbs)		Weight (lbs)		Weight (lbs)	
	2500	3000	2500	3000	2500	3000
140	35, 31	32, 34	28, 32	26, 29	23, 22	22, 25
160	31, 33	30, 28	29, 30	27, 28	25, 28	24, 26
180	28, 30	29, 29	28, 29	25, 27	22, 25	23, 21

In a fixed effects model, if the levels are quantitative and equally spaced, it can be examined whether the responses are linearly ordered for the levels with a positive or negative slope. Also of interest is whether the responses for the levels take a curvature giving maximum or minimum responses in the domain of tested levels. These can be determined by using appropriate coefficients in the contrast statement and the coefficients are given in any standard text book on experimental design.

Consider an experiment with three crossed factors: number of cylinders (4, 6, and 8), horse power (140, 160, and 180), and weight (2500 and 3000). Considering $3 \times 3 \times 2 = 18$ types of cars and taking two cars of each type, the approximate gas mileage delivered by the cars is given in Table 3.10.

The necessary program is given below:

```
Data a;
/***input data***/
Input hp cylinder weight response @@;  cards;
140 4 2500 35 140 4 2500 31 140 4 3000 32 140 4 3000 34 160 4
2500 31 160 4 2500 33 160 4 3000 30 160 4 3000 28 180 4 2500
28 180 4 2500 30 180 4 3000 29 180 4 3000 29 140 6 2500 28 140
6 2500 32 140 6 3000 26 140 6 3000 29 160 6 2500 29 160 6 2500
30 160 6 3000 27 160 6 3000 28 180 6 2500 28 180 6 2500 29 180
6 3000 25 180 6 3000 27 140 8 2500 23 140 8 2500 22 140 8 3000
22 140 8 3000 25 160 8 2500 25 160 8 2500 28 160 8 3000 24 160
8 3000 26 180 8 2500 22 180 8 2500 25 180 8 3000 23 180 8 3000
21
;
/***end of input data***/
proc glm;  class hp cylinder weight;
model response = hp cylinder weight hp*cylinder hp*weight
  cylinder*weight hp*cylinder*weight;
contrast "hp linear"  hp -1 0 1; * There are 3 levels of horse
  power and cylinders. The coefficients are given for linear
  and quadratic. For other levels one needs to input the
  coefficients as given in experimental design books.;
```

```
contrast 'hp quadratic' hp 1 -2 1;
contrast 'cylinder linear' cylinder -1 0 1;
contrast 'cylinder quadratic' cylinder 1 -2 1;run;
```

The output is as follows:

```
                                  ***
        Source       DF Type III SS  Mean Square  F Value  Pr > F (cc1)
HP                    2   29.3888889   14.6944444    5.29     0.0156
CYLINDER              2  299.5555556  149.7777778   53.92    <0.0001
WEIGHT                1   16.0000000   16.0000000    5.76     0.0274
HP*CYLINDER           4   30.6111111    7.6527778    2.75     0.0600
HP*WEIGHT             2    4.1666667    2.0833333    0.75     0.4866
CYLINDER*WEIGHT       2    4.6666667    2.3333333    0.84     0.4479
HP*CYLINDER*WEIGHT    4    6.1666667    1.5416667    0.55     0.6980
```

```
Contrast       DF Contrast SS Mean Square  F Value        Pr > F
hp linear       1   22.0416667   22.0416667    7.93     0.0114 (cc2)
hp quadratic    1    7.3472222    7.3472222    2.64     0.1213 (cc3)
cylinder        1  294.0000000  294.0000000  105.84    <0.0001 (cc4)
linear
cylinder        1    5.5555556    5.5555556    2.00     0.1744 (cc5)
quadratic
```

From the output the p-values in the column (cc1) of the Type III SS will be compared with the significance level 0.05. It is noted that none of the interactions are significant and each of the three factor effects are significant showing that the gas mileage differs for different horse powers, the number of cylinders, and weights.

The p-value at (cc3) of 0.12 is not significant but (cc2) of 0.01 is significant. This shows that the horse power has a linear effect and no quadratic effect indicating that the gas mileage is linearly related to horse power.

The p-value at (cc5) of 0.17 is not significant but (cc4), which is <0.0001 is significant. This shows that the cylinders have a linear effect and no quadratic effect indicating that the gas mileage is linearly related to cylinders.

If (cc3) or (cc5) are significant, we could have concluded that quadratic effects are significant for those factors.

3.5.2 Tukey 1 df for Nonadditivity

Consider an experiment with two factors at "a" and "b" levels, respectively. To get the interaction between these two factors with $(a-1)(b-1)$ degrees of freedom, we need to replicate all the $a * b$ treatment combinations at least twice. When it is not possible to replicate and we have only $a * b$ observations with one replicate per treatment combination, Tukey (1949) suggested an ingenious method for testing the interaction with only one degree of

TABLE 3.11

Artificial Data of Gas Mileage

Horse Power	Cylinders		
	4	6	8
140	35	28	23
160	31	29	25
180	28	28	22

freedom. Consider the data given in Table 3.11, which is a condensed version of the data in Table 3.10.

The following program gives the required test statistics to test the interaction with one degree of freedom.

```
data a;
/***input data***/
input HP CYL GAS @@; cards;
140 4 35 140 6 28 140 8 23 160 4 31 160 6 29 160 8 25 180 4 28
180 6 28 180 8 22
;
/***end of input data***/
proc glm;class cyl hp;
model gas = cyl hp/p;output out = pred p = pred;
data pred1;set pred; predsq = pred*pred;
proc glm;class cyl hp; model gas = cyl hp predsq; run;
```

The required output is

```
                            ***
Source    DF    Type III SS   Mean Square   F Value    Pr > F
CYL       2     1.86018206    0.93009103    0.20       0.8324
HP        2     1.69217925    0.84608962    0.18       0.8456
PREDSQ    1     3.03043323    3.03043323    0.64       0.4836(dd1)
```

The p-value for testing the interaction between cylinders and horse power is given at (dd1) of the output. Since this p-value of 0.4836 is greater than 0.05, we conclude that there is no interaction between the number of cylinders and horse power at 0.05 level of significance.

3.5.3 Nested Factors

Suppose the job satisfaction of employees in a chain departmental store setting had to be evaluated. One would like to know whether the satisfaction is different from state to state, between cities in a state, and between the stores in the same city. We randomly selected two states and in each selected state we chose three cities and in each selected city we chose three stores. In each of the selected stores a sample of five employees were given a questionnaire

TABLE 3.12

Data on Job Satisfaction of Five Employees in Select Stores

State	City	Store	Satisfaction	State	City	Store	Satisfaction
1	1	1	90, 89, 92, 93, 88	2	1	1	80, 89, 92, 93, 88
1	1	2	80, 87, 90, 83, 98	2	1	2	75, 89, 70, 60, 90
1	1	3	88, 86, 94, 82, 89	2	1	3	78, 89, 80, 85, 91
1	2	1	87, 81, 73, 83, 80	2	2	1	70, 72, 60, 50, 68
1	2	2	89, 82, 89, 93, 82	2	2	2	84, 77, 78, 81, 84
1	2	3	80, 89, 91, 97, 83	2	2	3	77, 75, 52, 78, 83
1	3	1	87, 83, 88, 83, 82	2	3	1	76, 81, 60, 81, 82
1	3	2	79, 79, 72, 73, 76	2	3	2	82, 89, 82, 91, 89
1	3	3	90, 89, 92, 93, 87	2	3	3	30, 59, 62, 63, 56

each on job satisfaction. Let the questionnaire indicate the job satisfaction on a 100-point scale. Artificial data are given in Table 3.12.

The employees' satisfaction data are analyzed in the program below:

```
data a;
/***input data***/
do state = 1 to 2;do city = 1 to 3;do store = 1 to 3;
  do employee = 1 to 5;
input response @@;output;end;end;end;end;cards;
90 89 92 93 88 80 87 90 83 98 88 86 94 82 89 87 81 73 83 80
89 82 89 93 82 80 89 91 97 83 87 83 88 83 82 79 79 72 73 76
90 89 92 93 87 80 89 92 93 88 75 89 70 60 90 78 89 80 85 91
70 72 60 50 68 84 77 78 81 84 77 75 52 78 83 76 81 60 81 82
82 89 82 91 89 30 59 62 63 56
;
/***end of input data***/
proc nested;class state city store; var response; run;
```

***

Nested Random Effects Analysis of Variance for Variable
response

Variance Source	DF	Sum of Squares	F Value	Pr > F (ee1)	Error Term	Mean Square
Total	89	11825				132.868414
state	1	2151.111111	6.23	0.0670	city	2151.111111
city	4	1380.977778	0.92	0.4861	store	345.244444
store	12	4525.200000	7.21	<0.0001	Error	377.100000
Error	72	3768.000000				52.333333

***

Looking at the p-values in column (ee1) it can be concluded whether the factors are significant or not. From the output the p-value (<0.0001) corresponding to the stores is significant, indicating that between the stores there is a variability in the employee job satisfaction. The p-value 0.0607 indicates a borderline nonsignificance between the states.

3.6 Variance Components

When doing the ANOVA, the levels of factors may be selected from a population of levels of that factor or they may be just a specific set of levels. When the levels of the factor are selected from a population of levels the researcher's interest is to test whether all the population levels give the same responses and also the researcher may like to estimate the variance of the responses for the population levels of factors. When the levels are specified, the interest is only to compare the tested levels of factors. When the levels are randomly selected it is called random effects factor, and when only the specific levels of factors are tested, then it is called a fixed effect factor. The interaction of factors when at least one factor is random is considered to be random. Usually the nested factors are considered to be random. With random factors the variance of the responses of effects for the levels can be estimated, and such an analysis is provided by the variance components. There are several methods of estimating the variance components, like restricted maximum likelihood, type 1 sums of squares, minimum variance quadratic unbiased estimators, and maximum likelihood. In this program the restricted maximum likelihood estimators (REML) is provided.

Consider testing the accuracy of stop watches. Randomly four stop watches of a particular brand are selected and each stop watch was tested by two randomly selected operators. Let these stop watches be used to find the time of running a mile. Consider five randomly selected runners in this experiment. The time measured by the four stop watches on the five runners is given in Table 3.13. In this setting operators are nested within stop watches.

```
Data a;
/***input data***/
Input watch oper runner time @@; cards;
1 1 1 54 1 2 1 52 1 1 2 55 1 2 2 57 1 1 3 51 1 2 3 52 1 1 4 55
1 2 4 59 1 1 5 50 1 2 5 49 2 1 1 49 2 2 1 51 2 1 2 65 2 2 2 57
2 1 3 56 2 2 3 54 2 1 4 55 2 2 4 59 2 1 5 57 2 2 5 59 3 1 1 49
3 2 1 49 3 1 2 58 3 2 2 62 3 1 3 51 3 2 3 52 3 1 4 59 3 2 4 56
3 1 5 51 3 2 5 49 4 1 1 58 4 2 1 53 4 1 2 57 4 2 2 56 4 1 3 56
4 2 3 59 4 1 4 54 4 2 4 57 4 1 5 60 4 2 5 62
;
/***end of input data***/
proc sort;by watch oper runner;
```

```
proc varcomp method = reml;  class watch oper runner;
  model time = watch oper(watch) runner watch*runner; run;
```

***

```
                Convergence criteria met.
                      REML Estimates
            Variance
            Component                       Estimate
            Var(WATCH)                    1.60833(ff1)
            Var(oper(watch))             0
            Var(RUNNER)                   3.92083(ff2)
            Var(WATCH*RUNNER)             7.44167(ff3)
            Var(Error)                    4.90000(ff4)
```

***

TABLE 3.13

Time by Four Stop Watches on Five Runners

	Stop Watch							
	1		**2**		**3**		**4**	
Runner	**Operators**		**Operators**		**Operators**		**Operators**	
	1	**2**	**1**	**2**	**1**	**2**	**1**	**2**
1	54	52	49	51	49	49	58	53
2	55	57	65	57	58	62	57	56
3	51	52	56	54	51	52	56	59
4	55	59	55	59	59	56	54	57
5	50	49	57	59	51	49	60	62

The REML estimate of 0 implies that the corresponding estimated variance is either negative or 0. The variance estimates are given in (ff1–ff4). (ff1) indicates the variance between the watches and is 1.61. (ff2) is the variance between the runners and is 3.9. (ff3) is the interaction between watch and runners and is 7.44. (ff4) is the unexplained variance due to random noise and is 4.9. The interaction variance given at (ff3) is high and the watch used affects the runner's time.

In the above program, by default all the terms in the model are assumed to be random effects. All the fixed effects must be specified in the model in the beginning and be indicated by *fixed* = *m* where the first *m* terms in the model are fixed effects. To this end, suppose only five specific runners are selected, without randomly selecting them from a group of runners then the runners would have been fixed. Update the program accordingly by placing the fixed effect after the equal sign and indicate the numbers of the fixed effects as an option.

```
proc varcomp method = reml;  class watch oper runner;
  model time = runner watch watch*runner oper(watch)/fixed = 1;
  * In this example only the first term (runner) in the model
  is a fixed effect;  run;
```

The output given below is similar to the earlier output in this section, excluding the variance for the fixed effects:

```
                            ***
                     REML Estimates
              Variance
              Component              Estimate
              Var(WATCH)             1.60833
              Var(WATCH*RUNNER)      7.44167
              Var(OPER(WATCH))       0
              Var(Error)            4.90000
                            ***
```

3.7 Split Plot Designs

Consider experiments with two factors. Sometimes the experimenter wants to test the levels of one factor less accurately compared to testing the other factor and the interactions. It is also possible that one of these factors may be requiring larger experimental unit compared to the levels of the other factors. In such cases Split Plot Designs are used.

The factor used on the larger experimental unit is called whole plot treatment and the factor used in smaller units and within the first factor is called subplot treatment. Consider an experiment in r replications or r blocks. The factor A with "a" levels is used randomly to the whole plots. Within each whole plot, levels of factor B are randomly assigned. In this case the levels of factor A are tested less accurately compared to the levels of factor B and the AB interaction. The difference in the analysis of the split plot designs compared to a two-factor design is that the blocks and factor A effects are tested using their mean squares against the block into factor mean square in the split plot design. There are many variations of the split plot design and the interested reader is referred to Federer and King (2007).

Consider an experiment where a farmer is interested in testing three different growth hormones denoted by GH_1, GH_2, and GH_3 on two breeds of chicken denoted by C_1 and C_2 for weight gain. The farmer is also interested in comparing the effects of the three hormones more accurately. He thus uses the hormones as subplot treatments and chicken as main-plot treatments. Let there be three replications that are taken as whole blocks. The artificial data of the growth of a chicken for a specified time period are given in Table 3.14.

The program is as follows:

```
Data a;
/***input data***/
```

```
Input block chicken gh wg@@;cards;
1 1 1 9 1 1 3 10 1 1 2 11 1 2 3 12 1 2 1 13 1 2 2 11 2 2 2 8 2
2 3 9 2 2 1 9
2 1 1 9 2 1 2 11 2 1 3 12 3 1 3 9 3 1 1 10 3 1 2 10 3 2 1 11 3
2 2 9 3 2 3 12
;
/***end of input data***/
proc glm; class block gh chicken;
  model wg = block chicken block*chicken gh gh*chicken;
  test h = chicken e = block*chicken;
  test h = block   e = block*chicken
;
means gh/snk; means chicken/snk e = block*chicken; * we can ask
  for multiple comparisons for the factors using earlier
  methods. The whole plots treatment will have the error
  block*whole plot treatment; run;
```

TABLE 3.14

Artificial Data of the Growth of Chicken for a Specified Time Period

Block 1 Chicken		Block 2 Chicken		Block 3 Chicken	
C_1	C_2	C_2	C_1	C_1	C_2
GH_1 (9)	GH_3 (12)	GH_2 (8)	GH_1 (9)	GH_3 (9)	GH_1 (11)
GH_3 (10)	GH_1 (13)	GH_3 (9)	GH_2 (11)	GH_1 (10)	GH_2 (9)
GH_2 (11)	GH_2 (11)	GH_1 (9)	GH_3 (12)	GH_2 (10)	GH_3 (12)

The output is as follows:

```
                    The GLM Procedure
                Dependent Variable: wg
                         Sum of        Mean         F
Source              DF    Squares       Square      Value    Pr > F
Model               9    27.38888889   3.04320988   3.91     0.0339
Error               8     6.22222222   0.77777778
Corrected Total    17    33.61111111

           R-Square    Coeff Var    Root MSE    wg Mean
           0.814876    8.580815     0.881917    10.27778

                            ***
Source          DF  Type III SS   Mean Square  F Value   Pr > F
block            2   5.44444444    2.72222222   3.50      0.0809
chicken          1   0.50000000    0.50000000   0.64      0.4458
block*chicken    2  13.00000000    6.50000000   8.36      0.0110
gh               2   1.44444444    0.72222222   0.93      0.4339 (gg3)
gh*chicken       2   7.00000000    3.50000000   4.50      0.0490 (gg4)
```

```
Tests of Hypotheses Using the Type III MS for block*chicken as
                        an Error Term
Source         DF  Type III SS  Mean Square  F Value    Pr > F
chicken        1    0.50000000   0.50000000   0.08    0.8075 (gg2)
block          2    5.44444444   2.72222222   0.42    0.7048 (gg1)
                      The GLM Procedure
                Student-Newman-Keuls Test for wg
```

Note: This test controls the Type I experiment-wise error rate under the complete null hypothesis but not under partial null hypotheses.

```
        Alpha                                   0.05
        Error Degrees of Freedom                8
        Error Mean Square                       0.777778
        Number of Means        2                3
        Critical Range         1.1741493        1.4549286
```

```
Means with the same letter are not significantly different.
        SNK Grouping(gg6)      Mean          N        gh
        A                      10.6667        6         3
        A
        A                      10.1667        6         1
        A
        A                      10.0000        6         2
```
```
                      The GLM Procedure
                Student-Newman-Keuls Test for wg
```

Note: This test controls the Type I experiment-wise error rate under the complete null hypothesis but not under partial null hypotheses.

```
        Alpha                            0.05
        Error Degrees of Freedom         2
        Error Mean Square                6.5
        Number of Means                  2
        Critical Range                   5.1711374
```

```
Means with the same letter are not significantly different.
        SNK Grouping(gg5)      Mean          N       chicken
        A                      10.444         9         2
        A
        A                      10.111         9         1
```

In the output, *p*-value (gg1) indicates the effectiveness of the blocking. The *p*-value given at (gg2) is used to test the difference in the means for the whole plot treatment, Factor A (chicken). These two are not significant in this example.

The p-values at (gg3) and (gg4) show the effectiveness of subplot treatment, Factor B (growth hormone) and the interaction of A*B (chicken*growth hormone). The p-value for the growth hormone given at (gg3) is not significant and the p-value 0.049 given at (gg4) indicates borderline significance of the interaction between chicken lines and the growth hormones. The SNK multiple comparison for testing the levels of factor A and factor B are given in (gg5) and (gg6). From (gg5) and (gg6) we note that the levels of chicken and growth hormones have homogeneous effects.

3.8 Latin Square Design

A Latin Square design is an arrangement of v treatments in a $v \times v$ square array where every treatment occurs exactly once in each row and in each column. While in an RBD design the source of variation in one direction coming from the blocking is removed, in a Latin square design two sources of variations coming from rows and columns are removed. This design is also used to test the effect of three factors and does not consider the interaction between the factors but only considers the main effects of the three factors used. When there are many sources of variation one can use orthogonal Latin squares to remove the variation. The disadvantage of the Latin square design is that more replications are needed for the treatment, when tested for several treatments. Usually, Latin square designs are recommended with four to six treatments.

Suppose a car manufacturer is interested in determining whether age groups of the drivers, the model, and speed have an effect on the stopping distance when brakes are suddenly applied. For this purpose the manufacturer wants to examine at four speeds: 30, 40, 50, and 60 mph. The models are denoted by A, B, C, and D and the four age groups of interest are: ≤30, 31–40, 41–50, and ≥51. The artificial data are given in Table 3.15.

In this experiment one subject of each age group is driving the car. The entry in cell (1, 1) implies that the driver in age group ≤30 is driving Model A

TABLE 3.15

Artificial Data on the Stopping Distance of Cars

	Age Groups			
Speed (mph)	**≤30**	**31–40**	**41–50**	**≥51**
30	A (25)	B (30)	D (30)	C (35)
40	D (30)	C (30)	B (35)	A (40)
50	C (35)	D (35)	A (35)	B (45)
60	B (40)	A (35)	C (40)	D (50)

car at 30 mph stopped at a distance of 25 ft when brakes are suddenly applied. The following program provides the required analysis.

```
Data a; Input agegroup speed model$ response @@; cards;
1 1 a 25 2 1 b 30 3 1 d 30 4 1 c 35 1 2 d 30 2 2 c 30 3 2 b 35
4 2 a 40
1 3 c 35 2 3 d 35 3 3 a 35 4 3 b 45 1 4 b 40 2 4 a 35 3 4 c 40
4 4 d 50
;
proc glm;  class agegroup speed model;
  model response = agegroup speed model; means agegroup/snk;
means speed/snk; means model/snk; run;
```

The output is as follows:

The GLM Procedure

Dependent Variable: RESPONSE

Source	DF	Sum of Squares	Mean Square	F Value	Pr > F
Model	9	581.2500000	64.5833333	31.00	0.0002
Error	6	12.5000000	2.0833333		
Corrected Total	15	593.7500000			

R-Square	Coeff Var	Root MSE	response Mean
0.978947	4.051581	1.443376	35.62500

***

Source	DF	Type III SS	Mean Square	F Value	Pr > F
AGEGROUP	3	268.7500000	89.5833333	43.00	0.0002 (hh1)
SPEED	3	281.2500000	93.7500000	45.00	0.0002 (hh2)
MODEL	3	31.2500000	10.4166667	5.00	0.0452 (hh3)

The GLM Procedure

Student–Newman–Keuls Test for RESPONSE

Note: This test controls the Type I experiment-wise error rate under the complete null hypothesis but not under partial null hypotheses.

Alpha	0.05
Error Degrees of Freedom	6
Error Mean Square	2.083333

Number of Means	2	3	4
Critical Range	2.4973691	3.1314168	3.5330886

Means with the same letter are not significantly different.

SNK Grouping (hh4)	Mean	N	AGEGROUP
A	42.500	4	4
B	35.000	4	3
B			
B	32.500	4	1
B			
B	32.500	4	2

```
                    The GLM Procedure
          Student-Newman-Keuls Test for RESPONSE
```

Note: This test controls the Type I experiment-wise error rate under the complete null hypothesis but not under partial null hypotheses.

```
Alpha                            0.05
Error Degrees of Freedom         6
Error Mean Square                2.083333


Number of Means   2              3              4
Critical Range    2.4973691      3.1314168      3.5330886
```

```
Means with the same letter are not significantly different.
     SNK Grouping(hh5)       Mean          N           SPEED
          A                 41.250          4             4
          B                 37.500          4             3
          C                 33.750          4             2
          D                 30.000          4             1
                    The GLM Procedure
          Student-Newman-Keuls Test for RESPONSE
```

Note: This test controls the Type I experiment-wise error rate under the complete null hypothesis but not under partial null hypotheses.

```
    Alpha                            0.05
    Error Degrees of Freedom         6
    Error Mean Square                2.083333


Number of Means    2              3              4
Critical Range     2.4973691      3.1314168      3.5330886
```

```
 Means with the same letter are not significantly different.
      SNK Grouping(hh6)       Mean          N           MODEL
              A              37.500          4             b
              A
  B           A              36.250          4             d
  B           A
  B           A              35.000          4             c
  B
  B                          33.750          4             a
```

In the output, the *p*-values (hh1), (hh2), and (hh3) are used to test the significance of age group, speed, and brand.

The outputs at (hh4), (hh5), and (hh6) show the SNK multiple comparisons for testing the levels of the three factors.

From (hh1), (hh2), and (hh3) the *p*-values are 0.0002, 0.0002, and 0.0452, respectively, indicating that each of the three factors is significant. The multiple comparisons at (hh4) for age group indicate that the effects of age groups 1, 2, and 3 are the same and 4 is different. All the four speeds are different indicated at (hh5). From (hh6) models B, D, and C are similar, as well as models D, C, and A.

To remove the heterogeneity of the experimental material in more than two directions, one can use orthogonal Latin squares and for the construction of these designs, we refer to Raghavarao (1971).

3.9 Two-Treatment Crossover Design

Variability between experimental units is the main source to test the significance of the applied treatments. It is desirable that the variability between the units is minimized to get a more effective comparison of the treatments. Latin square design provides an example of removing variability between units. Crossover designs are commonly used to remove unit variability. A sequence of treatments is applied on each unit in a crossover design. When the treatments are applied consecutively with no "wash out" period, each treatment produces a *direct effect* in the period the treatment is applied and a *carryover effect* (or *residual effect*) in the succeeding periods after its application. We consider designs where the carryover effect is for the immediate succeeding period only and such carryover periods are called the *first-order carryover effects*. The commonly used design in the pharmaceutical industry is a two-period, two-treatment carryover design applied in two sequences. Only these designs will be discussed in this section. A detailed discussion on all types of carryover designs can be found in Jones and Kenward (2003).

Suppose an experimenter is interested in comparing the area under the curve (AUC) for two drugs A and B. Then on one group of subjects the treatments A and B are given one after another and the sequence B and A in that order are given in another group of subjects. To compare two teaching methods A and B in some sections of a class, Method A is first given followed by B and vice versa for the other sections. Comparing two crops A and B, some farmers may harvest crop A in one year and crop B in another year while other farmers may harvest B in the first year and A in the second year. In this two-treatment two-period two-sequence design, the experimental units must be randomly selected.

To compare the direct effects of the two treatments using the crossover nature of the design, one needs to have equal carryover effects of the two treatments. If the carryover effects of the treatments are different, the equality of direct effects can be tested only by using the first-period data with

TABLE 3.16

Test Scores by Two Teaching Methods

Subject	Period 1	Period 2	Subject	Period 1	Period 2
1	A(78)	B (68)	11	B (72)	A (81)
2	A (80)	B (70)	12	B (74)	A (71)
3	A (82)	B (68)	13	B (78)	A (77)
4	A (86)	B (79)	14	B (78)	A (76)
5	A (78)	B (74)	15	B (76)	A (80)
6	A (83)	B (81)	16	B (79)	A (81)
7	A (88)	B (78)	17	B (74)	A (75)
8	A (79)	B (80)	18	B (80)	A (78)
9	A (80)	B (81)	19	B (77)	A (80)
10	A (81)	B (81)	20	B (82)	A (84)

reduced power. To get a large power in testing the equality of carryover effects, larger significance level, like $\alpha = 0.1$, are used.

Consider a situation where two teaching methods A and B are compared in two periods. Let us take a random sample of 10 students who are first taught A and then B and in another sample of 10 students where B was taught first and then A. The test scores with 100 as the maximum score in each test are given in Table 3.16.

The necessary program is given below:

```
data per1grp1;
/***input data***/
input subj resp1@@;cards;
1 78 2 80 3 82 4 86 5 78 6 83 7 88 8 79 9 80 10 81
;
/***end of input data***/
data pergrp1;set per1grp1; group = 1; proc sort;by subj;
data per2grp1;
/***input data***/
input subj resp2@@;cards;
1 68 2 70 3 68 4 79 5 74 6 81 7 78 8 80 9 81 10 81
;
/***end of input data***/
data per2grp1; set per2grp1; group = 1; proc sort;by subj;
data per1grp2;
/***input data***/
input subj resp1@@;cards;
11 72 12 74 13 78 14 78 15 76 16 79 17 74 18 80 19 77 20 82
;
/***end of input data***/
data per1grp2;set per1grp2; group = 2; proc sort;by subj;
data per2grp2;
/***input data***/
```

```
input subj resp2@@;cards;
11 81 12 71 13 77 14 76 15 80 16 81 17 75 18 78 19 80 20 84
;
/***end of input data***/
data per2grp2;set per2grp2; group = 2; proc sort; by subj;
data group1; set per1grp1 per1grp2; proc sort; by subj;
data group2; set per2grp2 per2grp1; proc sort; by subj;
data group;merge group1 group2;by subj;
sum = resp1 + resp2;diff = resp1-resp2;
proc ttest; var sum;class group;run;
proc ttest;var diff;class group;run;
proc ttest;var resp1;class group;run;
```

The output is as follows:

The TTEST Procedure

***

T-Tests

Variable	Method	Variances	DF	t Value	Pr > |t|
sum	Pooled	Equal	18	0.75	0.4647 (ii2)
sum	Satterthwaite	Unequal	17.1	0.75	0.4652 (ii3)

Equality of Variances

Variable	Method	Num DF	Den DF	F Value	Pr > F
sum	Folded F	9	9	1.60	0.4942 (ii1)

The TTEST Procedure

***

T-Tests

Variable	Method	Variances	DF	t Value	Pr > |t|
diff	Pooled	Equal	18	3.31	0.0039 (ii5)
diff	Satterthwaite	Unequal	15.6	3.31	0.0046 (ii6)

Equality of Variances

Variable	Method	Num DF	Den DF	F Value	Pr > F
diff	Folded F	9	9	2.28	0.2358 (ii4)

The TTEST Procedure

***

T-Tests

Variable	Method	Variances	DF	t Value	Pr > |t|
resp1	Pooled	Equal	18	3.14	0.0056 (ii8)
resp1	Satterthwaite	Unequal	17.9	3.14	0.0057 (ii9)

Equality of Variances

Variable	Method	Num DF	Den DF	F Value	Pr > F
resp1	Folded F	9	9	1.20	0.7937 (ii7)

The crossover design is effective when the carryover effects of the two treatments are the same. The equality of the two carryover effects is tested from the p-value given in (ii2) or (ii3) based on the p-value at (ii1). It may be recalled that if the p-value at (ii1) is more (less) than 0.05 then the p-value at (ii2), [(ii3)] is used to test the significance of the two carryover effects.

Note that the p-value at (ii1) is more than 0.05 and hence the p-value at (ii2) is used to test the equality of the carryover effects. Since the p-value at (ii2) is more than 0.1 it can be concluded that the two carryover effects are the same and the p-value at (ii5) or (ii6) is used to test the equality of the direct effects of the two treatments. Had the p-value at (ii2) been <0.1 one could have used (ii8) or (ii9) to draw the inference on the equality of the two direct effects.

The p-value at (ii4) is more than 0.05 and hence the p-value of 0.0039 given at (ii5) is used to draw conclusions of the equality of the direct effects. Since the p-value at (ii5) is <0.05 it can be concluded that the two teaching methods A and B are significantly different.

4

Nonparametric Methods

If the data are continuous and normally distributed, then tests from Chapter 3 should be used. However, if the data are continuous and are not normal or on an ordinal scale, then one would use nonparametric tests described in this chapter.

Nonparametric tests are used when the distribution of data is unknown. There are many nonparametric tests to choose from. These tests may be less powerful than their parametric counterparts, since less information is known about the distribution of the data, thus making it more difficult to detect smaller differences. However, an advantage of using nonparametric tests is that they are distribution free. Very mild assumptions are made on the data to draw statistical inferences. Sometimes different statistical procedures may lead to different inferences and the reader should make a judicious judgment to draw conclusions.

It may be noted that we may be able to use the methods from the last chapter by transforming the data using arcsine, square root, logarithm, and so on. Most nonparametric tests are based on ranks assigned to the data, and the real data values are ignored. Ties are broken, by giving mid-rank to the tied responses. For many of these tests, testing is done on the median of the distribution rather than on the mean.

4.1 One Sample

4.1.1 Sign Test

To test for a given median, the observations are measured from the hypothesized median and using the signs, the null hypothesis is rejected (retained). This test does not consider the importance of data values and only uses the signs of the data. Usually, one needs to have at least 12–15 data points for using the sign test. This test can be used on one sample for testing the median, or paired sample to test the equality of the distributions of both components in the pair.

Suppose a farmer was wondering which variety of plant A or B yield better crop during the year. He chooses 30 similar plots and divides them into 15 pairs of plots. In each pair he randomly chooses variety A for one plot and

TABLE 4.1

Yield from Variety A and B

Variety A Yield	Variety B Yield	Variety A Yield	Variety B Yield	Variety A Yield	Variety B Yield
30	33	37	41	35	40
43	40	45	39	42	35
40	45	43	40	30	40
33	31	50	42	33	39
35	40	37	41	40	47

variety B for the other. The artificial yield (in lbs) from the plants is given in Table 4.1.

The program is as follows:

```
data pair;
/***input data***/
input result1 result2@@;cards;
30 33 43 40 40 45 33 31 35 40 37 41 45 39 43
40 50 42 37 41 35 40 42 35 30 40 33 39 40 47
;
/***end of input data***/
data pair;set pair; diff = result1 - result2;
  proc univariate;var diff; run;
```

The output is as follows:

```
                              ***
                  Tests for Location: Mu0 = 0
    Test              -Statistic-              --p-Value--
    Student's t    t    -0.9156        Pr > |t|      0.3754
    Sign           M    -1.5           Pr >= |M|     0.6072 (a1)
    Signed rank    S    -16            Pr >= |S|     0.3812 (a2)
                              ***
```

From the output the *p*-value at (a1) is 0.6072, indicating that there is no difference in the yields of A or B.

The median and the CI for the median should be used as descriptive statistics. The following program gives the median at (b1) and the $(1 - \alpha)100\%$ CI of the median at [(b2), (b3)] of the output as described in Dunsmore (1974).

```
data pair;
/***input data***/
input result1 result2@@;cards;
30 33 43 40 40 45 33 31 35 40 37 41 45 39 43
```

```
40 50 42 37 41 35 40 42 35 30 40 33 39 40 47
;
/***end of input data***/
data pair; set pair; diff = result1 - result2;*for a single
  sample diff is the sample data; proc univariate
  noprint;var diff;
output out = median median = MEDIAN n = n;
data final1;set pair;a = 1; proc sort;by a; data
  median1;set median;
/***input data***/
alpha = .05;
/***end of input data***/
z = probit(1 - alpha/2); d = int((n/2) - .5 - (z*sqrt(n/4))) + 1; a = 1;
keep median n d a; proc sort; by a;
data final2; merge final1 median1; by a;
proc sort; by diff; data ll; set final2; by diff;
if _n_ = d then LL = diff; if ll = . then delete; keep ll a
  median; proc sort; by a;
data ul; set final2; by diff;
if _n_ = n - d + 1 then UL = diff; if ul = . then delete; keep ul a;
data final3; merge ll ul; by a; drop a; proc print;var ll
  median ul; run;
```

The output is as follows:

```
LL          MEDIAN     UL
-5 (b2)     -4 (b1)    3 (b3)
```

From the output we note that the median for the difference in yields of variety A and B is −4 and its 95% CI is (−5, 3).

This program can also be used for one-sample data to estimate the median and its confidence interval.

4.1.2 Wilcoxon Signed-Rank Test

This test can be used in the same setting as that of the sign test, but the sign test does not consider the magnitude of the positive and negative values. The Wilcoxon signed-rank test considers the magnitude of the positive and negative values of the data. For a one-sample case, we will be testing the median for a hypothesized value and for a paired sample that the median of the difference of the two variables is 0. For the data given in Table 4.1 in the output, we obtain the p-value for the signed-rank test as 0.3812 at (a2). To find the CI for the median of the differences, we can add the option CIPCTLDF after PROC UNIVARIATE to the program in Section 4.1.1:

```
proc univariate cipctldf; run;
```

This option provides the median and its CI based on the method described by Hahn and Meeker (1991).

```
                              ★★★
                    Quantiles (Definition 5)
                                95% Confidence Limits
        Quantile        Estimate        Distribution-free
        100% Max            8
        99%                 8                .              .
        95%                 8                6              8
        90%                 7                3              8
        75% Q3              3               -4              8

        50% Median        -4(c1)          -5(c2)          3(c3)  ★★★

        25% Q1            -5              -10             -4
        10%              -7              -10             -5
        5%              -10              -10             -6
        1%              -10                .              .
        0% Min          -10
                              ★★★
```

Based on this output, the estimate of the median is −4 given at (c1) and its 95% CI is (−5, 3) given at [(c2), (c3)]. This output also gives the estimates of the other percentiles and their confidence intervals.

4.1.3 Kolmogorov Goodness of Fit

Kolmogorov goodness of fit is used to test whether the sample data are coming from a specific distribution. It measures the difference between the distribution functions of the sample and hypothesized distribution. Desu and Raghavarao (2004) provide a program along with the 95% CI.

4.1.4 Cox and Stuart Test

Sometimes one may want to see whether the data are random or they follow a trend. The null hypothesis is that there is no trend versus the alternatives of an upward or downward trend (Cox and Stuart, 1955). This test is a type of extension of the sign test. For this test, the data from the first half are compared with the data from the second half to see whether the numbers are increasing or decreasing.

The sales of an item A over 12 months are given below:

45, 83, 41, 67, 66, 64, 45, 37, 52, 65, 73, 37

The following program provides the necessary information to draw inferences.

```
data group;
/***input data***/
input response@@;cards;
45  83  41  67  66  64  45  37  52  65  73  37
;
/***end of input data***/
proc univariate noprint; var response; output out=n n=n;
data group; set group; a=1; proc sort; by a;
data n;set n; a=1; proc sort; by a;
data group; merge group n; by a; c=round(n/2);
data group1; set group; if _n_<=c; resp1=response; cnt=_n_;
drop response; proc sort; by cnt;
data group2; set group; if _n_>c; resp2=response;
  data group2;set group2;
cnt=_n_; drop response; proc sort; by cnt;
data final; merge group1 group2; by cnt;
proc sort;by a cnt; data final;set final; by a cnt; retain
  counter 0;
if resp1=. or resp2=. then delete; if resp2>resp1 then
  counter+1;
proc sort;by a cnt counter; data counter;set final; by a cnt
  counter;
if last.a; t=counter; PVALUE1=probbnml(.5,c,t);
PVALUE2=1-probbnml(.5,c,t-1); PVALUE=min(pvalue1, pvalue2);
pvalue=2*pvalue; proc print; var pvalue pvalue1 pvalue2;run;
```

PVALUE	PVALUE1	PVALUE2
0.6875 (d1)	0.34375 (d2)	0.89063 (d3)

The p-value 0.6875 at (d1) is used to test against the alternative of no trend. The p-value 0.3438 at (d2) is used to test against the alternative of negative trend. The p-value 0.8906 at (d3) is used to test against the alternative of positive trend. Our data do not show any trend in the sales over the 12 months and the data are randomly distributed.

4.2 Two Samples

The commonly used tests to compare the distributions of two samples are the *Wilcoxon–Mann–Whitney test* and the *median test*. For some distributions the Wilcoxon–Mann–Whitney test is more efficient than the median test. We will discuss these two tests here and for other tests one can refer to any standard nonparametric method books by Conover (1980), Desu and Raghavarao (2004), or Lehman (1998).

4.2.1 Wilcoxon–Mann–Whitney Test

The Wilcoxon–Mann–Whitney test is similar to the two-sample *t*-test in the case of normally distributed data and can be used for equal or unequal sample sizes. This test is also commonly referred to as the Wilcoxon rank-sum test.

The data from both groups are lumped together and ranked disregarding the groups. The mean rank is provided for tied observations. After the ranking has been completed, the ranks are then summed for each group, and the statistic computed. Using this test statistic, the null hypothesis where the two distributions are the same versus the alternative where the two distributions are not the same, will be tested.

Suppose an epidemiologist was wondering if City 1 had more cases of a new disease than City 2 based on the data given in Table 4.2, from various randomly selected hospitals.

The following program provides the answer to the epidemiologist's problem:

TABLE 4.2

Frequency for New Disease at Various Hospitals

City 1	City 2	City 1	City 2
100	123	147	158
126	59	79	93
37	210	75	180
96	57	279	58
356	135		90
46	172		83
189	202		67

```
data group1;
/***input data***/
input response @@; cards;
100 126 37 96 356 46 189 147 79 75 279
;
/***end of input data ***/
data group1;set group1; group = 1; data group2;
/***input data**/
input response @@; cards;
123 59 210 57 135 172 202 158 93 180 58 90 83 67
;
/***end of input data ***/
```

```
data group2;set group2; group = 2; data final; set group1
  group2;
proc npar1way wilcoxon; class group; var response;
exact;* this maybe ignored for large data sets;run;
```

The NPAR1WAY Procedure
***

Wilcoxon Two-Sample Test

Statistic (S)	145.0000	
Normal Approximation		
Z	0.0821	
One-Sided Pr > Z	0.4673	(e4)
Two-Sided Pr > $\|Z\|$	0.9346	(e3)
t Approximation		
One-Sided Pr > Z	0.4676	
Two-Sided Pr > $\|Z\|$	0.9352	
Exact Test		
One-Sided Pr >= S	0.4679	(e2)
Two-Sided Pr >= $\|S - \text{Mean}\|$	0.9358	(e1)

***

The exact distribution of the statistic is used and the *p*-value for the test is provided at (e1) for a two-sided alternative. If we want to conclude that the first-sample observations are larger than the second sample probabilistically, the *p*-value at (e2) is used. If the observations in the first sample are larger than the observations in the second sample probabilistically, we say that the first population is stochastically larger than the second population. If we want to conclude that the first-sample observations are smaller than the second sample probabilistically, the *p*-value is 1 minus the *p*-value given at (e2). In our problem, the one-sided *p*-value is needed and is 0.4679, indicating equal distributions of the number of cases in the two cities.

The exact test takes a longer time with large data sets and we can suppress the exact option in the program. If the two sample sizes are large, then we can use the normal approximation and draw similar conclusions using (e3) or (e4) as discussed in the previous paragraph. In our example, the *p*-values with normal approximation and exact test are fairly close because the data are of reasonable size.

4.2.2 Mood's Median Test

This test is similar to the Wilcoxon–Mann–Whitney test and is used in the same context. However, this has less power than the Wilcoxon–Mann–Whitney test and needs a larger sample size to obtain the same power. For the Median test, the median is determined from the combined two samples and each of the observations in the two groups is dichotomized as greater than or less than this median. Using the number of observations greater than the median in the first group, the test statistic is formed and the *p*-value is determined. Let us consider the data given in Table 4.2. To obtain the *p*-value, one uses the median option in NPAR1WAY as shown below:

```
proc nparlway median; *the median option provides the results
  for a Moods Median test; class group; var response;
exact;*this maybe ignored for large data sets; run;
```

The output is given below:

```
                        ***
                Median Two-Sample Test
        Statistic (S)                      5.0000
        Normal Approximation
        Z                                 -0.2212
        One-Sided Pr < Z                   0.4124  (f4)
        Two-Sided Pr > |Z|                 0.8249  (f3)
        Exact Test
        One-Sided Pr <= S                  0.5704  (f2)
        Two-Sided Pr >= |S - Mean|         1.0000  (f1)
                        ***
```

The *p*-values given at (f1)–(f4) can be interpreted as in Section 4.2.1.

4.2.3 Kolmogorov–Smirnov

The *Kolmogorov–Smirnov test* is used in the case of two samples where one wants to see whether the two distributions are the same or not. As in the one-sample case, the *empirical distribution function* (EDF) from the first and the second sample is considered and the maximum difference from the two EDFs is determined and compared against a critical value. The null hypothesis is that the two distribution functions are the same. For further details, refer to Desu and Raghavarao (2004).

Let us consider 40 subjects receiving drug and 40 subjects receiving placebo. The patient global assessment score was applied to each subject (1 = poor, 2 = good, 3 = fair, 4 = excellent) and we are interested in comparing that the global assessment distributions are the same for placebo and drug. The following program will provide the Kolmogorov–Smirnov test and its *p*-value for the data given in Table 4.3.

```
data a1;
/***input data***/;
input trt $ resp freq @@; cards;
plac 4 14 plac 3 14 plac 2 7 plac 1 5 drug 4 4 drug 3 6
  drug 2 20 drug 1 10
```

```
;
/***end of input data***/
proc npar1way edf;   class trt; var resp; freq freq; run;
```

The output is as follows:

```
              The NPAR1WAY Procedure
                      ***
     Kolmogorov-Smirnov Two-Sample Test (Asymptotic)
     KS          0.225000            D          0.450000
     KSa         2.012461         Pr > KSa      0.0006 (g1)
                      ***
```

TABLE 4.3

Drug and Placebo Global Assessment Scores

	Drug				Placebo			
Response	1	2	3	4	1	2	3	4
Frequency	10	20	6	4	5	7	14	14

The asymptotic p-value of the Kolmogorov–Smirnov statistic is 0.0006, given at (g1), rejecting the null hypothesis that the distributions are identical in the two groups.

4.2.4 Equality of Variances

Let us consider two vending machines dispensing coffee and we would like to see that the amount of coffee dispensed from each machine has similar variability. In other words, we want to test that the variances are the same for the two populations. Levene's test discussed in Chapter 3 can be used for this purpose. However, Conover (1980, p. 239) uses a different test and we will give the necessary program for that test.

Artificial data are given in Table 4.4 showing the coffee dispensed from the two vending machines.

TABLE 4.4

Artificial Data for Coffee Dispensed

Machine 1	Machine 2	Machine 1	Machine 2
5.8	5.8	5.9	5.7
5.9	5.5	6.0	5.8
5.4	6.0	6.1	6.1
5.1	5.9	6.2	5.9
6.3	5.8	6.1	6.0

```
data a;
/***input data***/
input response @@; cards;
5.8 5.9 5.4 5.1 6.3 5.9 6.0 6.1 6.2 6.1
;
/***end of input data***/
data a;set a; group = 1; data b;
/***input data***/
input response @@; cards;
5.8 5.5 6.0 5.9 5.8 5.7 5.8 6.1 5.9 6.0
;
/***end of input data***/
data b; set b; group=2; data final; set a b;  proc sort; by group;
data final2;set final; proc sort; by group;
proc univariate noprint; output out = mean
  mean = mean;by group;var response;
data mean;set mean; proc sort; by group; run;
data final3;merge mean final2;by group; diff=abs(response – mean);
proc rank out = final4;  var diff; ranks rankdiff;run;
data final4; set final4; ranksq = rankdiff*rankdiff;
  ranksqsq = ranksq*ranksq;
proc univariate data = final4 noprint;output out = grpall
  n = totaln mean = meanrs;
var ranksq; run;
proc univariate data = final4 noprint;output out = grpall2
  sum = sumrsrs;var ranksqsq; run; data group1;set final4;
  if group = 1;
proc univariate noprint;output out = group1 sum = sum n=n;
  var ranksq;
data group1;set group1;a = 1;proc sort;by a;
data group;set grpall;a = 1;proc sort;by a;
data groupall;set grpall2;a = 1;proc sort;by a; data final;
merge group1 group groupall;by a; m=totaln – n;
  tnum = sum – n*meanrs;
tden = sqrt(((n*m*sumrsrs)/(totaln*(totaln – 1))) –
      (n*m*meanrs*meanrs/(totaln – 1)));
T = tnum/tden; PVALUE = 2*(1 – probnorm(t)); keep t pvalue;
  proc print; run;
```

T	PVALUE
1.47583	0.13999 (h1)

The *p*-value given at (h1) of 0.13999 indicates that we retain the null hypothesis of equal variances for the two vending machines. For a one-sided test, to conclude that the variance of the first population is more than the second sample, take half the *p*-value if *t* is positive and 1 minus half the *p*-value if *t* is negative.

Had we used Levene's test for this problem, the *p*-value would be 0.1265 drawing the same conclusion.

4.3 *k* Samples

The *Kruskal–Wallis test* is based on the ranks of all the observations and is discussed in Section 4.3.1 and the Median test is based on the median from all the samples and is discussed in Section 4.3.2.

4.3.1 Kruskal–Wallis Test

A nonparametric test analogous to the one-way ANOVA is the Kruskal–Wallis test. This test reduces to the Wilcoxon test described in Section 4.2.1, when we have two groups.

Random samples will be drawn from k populations and inferences are made on the equality of the k distributions, $F_1 = F_2 = \cdots = F_k$, whereas in the parametric setting we test the equality of all k means.

The global null hypothesis of primary interest is that the distributions are the same for all the response variables against the alternative that at least one pair of response variables have different distributions. The test is based on ranking the data from all the groups and seeing if the sum of the ranks is different between the groups. The p-value given at (i1) of the output is used to test the null hypothesis of equality of the k population distributions. If this p-value is less than the significance level, say 0.05, then the null hypothesis of equality of all distributions will be rejected.

Suppose the investigator is interested in testing that the ith and jth group have the same distributions for $i \neq j, j = 1, 2, \ldots, k$. This can also be done in this program. Sometimes the investigator may be interested in choosing the alternative hypothesis that all the distribution function are completely ordered and this can be done by using the Jonckheere test as given in Section 4.3.3.

Let us consider the data from Table 3.1 where the physician selects 11 subjects for each of the four groups and records the number of pounds lost in 12 weeks. Let him be interested in testing the global hypothesis that all the four regimens of weight loss programs have the same distribution. Further, he also wants to compare Regimen 1 with Regimen 2 and Regimen 1 with Regimen 3. The necessary program is given below:

```
data a;input response @@;cards;
5 2 2 3 3 2 5 3 2 2 1
;
data a;set a;group = 1; data b;input response @@;cards;
5 5 4 5 3 6 5 7 5 7 4
;
data b;set b;group = 2; data c;input response @@;cards;
7 5 6 8 5 7 5 6 5 6 6
;
data c;set c;group = 3; data d;input response @@;cards;
8 7 9 10 9 7 9 10 12 9 10
;
```

```
data d;set d;group = 4; data final;set a b c d;
data comb2;set final; ods trace on; ods results = on;
proc npar1way wilcoxon;  output out = stats; class group;var
  response;
ods output wilcoxonscores = all;run;
data all;set all;proc transpose out = allt;var meanscore n;run;
%macro groups(group); data mean;set allt;
if _label_ = 'Mean Score';
rename col1 - col&group = mean1 - mean&group;a = 1;
drop _name_ _label_;proc sort;by a;
data n;set allt; rename col1 - col&group = n1 - n&group;
  if _name_ = 'N';
a = 1;drop _name_ _label_; proc sort;by a;
data stats;set stats; a = 1; proc sort; by a; data final;
  merge mean n stats;by a;
%macro compare(group1,group2,title);
data compare;set final; n = sum(n1,n2,n3,n4);
  diff = mean&group1 - mean&group2;
absdiff = abs(diff); s2 = n*(n + 1)/12;
se = ((s2*(n - 1 - _kw_)/(n - &group))**.5)*
    ((1/n&group1 + 1/n&group2)**.5); *This is an approximation
  based on ANOVA of ranks without ties;
pvalue_2_sided = 2*(1 - probt(absdiff/se,n - &group));
keep diff pvalue_2_sided;title &title; proc print;run;
%mend compare;
/***call the macro for the groups of interest ***/;
%compare(1,2, 'group 1 vs group 2');
%compare(1,3, 'group 1 vs group 3');
%mend groups;
data a;%groups(4);run;
```

The output is as follows:

```
                           ***
            Average scores were used for ties.
                   Kruskal–Wallis Test
      Chi-square                        33.7937
      DF                                 3
      Pr > Chi-square                    <0.0001 (i1)

                 Group 1 versus Group 2
      diff                             pvalue_2_sided
      −11.6364                         0.000071663 (i2)

                 Group 1 versus Group 3
      diff                             pvalue_2_sided
      −17.4545                         5.919E-8 (i3)
```

The p-value for the Kruskal–Wallis test is given at (i1) and is <0.0001 indicating that not all groups have the same distribution. The p-value of <0.0001 given at (i2) indicates that groups 1 and 2 have different distributions. The *p*-value of <0.0001 given at (i3) indicates that groups 1 and 3 have different distributions.

It may be noted that the Kruskal–Wallis test may reject the global null hypothesis while no contrast shows significance, or vice versa.

4.3.2 Median Test

In Section 4.3.1 we discussed the Kruskal–Wallis test. The test was based on the ranks of all the observations and is a more powerful test than the median test, which will be described in this section. For the median test, from the combined sample, the median is determined and each of the observations in the *k* groups are dichotomized as greater than or less than this median. The chi-square test is then applied. The null hypothesis is H_0: All samples are from the populations with the same median. The alternative is H_A: at least a pair of distributions has different medians.

Let us consider the same data as in Table 3.1 of Section 3.3.1. The same program for the median test given in Section 4.2.2 can also be used in this context and the output is as follows:

```
                    ***
            Median One-Way Analysis
        Chi-Square            25.6412
        DF                    3
        Pr > Chi-Square       <0.0001(j1)
```

The *p*-value given at (j1) is used to draw the inference on the equality of the *k* distributions using the Median test. In this problem, the *p*-value is <0.0001 and we reject the null hypothesis of equal distribution for all the four groups.

4.3.3 Jonckheere Test

If the investigator is interested in concluding that the responses in Group 2 have larger values than Group 1, Group 3 has larger values than Group 2, and so on (i.e., *stochastic ordering*), we take the ordered alternative hypothesis and use the *Jonckheere test*. In the Kruskal–Wallis test, the alternative is that all the groups do not have the same distribution, while in the Jonckheere test, we take the completely ordered alternative.

If the investigator is interested in showing that with the regimen of diet and exercise, patients lose more pounds than patients exercising, and patients exercising lose more weight than the patients on diet pills, and the patients on diet pills lose more weight than the patients not exercising or on diet pills. In this case, we have the ordered alternative and we use the Jonckheere–Terpstra test (Jonckheere, 1954; Terpstra, 1952) and not the Kruskal–Wallis test.

The program for the Jonckheere test is given below using the data from Table 3.1.

```
Data a;
/***input data ***/
Input group wgtloss @@; cards;
1 5 1 2 1 2 1 3 1 3 1 2 1 5 1 3 1 2 1 2 1 1 2 5 2 5 2 4 2 5 2
3 2 6 2 5 2 7 2 5 2 7 2 4 3 7 3 5 3 6 3 8 3 5 3 7 3 5 3 6 3 5
3 6 3 6 4 8 4 7 4 9 4 10 4 9 4 7 4 9 4 10 4 12 4 9 4 10
;
/***end of input data***/
data a1;set a; proc freq;tables group*wgtloss/jt;run;
```

The output is as follows:

***

```
               Statistics for Table of Group by weight Loss
                        Jonckheere-Terpstra Test
               Statistic                         669.0000
               Z                                   6.4880
               One-sided Pr > Z                  <0.0001(k1)
               Two-sided Pr > |Z|                <0.0001(k2)
```

To conclude, the observations in Group 1 are smaller than the observations in Group 2, the group observations are smaller than Group 3, and so on, we take the p-value, $Pr > Z$, and in the other ordered scenario, we take the p-value, $Pr < Z$. The two-sided p-value indicates either ordering just discussed.

In our problem, we are interested in $Pr > Z$ and hence the p-value is <0.0001 given at (k1). If we were interested in either type of ordering, we will take the p-value <0.0001 given at (k2).

4.4 Transformations

Most of the nonparametric methods use the ranks of the observations to provide an appropriate test for making inferences. However, sometimes we can transform the data and use the transformed data to make the necessary tests as discussed in Chapter 3. Two commonly used transformations are: *Van der Waerden Scores* and *Savage Scores*. Van der Waerden Scores assume the underlying distribution to be normal and Savage score assumes the underlying distribution to be exponential. A variable with exponential distribution has positive values and its curve is elbow shaped dropping steeply with small

X values and tapers off with large X values. We can implement these scores in NPAR1WAY of SAS. Some researchers transform the data with the Van der Waerden scores and use the standard normal distribution methods in their analysis in more complicated settings.

Consider the data given in Table 4.2 and the VW and SAVAGE option in the NPAR1WAY procedure.

```
proc npar1way vw savage; class group; var response; run;
```

Output:

```
                           ***
           Van der Waerden Two-Sample Test
        Statistic                      0.2451
        Z                              0.1089
        One-Sided Pr > Z               0.4566
        Two-Sided Pr > |Z|             0.9132 (11)
                           ***
              Savage Two-Sample Test
        Statistic                      1.5171
        Z                              0.6506
        One-Sided Pr > Z               0.2576
        Two-Sided Pr > |Z|             0.5153 (12)
```

The p-values for a two-sided alternative for Van der Waerden and Savage scores are given in (11) and (12) and are not significant in this problem.

4.5 Friedman Test

Friedman's test is an extension of the Kruskal–Wallis test and is used when one has a two-way ANOVA or a randomized block design. The blocks are homogeneous groups such as oven temperatures, animal litters, gender, similar baseline disease characteristics, and so on. Sometimes the blocks may consist of subjects and on each subject we randomly assign all the treatments so that the subject is the block.

In this case, the observations in each block are ranked and the test statistic is constructed using these ranks. A two-way ANOVA using PROC GLM is performed for the groups and blocks, based on these ranks. The F-value corresponding to the groups is used to find the Friedman's test statistics and the p-value. The null hypothesis is that the treatment effects are equal against the alternative that there is at least one treatment difference.

Let us be interested in testing the lifetime of bulbs A, B, and C. We take 16 bulb stands where each stand can hold three bulbs. We randomly assign the

TABLE 4.5

Lifetime of Bulbs

Bulb Stand (Block)	A	B	C	Bulb Stand (Block)	A	B	C
1	155	192	212	9	133	123	210
2	153	115	214	10	135	102	155
3	154	145	135	11	124	205	193
4	184	225	193	12	197	141	163
5	206	147	142	13	181	171	160
6	187	175	166	14	201	136	171
7	196	186	171	15	130	120	110
8	165	192	112	16	135	130	120

bulbs A, B, and C at each stand and note the lifetime of the bulbs. The data are given in Table 4.5. Bulbs A and B were manufactured by one manufacturer and bulb C by another manufacturer. The researcher is interested in comparing the two manufacturers' products. For this purpose, the contrast of interest in A, B, and C brands is "1 1 − 2." This contrast will be approximately tested from PROC GLM in the following program.

We assume that the data are nonnormal and want to test the effects of bulbs A, B, and C. For this purpose, we use Friedman's test and the necessary program is as follows:

```
Data a;
/***input data***/
Input block trt$ response @@; cards;
1 A 155 1 B 192 1 C 212 2 A 153 2 B 115 2 C 214 3 A 154 3 B
145 3 C 135 4 A 184 4 B 225 4 C 193 5 A 206 5 B 147 5 C 142 6
A 187 6 B 175 6 C 166 7 A 196 7 B 186 7 C 171 8 A 165 8 B 192
8 C 112 9 A 133 9 B 123 9 C 210 10 A 135 10 B 102 10 C 155 11
A 124 11 B 205 11 C 193 12 A 197 12 B 141 12 C 163 13 A 181 13
B 171 13 C 160 14 A 201 14 B 136 14 C 171 15 A 130 15 B 120 15
C 110 16 A 135 16 B 130 16 C 120
;
/***end of input data***/
data a1;set a;
proc sort;by block; proc rank out=ranks; by block;
var response; ranks rresp;run; data final; set ranks;
  proc sort; by trt;
proc glm outstat=stat; class block trt;
model rresp=block trt;
contrast '1 and 2 vs 3' trt 1 1−2; *using the required
  contrast(s) to get approximate p-vlaue(s).; run;
data stat1;set stat;
```

```
/***input data***/
b = 16; *number of blocks; v = 3; *number of groups;
/***end of input data***/
if _source_ = 'trt' and _type_ = 'SS3'; f = f;
Friedman_test_statistic = b*(v - 1)*f/(b - 1 + f);df = v - 1;
pvalue = 1 - probchi(Friedman_test_statistic,df); proc print;
var friedman_test_statistic pvalue; run;
data contrast;set stat;
if _type_ = 'CONTRAST';
contrast = _source_;
p_value = prob;
proc print;var contrast p_value;run;
```

Friedman_test_statistic	pvalue
3.5	0.17377 (m1)
contrast	p_value
1 and 2 vs 3	0.21861 (m2)

The *p*-value given at (m1), 0.174 is used to test that all bulbs have the same lifetime. As this *p*-value is >0.05 we conclude that there is no difference between the bulbs' lifetime. The *p*-value given at (m2) 0.2186 can be used to test the significance of A and B brands versus C brand and this is nonsignificant at 0.05 level. Alternatively, one can use

```
proc freq;tables block*trt*response/chm2 scores = rank;run;
```

using the row mean square option.

4.6 Association Measures

We will now briefly discuss the measures of association between the two variables in a nonparametric setting. These measures are similar to the Pearson correlation discussed in Chapters 1 and 3.

4.6.1 Spearman Rank Correlation

Let us consider two random samples of size *n* each. The researcher may want to know if there is some sort of association between the two variables. This includes the height and weight of an individual, Test 1 and Test 2 scores in a class, families' annual income and the price of their home, and so on.

The *Spearman rank correlation* is used to measure this association when the data are nonnormally distributed, and ranges from –1 to 1, with correlation of 0 being no association. If the variables increase or decrease together, then there is a positive correlation. If the variables go in opposite directions, then there is a negative correlation. The Spearman rank correlation is the Pearson correlation of the two variables when the ranks are assigned for each variable.

Let us consider the annual salaries (in thousands of dollars) for a wife and husband in 12 households given in Table 4.6 and we like to find an association measure for the salaries of wives and husbands. Since the salary data may not be normally distributed, the association is measured by Spearman rank correlation. To obtain this correlation, the necessary program is given below.

```
data a;
input resp1 resp2 @@;cards;
80 70 67 70 85 82 87 73 75 81 94 81 78 87 80 74 86 79 85 75 80
81 90 82
;
proc rank out = ranks; var resp1 resp2; ranks rresp1 rresp2;
data final;set ranks; proc corr fisher (type = twosided);
  var rresp1 rresp2; run;
```

The output is as follows:

```
                                 ***
Pearson Correlation Statistics (Fisher's z Transformation)
                    With                 Sample          ***
Variable            Variable     N       Correlation
rresp1                rresp2      12      0.18360 (n1)

Pearson Correlation Statistics (Fisher's z Transformation)
              With                                     p Value for
Variable    Variable         95% Confidence Limits     H0: Rho = 0
rresp1      rresp2      - 0.443002 (n2)  0.680842 (n3)  0.5774 (n4)
```

The Spearman rank correlation is 0.1836 given at (n1) with the 95% CI, (–0.443, 0.681) given at [(n2), (n3)]. The two-sided *p*-value for testing the null hypothesis of no association is 0.5774 given at (n4). The correlation is not significant at a 0.05 level in this problem.

TABLE 4.6

Salaries of Wives and Husbands (Thousands of Dollars)

Wives	80	67	85	87	75	94	78	80	86	85	80	90
Husbands	70	70	82	73	81	81	87	74	79	75	81	82

4.6.2 Kendall's Tau

Kendall's Tau is a measure similar to the Spearman rank correlation between two variables ranging from –1 to 1. Given a pair of observations if both variables are increasing or decreasing, the pair is said to be a concordant pair and if they go in opposite directions, the pair is considered to be discordant. Kendall's tau is based on the chances of getting the difference between the concordant and discordant pairs. For the data considered in Table 4.6, the following program provides Kendall's tau as its output.

```
data a;
/***input data***/
input resp1 resp2 @@;cards;
80 70 67 70 85 82 87 73 75 81 94 81 78 87 80 74 86 79 85 75 80
81 90 82
;
/***end of input data***/
proc corr kendall; var resp1 resp2;run;
```

The output is as follows:

```
        Kendall Tau b Correlation Coefficients, N = 12
                  Prob > |r| under H0: Rho = 0
                          resp1                resp2
     resp1                1.00000              0.14635(o1)
                                               0.5272(o2)
     resp2                0.14635              1.00000
                          0.5272
```

Kendall's tau is 0.146 given at (o1) and the two-sided *p*-value for testing no association by this method is 0.5272 given at (o2). Incidentally, we can also calculate Spearman's correlation by changing the option from Kendall to Spearman in the above program. The *p*-value obtained by this method for the Spearman's correlation is based on the *t*-test, whereas it is based on normal approximation in Section 4.6.1.

4.6.3 Kappa Statistic

When *n* individual units are classified into categories by two methods, the agreement of these two methods is measured relative to the independent evaluations by using the *Kappa statistic*. When Kappa = 0, the agreement of the two rating scales is the same as that of an independent reader. This measure differs from the usual correlations in the sense that the agreement between the actual evaluations and that of independent evaluation is measured.

The difference between unweighted and weighted kappa is based on how the disagreements are handled. Weighted kappa penalizes disagreements, whereas with unweighted kappa, the disagreements are treated equally.

Usually when two clinicians rate the patients' disease level, the agreement between the two clinicians is measured by kappa. When two laboratories classify the samples in ordinal scale, the agreement of the two labs can also be measured by the Kappa statistic.

Refer back to Section 2.3.1 for further details on Kappa and Section 2.6.4 for weighted kappa.

4.7 Censored Data

Censored data are data that are incomplete due to subjects having an event before their inclusion in the study or events not happening until the completion of the study, machine equipment failing, and so on. In clinical trials, subjects may not be able to be followed till the end of the study, because the subjects may have withdrawn from the study, or the subjects may be lost to follow-up, and so forth. This type of censoring is called *right censoring*. Instead of throwing out these data because they are not complete, partial information on these observations can be used. For these types of data the parametric assumptions are not appropriate due to nonnormality and censoring. This type of analysis is called survival or time-to–an-event analysis where both censored and noncensored data points are used in the analysis.

Sometimes we may know that the subject has died 2 years from the onset of the study, but we are only interested in the subject's 1 year survival status. We truncate the information at the 1-year time point and consider the subject alive at 1 year. This type of censored data or truncated data is said to be right censored or truncated.

Sometimes the patients may be entering the study after the study starts and sometimes the patients entering the study already had an event. Such data are called *left censored* or left truncated. However, we will consider right censoring and truncation in this book and we will not consider left-censored or truncated data.

Let us consider 15 subjects who are monitored for 90 days after a TIA episode, for a stroke. The various time points are displayed as follows:

20+ 30 40 60 14 34 56 57+ 19 47 90+ 80 40 51+ 70

The + after 20, 57, 90, and 51 indicates that these are the censored observations and the event has not occurred until the given time. The other observations indicate the event time.

In survival analysis, we are interested in obtaining the survival (or endpoint of interest) probabilities at various time points. The *survivor function* is usually denoted by $S(t)$, where t represents the time point of interest and it indicates the probability that the person survived beyond the specified time t. Thus, if one wants to know the survival function at 50 days, it is represented as $S(50)$. These data are usually graphed as step functions as shown in Chapter 1, Figure 1.9. At the beginning of the study, $S(0)$, the *survival function* is 1 and as t goes to infinity the survival function goes toward 0. Some researchers also use the complement of the survival function, known as the failure function. This function starts with 0 at the beginning of the study and goes to 1 as t goes to infinity.

The *hazard function* is a rate and not a probability and is usually denoted by $h(t)$ and ranges from 0 to infinity. This function indicates the event occurring between t and $t + \Delta t$, where Δt would represent a small increment in time, given that the individual has not had the event until time t. Let us consider 100 subjects with 1 death in the first month. The hazard rate is 1/100 for the first month. For the next month, the hazard rate is the number dying over the number still alive $(100 - 1 = 99)$, and so on. With small intervals the hazard rate approximates a continuous function. This function focuses on the time of the occurrence of the event. This is also referred to as the conditional failure rate. A constant hazard implies that the data are distributed exponentially for the time between the events. The *exponential distribution*, as noted before, is an elbow-shaped continuous distribution going from 0 to infinity. Its mean is the same as the standard deviation. It should be noted that both the survival and hazard function go in opposite directions.

The survival function at a given time point t is the probability that an individual did not have an event until the time point t. The median survival time is a descriptive statistic where approximately 50% of the cohort had an event until the median survival time point.

4.7.1 Kaplan–Meier Survival Distribution Function

Let us consider the stroke event data given earlier. We would like to know the probability that the individual has not had a stroke at a give time, say 30 days after having the TIA episode. The survival function will usually be determined by using *Kaplan–Meier (KM) estimates*. Such probabilities will be plotted on the y-axis and the time of the events on the x-axis and are called survival curves. The KM estimates and the 95% confidence intervals for the survival probabilities will be obtained by the following program. Censored observations will be denoted by 0 and the events will be denoted by 1.

```
data a;
/***input data***/
input event time@@; cards;
0 20 1 30 1 40 1 60 1 14 1 34 1 56 0 57 1 19 1 47 0 90 1 80 1
40 0 51 1 70
;
/***end of input data***/
data final;set a;
proc lifetest method = km plots = (s) outserv = a1;
time time*event(0);run; data a2;set a1; proc print; run;
```

The output is as follows:

```
                               ***
          Summary Statistics for Time Variable time
                      Quartile Estimates
                  Point              95% Confidence Interval
Percent         Estimate            (Lower            Upper)
75              70.0000             47.0000              .
50              56.0000(p1)         34.0000(p2)       70.0000(p3)
25              34.0000             19.0000           56.0000


       Mean                    Standard Error
     51.2569(p4)                  6.0369
```

Note: The mean survival time and its standard error were underestimated because the largest observation was censored and the estimation was restricted to the largest event time.

```
                    The LIFETEST Procedure
   Summary of the Number of Censored and Uncensored Values
     Total            Failed          Censored       Percent Censored
     15                11                4                26.67


     time   _CENSOR_    SURVIVAL(p5)   SDF_LCL(p6)  SDF_UCL(p7)
     0         .          1.00000       1.00000      1.00000
     14        0          0.93333       0.61264      0.99033
     19        0          0.86667       0.56391      0.96488
     20        1          0.86667          .            .
     30        0          0.79444       0.48791      0.92887
     34        0          0.72222       0.41718      0.88592
     40        0          0.57778       0.28989      0.78425
     47        0          0.50556       0.23291      0.72666
     51        1          0.50556          .            .
     56        0          0.42130       0.16691      0.65878
     57        1          0.42130          .            .
     60        0          0.31597       0.09057      0.57541
     70        0          0.21065       0.03726      0.47836
     80        0          0.10532       0.00653      0.36533
     90        1             .             .            .
```

In column (p5) of the output, we have the survival probabilities at every given distinct time points (also see Figure 4.1). At time point 30, the survival probability is 0.7944 and the failure probability is $(1 - 0.7944) = 0.2056$. For any time point between two event times, the survival probabilities are the ones given at the early time event. For example, at time 32, the survival probability is the same as the survival probability at the time point 30 and is

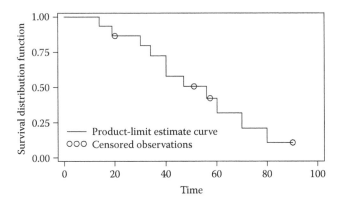

FIGURE 4.1
KM curve.

0.7944. In (p1) we have the median of the survival times. In our output we have 56 as the median which means nearly 50% of the patients having TIA episode will get a stroke on the 56th day. At (p2) and (p3), we have the lower and upper confidence limits for the median time as (34, 70). The mean survival time is given at (p4) and is 51.26. In column (p6) and (p7), we obtain the lower and upper confidence limits for the survival function at any given time point t. The confidence intervals are obtained using *Greenwood's formula* for the variance. For the time point 30, the lower and upper limits for the survival probability is (0.48791, 0.92887). The graph shown in the output is the survival function graph and also known as the *Kaplan–Meier curve*. This is a *step function* showing the survival probabilities at a given time point.

4.7.2 Wilcoxon (Gehan) and Log-Rank Test

Analogous to the Wilcoxon–Mann–Whitney test of comparing the two distributions, we would like to compare two survival curves. Gehan's versions of the Wilcoxon test and *Log-rank test* are commonly used for this purpose. The statistic is computed from the event times by considering the subjects at risk at the event times and giving appropriate scores. The p-value given is based upon the asymptotic chi-square test. These tests differ in terms of the weights attached to the event times. In the Gehan–Wilcoxon test, the weights depend on the number of people at risk at the event time, whereas in log-rank test, constant weight is attached for each event time. Since the Wilcoxon test gives more weight to earlier times than later time points, it is less sensitive than log-rank test to differences between groups that occur at later points in time. Log-rank test emphasizes failures at the end of the survival curve.

Let us assume that the data given in Section 4.6.1 are based on control group of patients. Let another sample of 15 patients be treated with a blood thinner coumadin. The event times for the treated patients are given below:

70 75 49+ 80 64 34+ 86 77 15 77 90+ 84 60 81+ 72

The following program provides the test for the homogeneity of the two distributions:

```
data group1; input event time@@; cards;
0 20 1 30 1 40 1 60 1 14 1 34 1 56 0 57 1 19 1 47 0 90 1 80 1
40 0 51 1 70
;
data group1;set group1; group = 1;
data group2; input event time@@; cards;
1 70 1 75 0 49 1 80 1 64 0 34 1 86 1 77 1 15 1 77 0 90 1 84 1
60 0 81 1 72
;
data group2;set group2; group = 2; data final;set group1 group2;
proc lifetest method = km plots = (s); time time*event (0);
  strata group;
*The strata statement the product limit estimator is
  calculated for each group and the the survival functions for
  the group are compared.;
symbol1 v = none color = black line = 1; symbol2 v = none
  color = black line = 2; run;
```

The output is as follows:

★★★

Test of Equality over Strata

Test	Chi-Square	DF	Pr > Chi-quare
Log-rank	3.4308	1	0.0640 (q1)
Wilcoxon	5.9947	1	0.0143 (q2)
−2Log (LR)	0.7059	1	0.4008

The p-value at (q1) of 0.0640 indicates that the two strata have similar survival times for treated and control patients based on the log-rank test. The p-value at (q2) of 0.0143 indicates that the two survival curves are different based on the Gehan–Wilcoxon test. The Figure 4.2 overlaying both the curves indicates the treatment groups has better survival rates compared to the control group, because the survival rate for the treated group is higher than the survival rate for the control group.

4.7.3 Life-Table (Acturial Method)

Sometimes, with a large number of observations we may be interested to get the survival and failure probabilities in different time intervals where the intervals need not have the same width. This can be achieved by using the option METHOD = LIFE in the LIFETEST procedure. For the data given in

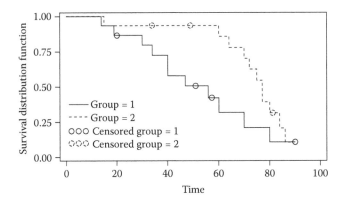

FIGURE 4.2
KM curves comparing two groups.

Section 4.7.1, if we want to get the survival and failure probabilities in 10-day intervals, the following program can be used:

```
data a;
/***input data***/
input event time@@; *With multiple observations we input the
  frequency at each time point; cards;
0 20 1 30 1 40 1 60 1 14 1 34 1 56 0 57 1 19 1 47 0 90 1 80 1
40 0 51 1 70
;
/***end of input data***/
data final;set a; proc lifetest method=life intervals=(0 to 90
  by 10) plots=(s); *int the parenthesis the first part is the
  range of the data and the last number is width of the interval;
time time*event(0); *Include frequency with multiple
  observations at a time point; run;
```

The output is as follows:

```
                    The LIFETEST Procedure
                 Life Table Survival Estimates
             Interval
    [Lower,    Upper)  ***    Survival(r1)  Failure(r2)
    0          10             1.0000        0
    10         20             1.0000        0
    20         30             0.8667        0.1333
    30         40             0.8667        0.1333
    40         50             0.7222        0.2778
    50         60             0.5056        0.4944
    60         70             0.4213        0.5787
    70         80             0.3160        0.6840
    80         90             0.2106        0.7894
    90         .              0.1053        0.8947
                        ***
```

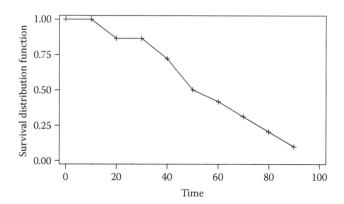

FIGURE 4.3
Survival curve by lifetest.

In columns (r1) and (r2), we have the survival and failure probabilities in the given time intervals. For example, in the time interval 30–40, the survival and failure probabilities are, respectively, 0.8667 and 0.1333. The survival curve using these time intervals is also provided in the output in Figure 4.3.

5

Regression

Correlation is used to measure the strength of linear relationship between two variables, whereas regression is used to model the response of one variable in terms of one or more other variables. The response variable is known as the dependent (endogenous) variable and the other variables used to predict the response are known as independent (exogenous) variables or predictors. This model can be linear, quadratic, Poisson, nonlinear, and so on, which best fits all the data points. Regression is useful to predict the future data points for the response variable, given the predictors.

Let us consider the example of height and weight of individuals. One would like to predict the weight of an individual, given the height of that individual. The predictor in this case is height which is the X variable, whereas we predict weight, which is the Y variable. For a given height, individuals have different weights. One can express the mean weight as a linear function of the height variable and predict the mean weight, given the X variable. The response Y is modeled as

$$Y = \beta_0 + \beta_1 X + \varepsilon,$$

where β_0 and β_1 are the intercept and the slope of the line, respectively, and ε is the random error. If β_0 is 0, the line passes through the origin and if β_1 is 0, there is no slope and the line is parallel to the X-axis. In certain situations, β_0 may not be meaningful to interpret. β_0 enables to predict the Y values in the domain of the X values in the study.

β_0 and β_1 need to be estimated from the given data. This is done by using the least-squares method by assuming that the Y variables for a given X are normally distributed and have a common variance. The common variance assumption is needed to estimate the parameters, whereas the normal distribution assumption is needed to test the significance and set confidence intervals (CIs) on the parameters. The distance between the Y values and the predicted Y values, $\hat{Y}$, is minimized by the method called least squares; refer to Draper and Smith (1981) to estimate the parameters.

The differences between the Y and $\hat{Y}$ for each of the data points are called statistical errors or residuals. Different assumptions may be made on the residuals based on the equation assumed to fit the $\hat{Y}$ values. For the simple linear regression case we assume the errors to be normally and independently distributed, with a mean of 0, and a common variance of σ^2. It may be noted that when we make a prediction $\hat{Y}$, the actual Y value need not be $\hat{Y}$ and it can be within some margin of error from $\hat{Y}$.

If these errors are not normally distributed, then one may perform the logistic or Poisson regression. The distribution of the errors can be obtained from the scatter plots by plotting the X and Y values for each data point. Usually, the X variables are taken as fixed constants, but may be random.

When we repeat the X values to obtain different Y values the variability of those Y values is called pure error. When we get pure error, we will be able to predict whether the model is fitting well for the data or we need to assume a different model or different or more independent variables, to predict the dependent variable.

We will consider different aspects of regression in the following sections. We will also review the diagnostics used to assess the various fits of the regression lines and determine the outliers in the data.

5.1 Simple Regression

The simplest and basic form of regression is known as simple linear regression. Here there is one response variable Y and one predictor variable X. The relationship between these two variables (X and Y) is expected to be linear based on the raw data or by some transformations (see Section 5.14) of the raw data. The equation for this is represented as

$$Y = \beta_0 + \beta_1 X + \varepsilon,$$

where β_0 and β_1 are unknown and are the parameters of the population, and ε is the random error. β_0 and β_1 are estimated for this equation based on the least-squares approach from the observed data.

The slope of the line is β_1 and tells us how much Y changes, when X is increased by one unit. The Y-intercept of the line is β_0 and is the value of Y when $X = 0$.

Let us consider an example of repairing the roof, where X represents the number of bids made and Y represents the cost for the repair given in Table 5.1.

The following program provides the necessary output to draw inferences on the model and parameters.

```
data a1;
/***input data***/
input X Y @@; cards;
3 10000 1 10000 4 15000 7 8000 5 7000 6 7000 11 8000 3 9000 8
   9000 10 5000 7 9000 2 8500 9 7000 12 6000
;
/***end of input data***/
ods trace on;
```

```
proc glm; model y=x/clparm; ods output
  overallANOVA = overallanova;
run; ods trace off; proc rsreg data = a1; model y = x/lackfit;
ods output errorANOVA = errorANOVA; run;
data error11; set erroranova; if source = 'Pure Error'; keep
  source df ss;
data error1; set erroranova; if source = 'Pure Error';
  source1 = source; df1 = df; ss1 = ss; a = 1; keep source1 df1 ss1
  a; proc sort;by a;
data error2;set overallanova;
if source = 'Error';a = 1; keep source df ss a; data lackfit;
  merge error1 error2;by a;
source = 'Lack of Fit'; df = df - df1; ss = ss - ss1; keep df ss
  source;
data final; set error11 lackfit error2;drop a; MS = ss/df;
  F = ms/lag(ms); dflag = lag(df); if source = 'Error' then f = .;
  PVALUE = 1 - probf(f,df,dflag);
drop dflag; proc print;run;
```

TABLE 5.1

Artificial Data on the Cost of Roof Repair

X	Y($)	X	Y($)
3	10,000	3	9000
1	10,000	8	9000
4	15,000	10	5000
7	8000	7	9000
5	7000	2	8500
6	7000	9	7000
11	8000	12	6000

The output is

```
                    The GLM Procedure
                 Dependent Variable: Y
                    Sum of
Source        DF    Squares      Mean Square   F Value    Pr > F
Model         1     23136663.15 23136663.15      5.54   0.0364 (a2)
Error      12(a9) 50095479.70 4174623.31(a10)
Corrected 13      73232142.86
  total
```

R-Square	Coeff. Var	Root MSE	Y Mean
0.315936 (a3)	24.13895	2043.189	8464.286

Source	DF	Type I SS	Mean Square	F Value	Pr > F
X	1	23136663.15	23136663.15	5.54	0.0364

Source	DF	Type III SS	Mean Square	F Value	Pr > F
X	1	23136663.15	23136663.15	5.54	0.0364

Parameter	Estimate	Standard Error	*t* Value	Pr > |t|	95% Confidence Limits	
	(a4)	(a6)	(a5)		(a7)	(a8)
Intercept	10893.91144	1167.604168	9.33	< 0.0001	8349.92050	13437.90238
X	−386.53137	164.188610	−2.35	0.0364	−744.26761	−28.79512

***

Source	DF	SS	MS	F	PVALUE
Pure error	2	1000000	500000.00	.	.
Lack of fit	10	49095480	4909547.97	9.81910	0.095903 (a1)
Error	12	50095480	4174623.31	.	.

Using the estimates given in column (a4) the predicting equation can be written as

$$\hat{Y} = 10893.91 + (-386.53)X$$

First we will test the model adequacy. This is possible because the data consist of repeated X-values. The p-value at (a1) is used to test the lack of fit of the model. If this p-value is greater than 0.05, we assume that there is no lack of fit and the model is adequate to make the predictions. If this p-value is less than 0.05, then the model is inadequate and we may need to add more independent variables for the prediction, or use a different model to draw the inferences. The p-value in this problem at (a1) is 0.0959; hence, we assume that the linear equation fit is adequate. It is important to use multiple observations on the Y variable for the same value of the X variable, to test the adequacy of the model by getting the p-value at (a1).

The p-value for the F statistic given at (a2) is used to test the significance of the slope in the model. If this p-value is less than 0.05, we conclude that the slope is significantly different from zero; otherwise, the slope in the model is zero. In our problem this p-value is 0.036 and the slope is significant.

R^2 given at (a3) lets us determine the strength of the relationship between X and Y and is the same as the sample squared correlation between the X and Y variables. R^2 ranges from 0 to 1, where 1 is a perfect fit. Usually, this value should be at least 0.7 so that the model is considered to give a reasonable fit. The R^2 value at (a3) is 0.3159, indicating that the percentage of variation of the Y variable explained by the linear regression is 31.59%. Although the model is significant, we are only able to express 31.59% of the variation in the Y variable by our fitted equation. It may be noted that sometimes the slope may be significant with a small R^2 value or vice versa. In such cases the experimenter should examine the estimated slope parameter and make a judicious judgement in using the regression equation for making predictions.

The estimates of the regression coefficients are given in column (a4) for the intercept β_0 and slope β_1. The significance of the coefficients can be tested by using the p-values in the column given by (a5). The standard errors of the estimated parameters are given in column (a6). Columns (a7) and (a8) give the confidence limits for the parameters. In our problem, the slope is –386.53 with a standard error of 164.19 and a *p*-value for testing that the slope is zero is 0.0364. It may be noted that this *p*-value is the same as the *p*-value in (a2) for simple regression. This value is significant and there is a significant slope in the linear equation predicting Y based on X. The 95% CI for the slope is (–744.27, –28.80). The negative slope in this problem indicates that the cost of the roof decreases as the number of bids increase. When appropriate, the *p*-value corresponding to the intercept is more than the level of significance, we interpret that the Y value is zero when X is zero.

To test for hypothesized values other than zero, for β_1, the *p*-values for one-sided and two-sided tests are given by (a11) and (a12) using the following additional programming lines:

```
data a1;
/***input data***/
Estimate =-386.53137; *(a4) for the variable of interest;
Se = 164.188610; * (a6) for the variable of interest;
Hypslope =-300;*hypothesized slope; Df = 12;*(a9) for the error
  df;
/***end of input data***/
T = (estimate - hypslope)/se; PVALUE1 = 1 - probt(t,df);
t = abs(t); PVALUE2 = 2*(1 - probt(t,df)); proc print; var pvalue1
  pvalue2;run;
```

PVALUE1	PVALUE2
0.69611 (a11)	0.60778 (a12)

The *p*-values at (a11) and (a12) indicate that the hypothesized slope is not rejected from the data for a one-sided or two-sided test for the slope equal to –300.

Sometimes we may be interested in predicting the Y value for a given X value not included in the data. The interval estimate is known as the prediction interval and the following lines provide the necessary program when the prediction is made at $X = X_0$. At (a13), the point estimate of the predicted value is given and its 95% prediction interval is given in [(a14), (a15)].

```
data a1;
/***input data***/
input x y @@; cards;
3 10000 1 10000 4 15000 7 8000 5 7000 6 7000 11 8000
3 9000 8 9000 10 5000 7 9000 2 8500 9 7000 12 6000
;
/***end of input data***/
proc univariate noprint;output out = stats n = n mean = xbar;
  var x;run;
data stats;set stats;
/***input data***/
inter = 10893.91144; *intercept of the line(a4);
```

```
slope = -386.53137; *slope of the line (a4);
s2 = 4174623.31; *mean square for error (a10);
seslope = 164.188610;*standard error for slope(a6); alpha = .05;
x0 = 3;*New X value;
/***end of input data***/
varslope = seslope**2; t = tinv((1 - alpha/2),n - 2); sxx = s2/
  varslope;
YHAT = inter + slope*x0; seyhat = sqrt(1 + (1/n) + (((x0 - xbar)**2)/
  (sxx)));
UPPER_CI = yhat + t*seyhat*sqrt(s2); LOWER_CI = yhat - t*
  seyhat*sqrt(s2);
proc print; var lower_ci yhat upper_ci; run;
```

LOWER_CI	YHAT	UPPER_CI
4978.79(a14)	9734.32(a13)	14489.85(a15)

If we want to predict the cost when three bids are collected, the estimate of the predicted value is 9734.32, given at (a13) and the prediction interval is (4978.79, 14489.85), given at [(a14), (a15)]. For further details and examples see Raghavarao (1988). In the case of confidence intervals for X_0, remove the 1 in the variable seyhat. The prediction and confidence intervals length is minimum when $X_0 = \bar{X}$.

5.2 Polynomial Regression

An extension of the simple linear regression discussed in Section 5.1 is polynomial regression where we predict Y, given the predictor X using the following form:

$$Y = \beta_0 + \beta_1 X + \beta_2 X^2 + \cdots + \beta_k X^k + \varepsilon,$$

where β_is are the unknown parameters and ε is random error. When $k = 1$, we obtain the simple linear regression, when $k = 2$, the quadratic regression, and when $k = 3$, the cubic regression. In the quadratic model depending on the sign of the β_2 coefficient, we can determine whether the *minimum* or *maximum* of the Y values is attained. If β_2 is positive, the curve provides a minimum value for Y and when β_2 is negative, it provides a maximum value for Y. In a cubic model the curve changes its orientation in two places. We assume that the variance of the Y values is the same at all X values.

Consider the data in Table 5.2 showing the average speed of the car (X) and the gas mileage (Y) obtained at that speed. We expect a quadratic regression equation providing the optimum speed to get maximum gas mileage.

The following program provides the necessary output:

```
Data a1;
/***input data***/
```

```
Input speed gasmil @@; cards;
40 20 40 22 35 18 50 25 55 30 55 31 60 29 65 25 65 26 70 20
;
/***end of input data***/
data a;set a1;
proc rsreg;model gasmil = speed/lackfit;run;
proc glm;model gasmil = speed speed*speed/clparm;
*clparm is used to obtain confidence intervals for the
  parameters;run;
```

TABLE 5.2

Artificial Data on Car Speed and Gas Mileage

X	Y	X	Y
40	20	55	31
40	22	60	29
35	18	65	25
50	25	65	26
55	30	70	20

**

Response Surface for Variable gasmil
***

Root MSE	1.904356
R-Square	0.8623 (b3)

***

Regression	DF	Type I Sum of Squares	*R*-Square	*F* Value	Pr > *F*
Linear	1	33.536276	0.1819	9.25	0.0188
Quadratic	1	125.477730	0.6805	34.60	0.0006

***

Residual	DF	Sum of Squares	Mean Square	*F* Value	Pr > *F*
Lack of fit	4	22.385994	5.596499	5.60	0.0944 (b1)
Pure error	3	3.000000	1.000000		
Total error	7	25.385994	3.626571		

***

The RSREG Procedure

Canonical Analysis of Response Surface Based on Coded Data

Critical Value

Factor	Coded	Uncoded
speed	0.119998	54.599960 (b10)

Predicted value at stationary point: 28.929931 (b11)

```
              Stationary point is a maximum.  (b9)
                         The GLM Procedure
                   Dependent Variable: gasmil
                       Sum of Source    DF    Squares    Mean Square  F Value    Pr > F
Model              2   159.0140060   79.5070030   21.92   0.0010(b2)
Error              7    25.3859940    3.6265706
Corrected total    9   184.4000000

                               ****

Parameter       Estimate      Std Error   t Value  Pr>|t|    95% Confidence Limits
                  (b4)          (b5)                 (b6)      (b7)         (b8)
Intercept    -69.26120146   14.78211105  -4.69    0.0022  -104.2153397  -34.30706317
Speed          3.59674743    0.58656825   6.13    0.0005     2.20973393   4.98376093
Speed*speed   -0.03293727    0.00559954  -5.88    0.0006    -0.04617808  -0.01969646
```

When the predictor variable X is repeated, we have the pure error, and the lack of the fit of the model can be assessed. The p-value for testing the lack of fit is given at (b1). In our example, this p-value is 0.0944 and is not significant. Hence, we assume that the lack of fit of the quadratic model is not significant. The significance of all the parameters of the quadratic model can be tested by using the p-value at (b2), and in this example it is 0.0010, indicating significance. The R^2 value 0.8623 given at (b3) shows that 86.23% of the variability in the Y variable is explained by the quadratic regression equation. The estimated intercept and regression coefficients are given in column (b4) and their standard errors are given in column (b5). The significance of these coefficients can be judged by the p-values given in column (b6). The CIs for the parameters are given in columns [(b7), (b8)].

In our example, the p-value for testing the significance of the parameter β_1 is 0.0005 and the p-value for testing the significance of β_2, the coefficient of the squared independent variable term, is 0.0006. Both these parameters are significant. From (b9) we see whether the graph gives a maximum or minimum value. At (b10), the X value where the maxima or minima occur is given and at (b11), the maximum or minimum predicted value is given. From our example, the gas mileage is maximum when speed $= 54.6$ and the optimum gas mileage attained is 28.9.

Using the estimates given in column (b4) we write our estimated response variable

$$\hat{Y} = -69.26 + 3.60X - 0.03X^2$$

5.3 Multiple Regressions

For many problems, more than one predictor variable (exogenous) is necessary to model the response variable (endogenous). Let us assume that we

TABLE 5.3

Artificial Data on Roof Cost with Additional Variables

Y—Minimum Cost	X₁—Number of Bidders	X₂—Area of the Roof	House Type	Z_1	Z_2
10,000	3	1500	Colonial	0	0
10,000	1	1400	Ranch	1	0
15,000	4	2000	Split	0	1
8000	7	1200	Split	0	1
7000	5	800	Split	0	1
7000	6	900	Colonial	0	0
8000	11	1000	Ranch	1	0
9000	3	1300	Ranch	1	0
9000	8	1700	Colonial	0	0
5000	10	700	Split	0	1
9000	7	1700	Ranch	1	0
8500	2	1600	Colonial	0	0
7000	9	800	Split	0	1
6000	12	900	Colonial	0	0

have p predictors (independent variables) to predict a response variable Y. The model for this is

$$Y = \beta_0 + \beta_1 X_1 + \cdots + \beta_p X_p + \varepsilon,$$

where β_is are parameters estimated from the data and ε is the random error. $\beta_1, \beta_2, \ldots, \beta_p$ are known as regression coefficients.

The least-squares method is used to estimate β_is. The estimate β_i tells us how much Y changes, when X_i is increased by one unit, while all the other X variables are held constant. This model reduces to simple linear regression if we have one predictor ($p = 1$).

Consider the example discussed in Table 5.1, where we predict the minimum cost for repairing the roof, and the predictor variable is the number of bids for the job. The minimum cost on repairs may also depend on the roof size and hence, we use two predictors: the number of bids X_1 and the roof size X_2. The data are shown in the first three columns of Table 5.3.

The necessary program to get the estimated model and test the appropriate parameters is given below:

```
data a1;
/***input data***/
input x1 x2 y @@; cards;
3 1500 10000 1 1400 10000 4 2000 15000 7 1200 8000 5 800 7000
6 900 7000 11 1000 8000 3 1300 9000 8 1700 9000 10 700 5000 7
1700 9000 2 1600 8500 9 800 7000 12 900 6000
;
```

```
/***end of input data***/
proc glm; model y=x1 x2/clparm; run;
```

The output is as follows:

```
                          The GLM Procedure
                        Dependent Variable: y
Source        DF   Sum of Squares  Mean Square  F Value     Pr > F
Model          2      54231193.42  27115596.71   15.70   0.0006(c1)
Error         11      19000949.44   1727359.04
Corrected     13      73232142.86
  total
```

```
          R-Square              Coeff. Var     Root MSE      y Mean
          0.740538(c2)           15.52748      1314.290     8464.286
                                    ***
```

```
Parameter    Estimate   Std Error     t    Pr>|t|  95% Confidence Limits
                                     Value
                (c3)        (c4)            (c5)       (c6)         (c7)
Intercept  3619.004794 1871.935411   1.93  0.0793  -501.097265 7739.106854
x1         - 109.302630  124.193453 -0.88  0.3976  -382.650576  164.045317
x2            4.425861    1.043151   4.24  0.0014     2.129902    6.721820
```

The predicting equation can be written, by using the estimates given in column (c3), as

$$\hat{Y} = 3619.0 + (-109.3)X_1 + (4.4)X_2$$

To test the lack of fit of the model we need to have data points with the same values for the predictor variables. A program similar to the one in Section 5.1 can be used to separate out the lack of fit and pure error sums of squares and test the significance of the lack of fit. In our data set we do not have repeated predictor variables data and hence we cannot test the lack of fit in this case.

The p-value for the F statistic given at (c1) is used to test the significance of all the model parameters, that is, $\beta_1 = 0$, $\beta_2 = 0$. If this p-value is less than 0.05, we conclude that at least one of the model parameters is significant. If this p-value is greater than 0.05, none of the model parameters are significant. In our problem, this p-value is 0.0006 and at least one of the model parameters is significant.

R^2 given at (c2) indicates the strength of the relationship between the predictors X_1, X_2 and the response variable Y. The R^2 value at (c2) is 0.7405, indicating that the percentage of variation of the Y variable explained by the linear regression by using the independent variables X_1, X_2, is 74.05. Note that the R^2 of 31.59% at (a3) given in Section 5.1 with 1 predictor variable X_1 has significantly improved to 74.05% with two predictor variables X_1 and X_2. PROC REG provides adj R^2 values which can be used to compare models with different number of predictor variables.

The estimates of the regression coefficients are given in column (c3). The standard errors of these estimated parameters are given in column (c4). The significance of the coefficients can be tested by using the p-values given in column (c5). Columns (c6) and (c7) give the confidence limits for the parameters. In our problem the estimate of β_1 is –109.3 with a standard error 124.19. The p-value for testing that this slope is zero is 0.3976. This value is not significant, and there is no evidence that X_1 variable provides contribution to the response variable Y when X_2 variable is added to the model. The 95% CI for the slope β_1 is (–382.7, 164.0). The interpretation of the estimated slope β_1 is that for every increase of 1 bidder, the cost goes down by $109.30 for the same roof size. The other parameters can be interpreted in the same way.

To test for hypothesized values other than 0, for β_1, the p-values for one-sided and two-sided tests are given by (c8) and (c9) using the same program given in Section 5.1 and updating with the present data and the hypothesized value of –100 for β_1. Similarly, one can do this for other parameters of interest.

```
PVALUE1              PVALUE2
0.52918(c8)          0.94164(c9)
```

Sometimes we may be interested to predict the Y value, given the values of the predictors for a new observation. The interval estimate is known as the prediction interval and the following lines provide the necessary program when the prediction is made at $x = x^*$, where the vector x^* has one in the first component and the chosen predictor variables in components 2, 3, ..., $p + 1$. In our example, we would like to predict the cost for the roof using the predictors $X_1 = 5$ and $X_2 = 1000$. The following program provides the necessary output:

```
data a1;
proc iml;
/***input data***/
* Input the X variables in the X matrix after the 1st column
  of ones. The commas separate each row of the matrix;
x = {1 3 1500, 1 1 1400, 1 4 2000, 1 7 1200, 1 5 800,
     1 6 900, 1 11 1000, 1 3 1300, 1 8 1700,
     1 10 700, 1 7 1700, 1 2 1600, 1 9 800, 1 12 900};
*input the response variable data;
y = {10000, 10000, 15000, 8000, 7000, 7000, 8000, 9000, 9000,
     5000, 9000, 8500, 7000, 6000};
n = 13;* number of observations;
p = 3;*number of columns of X matrix, including the column of
  1s;
alpha = .05; xstar = {1,5,1000};* the 1st input is always one,
  and the remaining variables are values of the predictors for
  predicting future response;
/***end of input data***/
```

```
xt = x`; yt = y`; xtx = xt*x; xtxinv = inv(xtx); xy = xt*y;
  beta = xtxinv*xy;
betat = beta`; rss = yt*y - betat*xy; df = n - p - 1; var = rss/(n - p - 1);
xstart = xstar`; sepred = sqrt(var)*sqrt(1 + xstart*xtxinv*xstar);
YHAT = xstart*beta; t = tinv((1 - alpha/2), df);
  LOWER_CI = yhat - sepred*t;
UPPER_CI = yhat + sepred*t; print lower_ci yhat upper_ci;run;
  quit;
```

The output is as follows:

```
  LOWER_CI                    YHAT                    UPPER_CI
  3972.1007(c11)          7498.3525(c10)        11024.604(c12)
```

At (c10) the point estimate of the predicted value is given as \$7498.35 and its 95% prediction interval is given in [(c11), (c12)] as (\$3972.10, \$11024.60).

5.3.1 Multicollinearity

Multicollinearity exists when there is a strong correlation among the predictor variables. Although this does not bias the coefficients, it makes them unstable. One way of checking for the multicollinearity is to look at the variance inflation factor. The variance inflation factor indicates the increase in the variance of the parameter due to the correlation between the predictors; hence, a variance inflation factor greater than 10 (see Der and Everitt, 2006, p. 165) indicates the multicollinearity of the predictor variables. If multicollinearity exists, one can combine some predictor variables or drop some predictor variables to remove the correlated predictors and form the necessary model. Alternatively, one may do the principal component regression. The significant number of principal components will be computed for the predictor variables and the response variable will be modeled using the principal components as the predictors. For the data given in Section 5.3, by using PROC REG with the option VIF produces the variance inflation factors and the modification to the programming line and output is as follows:

```
proc reg;model y = x1 x2/vif;run;
```

```
                        ***
                Parameter Estimates
        Variable ***                Variance Inflation
        Intercept                            0
        x1                                1.38276
        x2                                1.38276
```

In our problem the variance inflation factor for each of X_1 and X_2 is 1.38 which is less than 10, and we conclude that there is no multicollinearity in our data.

5.3.2 Dummy Variables

Sometimes a predictor variable may be a categorical variable with several levels. For example, three brands of a car tire, four different treatments, five different computer brands, and so on. For the categorical predictor variable, the change in response between adjacent levels may not be the same. In such cases we need to introduce dummy variables to account for the difference in the responses between the categorical levels of the predictor variables. If the categorical variable has k levels (0, 1, 2, ..., $k-1$), we use $k-1$ dummy variables. The $k-1$ dummy variables are denoted by Z_1, Z_2, ..., Z_{k-1}, where the dummy variable Z_i is given the value 1 for the ith categorical level of the predictor and 0s for other values, $i = 1, 2, ..., k-1$. Note that the 0 level of the categorical variable is given "0" value for each of Z_1, Z_2, ..., Z_{k-1}. The significance of the difference between the ith level and the 0th level of the categorical variable is concluded by testing the significance of the coefficient Z_i. The significance between the categorical levels i and j of the predictor variables is determined by testing the difference of the regression coefficients of Z_i and Z_j, $i \neq j = 1, 2, ..., k-1$.

Let us return to our example of repairing the roof and let us consider an extra predictor variable of the house type, such as ranch, colonial, and split level. This extra information was provided in Table 5.3 and two dummy variables Z_1, Z_2 are introduced.

The two dummy variables Z_1 and Z_2 represent the house types: "Ranch," "split," and "colonial." Ranch is denoted by $Z_1 = 1$, $Z_2 = 0$; Split is denoted by $Z_1 = 0$, $Z_2 = 1$; Colonial is denoted by $Z_1 = 0$, $Z_2 = 0$. The following program similar to the one given earlier with four predictor variables, X_1, X_2, Z_1, Z_2, provides the necessary output to compare the roof cost with the house types.

```
data a1;
/***input data***/
input x1 x2 x3$ y @@; cards;
3 1500 Colonial 10000 1 1400 Ranch 10000 4 2000 Split 15000 7
1200 Split 8000 5 800 Split 7000 6 900 Colonial 7000 11 1000
Ranch 8000 3 1300 Ranch 9000 8 1700 Colonial 9000 10 700 Split
5000 7 1700 Ranch 9000 2 1600 Colonial 8500 9 800 Split 7000
12 900 Colonial 6000
;
/***end of input data***/
data a2;set a1; if X3 = 'Ranch' then Z1 = 1;
else Z1 = 0; if X3 = 'Split' then Z2 = 1;
else Z2 = 0; proc glm; model y = x1 x2 z1 z2/clparm; run;
```

```
estimate 'Z1 - Z2' z1 1 z2 - 1;
* this statement is used to compare ranch vs split level
  houses; run;
```

                                    ***
       R-Square   Coeff. Var   Root MSE   *y* Mean
       0.807579(d1)   14.78309   1251.283   8464.286
                                    ***

Parameter	Estimate	Std Error	t Value	Pr > |t|	95% Confidence Limits	
	(d2)			(d3)	(d4)	(d5)
Intercept	2387.846096	1918.663471	1.24	0.2447	−1952.472217	6728.164409
x1	−104.234223	118.632621	−0.88	0.4024	−372.599856	164.131410
x2	4.816974	1.022114	4.71	0.0011	2.504791	7.129157
Z1	682.526815	842.509424	0.81	0.4388	−1223.361913	2588.415543
Z2	1443.121726	814.986663	1.77	0.1104	−400.506190	3286.749642

Parameter	Estimate	Std Error	t Value	Pr > |t|	95% Confidence Limits	
	(d6)			(d7)	(d8)	(d9)
Z1 − Z2	−760.594911	869.135412	−0.88	0.4043	−2726.715809	1205.525987

The regression equation for the different types of houses, using the estimates given in column (d2), is

$$\hat{Y} = 2387.85 + (-104.23)X_1 + (4.82)X_2 + 682.53\ Z_1 + (1443.12)\ Z_2.$$

Note that with the four predictor variables X_1, X_2, Z_1, and Z_2, R^2 has increased to 0.8076 given at (d1) from 0.7405 using X_1, X_2 predictors. It may be noted that R^2 increases with additional independent variables. The p-value given in column (d3) for Z_1 is 0.4388 and is not significant. Thus, the ranch and colonial types do not differ in the roof cost. In column (d3), Z_2 has a p-value of 0.1104 and is not significant. Thus, the colonial and split levels have the same cost. The CIs for the parameters are given in columns (d4) and (d5). The estimate for $Z_1 - Z_2$ is given in (d6). In column (d7), the p-value is 0.4043, indicating that the cost is not significant for the ranch and split levels. The confidence limits for the difference in the cost of ranch and split levels are given in columns (d8) and (d9).

This is one way of representing the dummy variables. It may be noted that the dummy variables can be defined in different ways to meet the objectives; refer to Draper and Smith (1981).

For the ranch type putting $Z_1 = 1$ and $Z_2 = 0$, we obtain the estimated ranch roof cost from the regression equation given above:

$$\hat{Y} = 2387.846 + (-104.234)X_1 + (4.817)X_2 + 682.527$$
$$= 3070.37 + (-104.23)X_1 + (4.82)X_2.$$

For split type of housing by setting $Z_1 = 0$ and $Z_2 = 1$, the estimated repair cost is

$$\hat{Y} = 2387.846 + (-104.234)X_1 + (4.817)X_2 + 1443.122$$
$$= 3830.97 + (-104.23)X_1 + (4.82)X_2.$$

The regression equation for the colonial type of house by setting $Z_1 = 0$ and $Z_2 = 0$ is

$$\hat{Y} = 2387.85 + (-104.23)X_1 + (4.82)X_2.$$

The three equations are parallel except that the intercepts are different.

5.3.3 Interaction

Consider two predictor variables X_1 and X_2 and a response variable Y. If we regress Y on X_1 and Y on X_2, separately, the sum of the two regression coefficients indicates the change in the response variable when each of X_1 and X_2 are increased by 1 unit. However, if X_1 and X_2 are considered as predictors to predict Y, the sum of the two regression coefficients may not be equal to the quantity considered earlier. This is because the two variables X_1 and X_2 interact to provide the response Y. This interaction may be positive or negative, when both variables jointly increase or decrease the response. In such cases the model with p predictor variables can be written as

$$Y = \beta_0 + \beta_1 X_1 + \beta_2 X_2 + \cdots + \beta_p X_p + \beta_{12} X_1 X_2 + \beta_{13} X_1 X_3 + \cdots + \beta_{p-1,p} X_{p-1} X_p + \varepsilon.$$

As we defined the two-factor interaction we may have three- or higher-factor interactions. The i factor interactions usually will be less than $i-1$ factor interactions and so on. The programming aspect of this interaction is to indicate the model as follows by placing the necessary main effects and interactions:

```
Proc glm;model Y = X1 X2 X1*X2 X3 X1*X3 X2*X3 X1*X2*X3...
```

It may be noted that the introduction of an interaction term requires the corresponding main effects to be included in the model statement.

5.3.4 Variable Selection

Sometimes there may be several predictors available to predict the response, and one needs to choose either all or some of the predictors, which explain the response variable. If all possible regressions with p predictors are considered, then we will have $2^p - 1$ different models and we may choose the best model of these $2^p - 1$ models. This can be done by using the adjusted R^2 value or Mallow's C_p statistic. The model with the smallest C_p closer to p is recommended (Mallows, 1973), where p is the number of parameters in the model including the intercept. Alternatively, the model with the largest adjusted R^2 value is selected. The adjusted R^2 value may not increase with additional predictor variables like R^2. Since C_p is closely related to adjusted R^2 (Kennard, 1971), we will illustrate the selection process using adjusted R^2. However, the adjusted R^2 option can be changed to the C_p option by using *selection = Cp* instead of *selection = adjrsq* in the program.

Let us consider a graduate-level course, where Y is the final grade for the class, X_1 is the age of the student, X_2 is the gender of the student (1 = female, 0 = male), X_3 is the grade point average (GPA), X_4 is the number of credit hours registered, and X_5 is the midterm grade see the data in Table 5.4.

The following are the programming lines:

```
data a;
/***input data***/
input x1 x2 x3 x4 x5 y @@; cards;
35 1 2 9 50 60 40 1 3 15 85 89 25 1 3 13 69 70
30 0 2.9 12 73 70 42 0 2.7 15 76 80 29 0 3.5 16 80 85
33 1 3 9 59 57 39 1 3.5 12 92 95 45 1 2.8 17 70 79
51 1 3.5 12 73 79 22 0 2.9 15 75 70 49 0 3.7 16 95 99
45 1 3.6 18 80 85 40 1 3.4 10 85 85 35 1 3.2 18 85 77
23 1 2.9 12 59 63 42 1 2.5 15 75 70 27 0 3 15 80 85
;
/***end of input data***/
proc reg; model y = x1 x2 x3 x4 x5 /selection = adjrsq; * the
  adjusted R2 may be replaced by Cp; run;
```

The REG Procedure

Model: MODEL1

Dependent Variable: y

Adjusted R-Square Selection Method

Number of observations read   18

Number of observations used   18

Number in Model	Adjusted R-Square	R-Square	Variables in Model
2	0.8362(e1)	0.8555	x1 x5
3	0.8306	0.8605	x1 x2 x5
3	0.8284	0.8587	x1 x3 x5
3	0.8247	0.8556	x1 x4 x5
4	0.8233	0.8649	x1 x2 x3 x5
4	0.8175	0.8605	x1 x2 x4 x5
4	0.8157	0.8590	x1 x3 x4 x5
1	0.8147	0.8256	x5
5	0.8086	0.8649	x1 x2 x3 x4 x5
2	0.8072	0.8299	x3 x5
2	0.8025	0.8258	x4 x5

2	0.8024	0.8256	x2 x5
3	0.7939	0.8303	x3 x4 x5
3	0.7935	0.8299	x2 x3 x5
3	0.7884	0.8258	x2 x4 x5
4	0.7781	0.8303	x2 x3 x4 x5
4	0.5835	0.6815	x1 x2 x3 x4
3	0.5701	0.6460	x1 x2 x3
3	0.5594	0.6371	x1 x3 x4
2	0.5118	0.5693	x1 x3
2	0.5048	0.5630	x3 x4
3	0.4836	0.5747	x2 x3 x4
1	0.4438	0.4766	x3
2	0.4418	0.5075	x2 x3
3	0.3549	0.4688	x1 x2 x4
2	0.3200	0.4000	x1 x4
2	0.3015	0.3837	x1 x2
1	0.1952	0.2425	x1
1	0.1863	0.2341	x4
2	0.1482	0.2484	x2 x4
1	−0.0014	0.0576	x2

The adjusted R^2 given at (e1) is the largest value with the predictor variables X_1 and X_5 and is 0.8362. Thus, the variables selected to predict Y are X_1 (age) and X_5 (midterm grade).

One can also select the predictors by using

Forward selection or

Backward selection, or

Stepwise selection.

TABLE 5.4

Artificial Data for Final Test Scores

Y	X_1	X_2	X_3	X_4	X_5	Y	X_1	X_2	X_3	X_4	X_5
60	35	1	2.0	9	50	79	51	1	3.5	12	73
89	40	1	3.0	15	85	70	22	0	2.9	15	75
70	25	1	3.0	13	69	99	49	0	3.7	16	95
70	30	0	2.9	12	73	85	45	1	3.6	18	80
80	42	0	2.7	15	76	85	40	1	3.4	10	85
85	29	0	3.5	16	80	77	35	1	3.2	18	85
57	33	1	3.0	9	59	63	23	1	2.9	12	59
95	39	1	3.5	12	92	70	42	1	2.5	15	75
79	45	1	2.8	17	70	85	27	0	3.0	15	80

In forward selection, the variables are included in the model one after another based on a preassigned SLENTRY value of the F statistic. If the SLENTRY value is not specified, the default value is 0.50 in SAS.

In backward selection, all the variables are first included in the model and the variables are deleted based on a preassigned SLSTAY value of the F statistic. If the SLSTAY is not specified, the default value is 0.10.

In the stepwise method, at every step, variables are added and/or deleted based on the preassigned SLENTRY and SLSTAY values of the F statistic. The SLENTRY and SLSTAY default values are both 0.15.

The successful inclusion of all the predictor variables depends on the appropriate choice of SLENTRY and SLSTAY values. The programming lines for a stepwise method are provided below and the output indicates the selected variables for the prediction. We will use the data given in Table 5.4 and we will choose which of the five variables best predict the final test score. The forward and backward selection methods can be used by replacing the stepwise selection in the program.

```
proc reg; model y = x1 x2 x3 x4 x5 /selection = stepwise; run;
```

The REG Procedure
Model: MODEL1

Dependent Variable: y

Number of observations read   18
Number of observations used   18

Stepwise Selection: Step 1
Variable x5 Entered: R-Square = 0.8256 and $C(p)$ = 1.4921

Analysis of Variance

Source	DF	Sum of Squares	Mean Square	F Value	Pr > F
Model	1	1897.27036	1897.27036	75.75	<0.0001
Error	16	400.72964	25.04560		
Corrected total	17	2298.00000			

Variable	Parameter Estimate	Std Error	Type II SS	F Value	Pr > F
Intercept	8.45403	8.03920	27.69708	1.11	0.3086
x5	0.91538	0.10517	1897.27036	75.75	<0.0001

Bounds on condition number: 1, 1

Stepwise Selection: Step 2
Variable x1 Entered: R-Square = 0.8555 and $C(p)$ = 0.8391
Analysis of Variance

Source	DF	Sum of Squares	Mean Square	F Value	Pr > F
Model	2	1965.89444	982.94722	44.40	<.0001
Error	15	332.10556	22.14037		
Corrected total	17	2298.00000			

```
                    The REG Procedure
                     Model: MODEL1
                 Dependent Variable: y
                Stepwise Selection: Step 2
```

Variable	Parameter Estimate	Std Error	Type II SS	F Value	Pr > F
(f1)					
Intercept	4.77986	7.84138	8.22676	0.37	0.5513
x1	0.24387	0.13852	68.62408	3.10	0.0987
x5	0.84714	0.10621	1408.54419	63.62	<0.0001

```
        Bounds on condition number: 1.1536, 4.6145
-----------------------------------------------------------------
```

All variables left in the model are significant at the 0.1500
  level.
No other variable met the 0.1500 significance level for entry
  into the model.

```
                Summary of Stepwise Selection
```

Step	Variable Entered	Variable Removed	Number of Vars In	Partial R-Square	Model R-Square	C(p)	F Value	Pr > F
1	x5		1	0.8256	0.8256	1.4921	75.75	<0.0001
2	x1		2	0.0299	0.8555	0.8391	3.10	0.0987

The model selected using the Stepwise selection from column ($f1$) includes the variables X_1 and X_5. In this example, the variables selected using stepwise and adjusted R^2 selection methods are the same.

5.4 Diagnostics

The assumptions used in building the regression model, such as the normality and constant variance for the error terms, need to be checked. There are several diagnostic methods used in this context. If these assumptions are violated, then the estimates and tests may not be correct.

The residual plots are used to check the normality of the response variable. For this purpose, we create a pp-plot and if the points are nearly on a straight line the response variable is following a normal distribution and if the points are widely spread out, the response variable is not normally distributed. The necessary program to construct the pp-plot and the graph is given below for the data of Table 5.4.

```
data a;
/***input data***/
input x1 x2 x3 x4 x5 y @@; cards;
```

```
35 1 2 9 50 60 40 1 3 15 85 89 25 1 3 13 69 70 30 0 2.9 12 73
70 42 0 2.7 15 76 80 29 0 3.5 16 80 85 33 1 3 9 59 57 39 1 3.5
12 92 95 45 1 2.8 17 70 79
51 1 3.5 12 73 79 22 0 2.9 15 75 70 49 0 3.7 16 95 99 45 1 3.6
18 80 85 40 1 3.4 10 85 85 35 1 3.2 18 85 77 23 1 2.9 12 59 63
42 1 2.5 15 75 70 27 0 3 15 80 85
;
/***end of input data***/
proc reg data = a;model y = x1 x2 x3 x4 x5/noprint;
plot npp.*r./nostat;run;
```

The plot in Figure 5.1 indicates a straight line pattern and hence we assume that the response variable is normally distributed.

Plotting the residuals against the predicted response of the variable will enable us to see whether the equality of the error variances assumption is satisfied. If the points in the graph are horizontal and evenly spread out showing no pattern, then the errors have the same variance. If the residuals increase (decrease) with the increased (decreased) predicted values, the equality of the variances assumption is not satisfied and one should make some transformation on the data or use the weighted least-squares regression method to draw the inferences. If the plot is U or an inverted U shape, then the model needs to be modified and a polynomial regression may be needed. For further details, refer to Draper and Smith (1981) and Weisberg (1985). The data considered earlier are used with the following modification to the program:

```
plot r.*p./nostat;run; .
```

The plot in Figure 5.2 indicates that the residuals are approximately spread out evenly, and hence the equality of the variance assumption is supported.

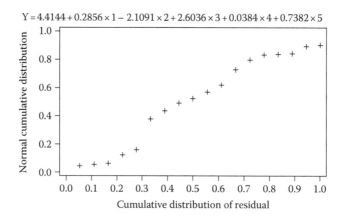

$Y = 4.4144 + 0.2856 \times 1 - 2.1091 \times 2 + 2.6036 \times 3 + 0.0384 \times 4 + 0.7382 \times 5$

FIGURE 5.1
Q–Q plot.

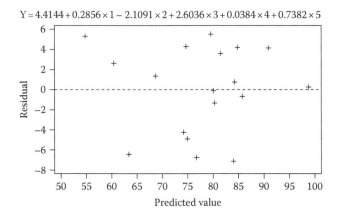

$$Y = 4.4144 + 0.2856 \times 1 - 2.1091 \times 2 + 2.6036 \times 3 + 0.0384 \times 4 + 0.7382 \times 5$$

FIGURE 5.2
Plot of predicted values vs. residuals.

We will now discuss the methods of identifying the outliers, and determining influential observations.

5.4.1 Outliers

The determined model should fit most of the data. However, there are some data points that will not fit the model. These data points are called outliers and are subject to the identified model. Some outliers may affect the regression equation and are influential observations discussed in Section 5.4.2. Large residuals are candidates for being outliers. Once the outliers have been identified, in certain situations, these can be dropped. We will now discuss the studentized residuals, which are residuals divided by their standard errors. To identify the outliers, the following programming line will be used after the model statement discussed earlier.

```
output out = a1 student = std_residual; proc print;run;
```

The output is as follows:

x1	x2	x3	x4	x5	y	std_residual (g1)
35	1	2.0	9	50	60	1.48150
40	1	3.0	15	85	89	0.92752
25	1	3.0	13	69	70	0.29352
30	0	2.9	12	73	70	−1.09517
42	0	2.7	15	76	80	−0.02771
29	0	3.5	16	80	85	0.83021
33	1	3.0	9	59	57	−1.54050
39	1	3.5	12	92	95	1.03605
45	1	2.8	17	70	79	1.01277

51	1	3.5	12	73	79	−0.34681
22	0	2.9	15	75	70	−0.97080
49	0	3.7	16	95	99	0.05625
45	1	3.6	18	80	85	0.18533
40	1	3.4	10	85	85	−0.17614
35	1	3.2	18	85	77	−1.68765
23	1	2.9	12	59	63	0.61539
42	1	2.5	15	75	70	−1.61122
27	0	3.0	15	80	85	1.20718

In the above table, the studentized residuals greater than 2 or less than −2 are usually considered to be outliers and in certain situations may be dropped and inferences can be drawn with fewer observations or one can use robust methods to analyze the data. In our problem, the studentized residuals given in column (g1) are all between −2 to 2 and hence, we have no outliers in the data.

5.4.2 Influential Observations

Influential observations have a high influence on the parameter estimates. The model is assumed to be correct, and the residuals are used to determine the influential observation. The model is fitted with and without the data points and those with large changes in the estimated parameters are called influential data points. Cook's distance is used to determine the influential observations, which with values more than 1 indicate the observations to be influential. The following programming lines give Cook's distance:

```
proc reg; model y = x1 x2 x3 x4 x5;
output out = out cookd = cookd;
data out; set out; proc print; run;
```

The output is

x1	x2	x3	x4	x5	y	cookd
35	1	2.0	9	50	60	0.39083
40	1	3.0	15	85	89	0.04266
25	1	3.0	13	69	70	0.00423
30	0	2.9	12	73	70	0.06066
42	0	2.7	15	76	80	0.00007
29	0	3.5	16	80	85	0.05005
33	1	3.0	9	59	57	0.19044
39	1	3.5	12	92	95	0.12052
45	1	2.8	17	70	79	0.08251
51	1	3.5	12	73	79	0.01530
22	0	2.9	15	75	70	0.06148
49	0	3.7	16	95	99	0.00037
45	1	3.6	18	80	85	0.00389

40	1	3.4	10	85	85	0.00310
35	1	3.2	18	85	77	0.22559
23	1	2.9	12	59	63	0.03095
42	1	2.5	15	75	70	0.20573
27	0	3.0	15	80	85	0.06704

All the values for the Cook's distance given in the last column of the output are less than 1 and hence there is no influential observation.

5.4.3 Durbin–Watson Statistic

When the predicted variable is time, the correlation between residuals that are 1, 2, 3, and so on observations apart is called auto (serial) correlation. This serial correlation can be either positive or negative. One can plot the ith residuals to the $(i - 1)$th residuals to see whether the serial correlation is positive or negative. To check for the serial correlations in a time series data or data obtained in a sequence, the Durbin–Watson test is used.

A fundamental assumption for the residuals is that they are normally and independently distributed with a common variance. If this occurs, the serial correlation is 0. The serial correlation, ρ_0, is between –1 and 1. Thus, to test for the serial correlation 0 against the alternative that the serial correlation is not 0, the Durbin–Watson test is used (Durbin and Watson, 1951). Let us consider the data given in Table 5.4 and assume that the data give the final test scores for the students sitting next to one another. It may be noted that the responses in a sequence are like responses over time. The following programming line will provide the necessary test:

```
proc reg data = a; model y = x1 x2 x3 x4 x5/dwprob;run;
```

```
                    The REG Procedure
                      Model: MODEL1
                  Dependent Variable: y
Durbin–Watson D                              2.327
Pr < DW                                      0.7929 (h1)
Pr > DW                                      0.2071 (h2)
Number of observations                       18
First-order autocorrelation                 −0.255 (h3)
```

Note: Pr < DW is the p-value for testing positive autocorrelation and Pr > DW is the p-value for testing negative autocorrelation.

To test for H_0: $\rho_0 = 0$ against the alterative $\rho_0 < 0$, the p-value given at (h2) is used and in this case it is 0.2071 and is not significant. To test for H_0: $\rho_0 = 0$ against the alterative $\rho_0 > 0$, the p-value given at (h1) of 0.7929 is used and in this case it is not significant. The first-order autocorrelation, the correlation between two adjacent residuals, is given at (h3) and is −0.255. An alternative runs test is available; see Draper and Smith (1981).

5.5 Weighted Regression

So far we used the linear, polynomial, and multiple regressions to estimate the regression parameters using the assumption that the errors are independently distributed with mean 0 and variance σ^2. Situations arise where the variances are not all the same and the observations may be correlated. Usually, different variances with independent errors occur and the weighted regression is considered in this setting only in this book. In this case we give weights, w to the observations, where they are the reciprocals of the variances of the observations. If the response is an average of n observations, the weight, w, given for that response is $w = n$, when the individual observations considered in the mean have the same variance. If there are multiple observations at the same independent variable, the variances of the dependent variable may be taken and w will be the reciprocal of that variance. When the observations have different variances and if ordinary regression is used, the estimated parameters will still be unbiased estimators of the parameters with standard errors, different from the standard errors of the parameters estimated by weighted least squares. However, the standard errors of the parameters obtained from the weighted least squares will usually be smaller than the standard errors of the parameters estimated by ordinary least squares.

Let us consider the data given in Table 5.4 with X_3 as an independent variable and Y as a dependent variable. Let us also assume that for the same X_3, the Ys have different variances. In this case, we need to consider the standard deviation of $\hat{Y}$; as different and regress the mean of Y on the same X_3. Other types of weights as needed may be used in the program.

```
data a1;
/***input data***/
input X3 Y @@; cards;
2 60 3 89 3 70 2.9 70 2.7 80 3.5 85 3 57 3.5 95 2.8 79 3.5 79
2.9 70 3.7 99 3.6 85 3.4 85 3.2 77 2.9 63 2.5 70 3 85
;
/***end of input data***/
data a2; set a1; proc sort; by x3;
proc univariate noprint; var y; by x3; output out = stats n
  = n var = var mean = MEAN; data stats;set stats; WEIGHT = n/
  var;*other weights can be similarly used as needed;
  if weight = . then weight = 1;
keep mean x3 weight; proc glm;model mean = x3/clparm;weight
  weight; run;
```

The GLM Procedure
Dependent Variable: MEAN the mean, Y
Weight: WEIGHT

Source	DF	Sum of Squares	Mean Square	F Value	Pr > F
Model	1	763.8142729	763.8142729	37.91	0.0002 (i1)

```
Error          9     181.3383464    20.1487052
Corrected     10     945.1526193
  total
```

	R-Square	Coeff. Var	Root MSE	Mean
	0.808139	5.671621	4.488731	79.14370

***

Parameter	Estimate	Std Error	t Value	Pr > |t|	95% Confidence Limits	
	(i2)	(i3)	(i4)		(i5)	(i6)
Intercept	26.29362576	8.72484817	3.01	0.0146	6.55664799	46.03060353
X3	17.68488091	2.87231341	6.16	0.0002	11.18725656	24.18250527

The p-value given at (i1) is used to test the null hypothesis that all regression coefficients are 0 against the alternative that at least one regression coefficient is not 0. The values in column (i2) provide the estimated parameters and the values in column (i3) are the standard errors of the estimated parameters. In column (i4) we obtain the p-values to test the significance of the individual regression coefficients. Columns (i5) and (i6) provide 95% CI of the parameters, which is (11.19, 24.18). In our example, the regression coefficient is significant and is 17.68 with a standard error of 2.87.

Had we regressed Y on X_3 using the ordinary least-squares method, the estimate of the regression coefficient would be 18.67 with a standard error of 4.89. Thus, we see that the weighted least-squares estimate has a smaller standard error compared to the ordinary least-squares estimate.

5.6 Logistic Regression

5.6.1 Dichotomous Logistic Regression

Often we come across scenarios where the response variable is dichotomized as having an event (1) or not having an event (0), and we would like to see which of the independent variables are significant in predicting the event. The events such as death (1) or no death (0) for subjects with a given disease within 5 years after the onset of the disease are modeled using the independent variables such as treatment, age, cholesterol level, blood pressure, and gender, and determine the significant independent variable in predicting the death. Another example is the passing (1) or failing (0) of a student in a course and we would like to see which of the variables such as age, number of hours worked, gender, and so on are significant in predicting whether the student will pass or fail. By using the linear regression model when the response is dichotomized, the estimated response variables are not necessarily bounded between 0 and 1. Let Y_i be the response variable and $X_{1i}, X_{2i}, ..., X_{ki}$ are the independent variables on the ith subject. Estimation of the probability of getting the event for given X_1, X_2, ... X_k values is achieved by the logistic regression method. We assume

$$\Pr(Y = 1) = p = \exp(\beta_0 + \beta_1 X_1 + \cdots + \beta_k X_k)/(1 + \exp(\beta_0 + \beta_1 X_1 + \cdots + \beta_k X_k))$$

and consider the log of the odds ratio $\{p/(1 - p)\}$

$$\ln (p/(1 - p)) = \beta_0 + \beta_1 X_1 + \cdots + \beta_k X_k,$$

where β_0, β_1, ..., β_k are unknown parameters. The parameters are estimated using the maximum likelihood method. Diagnostics and goodness of fit for this model are not included here, and the interested reader may refer to Allison (1999). Let us consider the data given in Table 5.4 of Section 5.3.4 and assume that students with a final test score of at least 80 are considered as having passed and those with a final test score of less than 80, as having failed. Let us consider the independent variables X_1, X_2, and X_3 to estimate the probability of the student passing the course.

Entering the response variable as 1 for pass and 0 for fail and using the same X_1, X_2, and X_3 variables, the following programming lines provide the necessary output.

```
data a;
/***input data***/
input X1 X2 X3 Y @@; cards;
35 1 2 60 40 1 3 89 25 1 3 70 30 0 2.9 70
42 0 2.7 80 29 0 3.5 85 33 1 3 57
39 1 3.5 95 45 1 2.8 79 51 1 3.5 79 22 0 2.9 70 49 0 3.7 99
45 1 3.6 85 40 1 3.4 85 35 1 3.2 77
23 1 2.9 63 42 1 2.5 70 27 0 3 85
;
/***end of input data***/
data a1;set a; if Y >= 80 then YNEW = 1; else YNEW = 0;
proc logistic descending;* The descending option predicts the
  probability that the dependent variable is equal to the
  highest value, one, in the dichotomous case; model ynew = x1
  x2 x3 /lackfit rsq clparm = wald; run;
```

The output is as follows:

$$\star\star\star$$

Probability modeled is ynew = 1.

Model Convergence Status

Convergence criterion (GCONV = 1E-8) satisfied.

$\star\star\star$

| R-Square | 0.4025 (j5) | Max-rescaled | R-Square | 0.5388 (j6) |

Testing Global Null Hypothesis: BETA = 0

Test	Chi-Square	DF	Pr > ChiSq
Likelihood ratio	9.2686	3	0.0259 (j2)
Score	6.8924	3	0.0754 (j3)
Wald	4.1545	3	0.2453 (j4)

The LOGISTIC Procedure

Analysis of Maximum Likelihood Estimates

Parameter	DF	Estimate (j11)	Std Error	Wald Chi-Square	Pr > ChiSq (j12)
Intercept	1	−14.4899	7.6783	3.5613	0.0591
x1	1	0.0966	0.0961	1.0103	0.3148
x2	1	−2.7181	1.6916	2.5818	0.1081
x3	1	4.0512	2.4471	2.7407	0.0978

Odds Ratio Estimates

Effect	Point Estimate (j15)	95% Confidence (j16)	Wald Limits (j17)
x1	1.101	0.912	1.330
x2	0.066	0.002	1.817
x3	57.467	0.475	>999.999

Association of Predicted Probabilities and Observed Responses

Percent concordant	88.8	Somers' D	0.775 (j7)
Percent discordant	11.3	Gamma	0.775 (j8)
Percent tied	0.0	Tau-a	0.405 (j9)
Pairs	80	c	0.888 (j10)

Wald's CI for Parameters

Parameter	Estimate	95% Confidence (j13)	Limits (j14)
Intercept	−14.4899	−29.5391	0.5592
x1	0.0966	−0.0918	0.2850
x2	−2.7181	−6.0336	0.5974
x3	4.0512	−0.7450	8.8475

***

Hosmer and Lemeshow goodness-of-fit test

Chi-Square	DF	Pr > ChiSq
7.4061	7	0.3879 (j1)

The Hosmer and Lemeshow (2000) goodness-of-fit test is used to test the lack of fit for the model with binary data. The p-value for the lack of fit is given at (j1) and if this p-value is >0.05 the fit is good and if it is ≤0.05, the fit is not satisfactory. In our problem, this p-value is 0.3879 and the fit is good.

The global null hypothesis that all the regression coefficients β_i for $i = 1$, 2, ..., k are zero against the alternative that at least one of these coefficients is nonzero is tested by using the likelihood ratio test, Score test, or Wald test. For large sample sizes the three tests are asymptotically equivalent and for small sample sizes the likelihood ratio test is recommended. The p-value for the global null hypothesis for these three tests is given in (j2), (j3), and (j4). If the p-values are >0.05, the global null hypothesis is not rejected and if the p-values are ≤0.05 at least one of the β_is, $i = 1, 2, ..., k$ is not zero. In this problem, the p-value for the likelihood ratio test is 0.0259, the Score test is 0.0754, and the Wald test is 0.2453. Thus, the global null hypothesis is retained by Wald and Score tests and is rejected by the likelihood ratio test.

The R^2 given at (j5) is not suitable to study the relationship between the indicator variables and the response variable as in the linear regression. Its upper bound is <1 and R^2 is rescaled (R^2 divided by its upper bound) to give the value (j6), which is an appropriate measure to see the strength of the independent variables in predicting dependent variables. For further details on the maximum rescaled R^2, refer to Nagelkerke (1991). The maximum rescaled R^2 in our problem is 0.5388 and does not indicate great strength of prediction of Y by the X_1, X_2, and X_3 variables.

The measures of association between the predicted probabilities and the observed responses by different statistics are given at (j7), (j8), (j9), and (j10). These measures are between 0 and 1, where the larger value indicates great strength of the independent variables in predicting the response. The c statistic 0.888, given in (j10) shows great strength of the independent variables in predicting the dichotomous response.

The maximum likelihood estimates of all the regression coefficients are given in column (j11), the p-values for testing each of these coefficients is given in column (j12), and the 95% confidence limits of the parameters are given in columns (j13) and (j14). The individual estimates have no practical interpretation and only the p-values indicate whether those coefficients are not zero. In our problem, none of these coefficients are significant.

The meaningful quantity for interpretation is the odds ratios and their point estimates are given in column (j15) with their 95% confidence limits given in columns [(j16), (j17)]. In our problem, this odds ratio for the variable X_1 is 1.101. When the odds ratio is more (less) than 1, then the odds of obtaining the final test score of at least 80 increase (decrease) for each year of increasing age.

In the problem, the odds of obtaining at least 80 points in the final test score increases with increasing age and GPA. The odds of obtaining at least 80 points in the final test are smaller for females than males as this odds ratio is less than 1.

5.6.2 Multinomial Logistic Model

Sometimes the categorical response variable may have more than two unordered classes. If the categories of the response variables are ordered, we have to use the cumulative logistic model, as discussed in Section 5.6.3. In the unordered case, we model this using the multinomial logistic regression. Let us assume that there are k categories for the response variable denoted by 1, 2, ..., k. Let p_i be the probability of the response belonging to the ith category. Let the independent variables in the prediction be $X_1, X_2, ..., X_k$. We assume

$$p_i = \frac{\exp(\beta_0 + \beta_{i1}X_1 + \beta_{i2}X_2 + \cdots + \beta_{ik}X_k)}{1 + \exp(\beta_0 + \beta_{i1}X_1 + \beta_{i2}X_2 + \cdots + \beta_{ik}X_k)}.$$

The independent variables may be continuous or categorical. Instead of estimating one set of parameters as in the dichotomous case, we estimate more than one set of parameters for the multinomial logit model. While using the PROC CATMOD it is essential that the continuous variables be denoted by the DIRECT statement.

Let us consider the situation where three candidates (1 = Democart, 2 = Republican, and 3 = Independent) are contesting for presidentship. The response of the voters to vote for a candidate may be dependent on gender (1 = female, 0 = male), ethnicity (1 = White, 2 = African American, 3 = Hispanic, 4 = Others), age, and education level (1 = high school, 2 = undergraduate, 3 = graduate or professional). Table 5.5 gives artificial data on the voting preferences of different voters.

The following program provides the output to interpret the role of the explanatory variables in predicting the voting preference of different voters:

```
data a;
input y x1 x2 x3 x4 @@;
cards;
1 1 3 41 3 1 1 4 25 2 1 1 4 56 3 1 1 3 45 3 1 1 4 35 2 1 1 4 21 3
1 0 2 54 1 1 0 2 49 3 1 1 4 34 3 1 1 1 47 2 1 1 3 23 3 1 1 3 67 3
2 0 4 45 1 2 1 4 30 1 2 0 1 28 1 2 0 2 34 1 2 0 2 49 3 2 0 4 44 2
2 0 3 37 1 2 0 3 53 1 2 1 3 62 1 3 0 4 65 3 3 0 1 55 2 3 0 1 37 1
3 0 2 51 1 3 0 2 41 1 3 0 4 39 3 3 0 4 27 2 3 0 3 29 1 3 1 3 57 2
2 1 2 71 1 2 0 2 80 1 2 0 4 42 1 2 0 2 78 1 2 0 2 76 1 2 0 4 51 1
2 0 2 36 1 2 0 2 46 1 2 0 4 43 1 2 0 2 48 1
;
proc catmod; direct x3; model y = x1 x2 x3 x4; run;
```

Maximum Likelihood Analysis
Maximum likelihood computations converged.

```
                    Maximum Likelihood ANOVA
          Source                    DF    Chi-Square   Pr > ChiSq
                                                         (k1)
          Intercept                  2       1.40       0.4959
          x1                         2       6.82       0.0330
          x2                         6       4.79       0.5709
          x3                         2       1.46       0.4812
          x4                         4      10.42       0.0339

          Likelihood ratio          62      39.22       0.9895
```

```
              Analysis of Maximum Likelihood Estimates
Parameter              Function  Estimate    Std    Chi-Square Pr > ChiSq
                        Number              Error
(k2)                     (k3)                                    (k4)
Intercept                 1        2.3423   3.1178     0.56      0.4525
                          2       -1.3405   2.2321     0.36      0.5481
x1            0           1       -3.0306   1.1973     6.41      0.0114
              0           2       -0.9100   0.9735     0.87      0.3499
x2            1           1        0.2794   2.0842     0.02      0.8934
              1           2       -0.9789   1.1516     0.72      0.3953
              2           1        2.2290   1.5528     2.06      0.1511
              2           2        0.3239   0.9226     0.12      0.7255
              3           1       -2.0834   1.6547     1.59      0.2080
              3           2       -0.7346   0.9679     0.58      0.4478
x3                        1       -0.0475   0.0662     0.51      0.4731
                          2        0.0272   0.0416     0.43      0.5139
x4            1           1       -0.8027   1.2324     0.42      0.5148
              1           2        2.2685   0.9962     5.19      0.0228
              2           1       -0.8142   1.2984     0.39      0.5306
              2           2       -1.1612   1.0590     1.20      0.2728
```

In the maximum likelihood ANOVA of the output, column (k1) gives the *p*-values for the global test of the inclusion of all the levels of the explanatory variable in predicting the outcome, adjusting for the other variables. We have here two *p*-values that are <0.05 corresponding to the variables gender and education level, which implies that gender and education level are significant in predicting the preference of the candidate and the explanatory variables, age and race, are not significant in the prediction.

In the analysis of maximum likelihood estimates, the parameters shown in column (k2) refer to the independent variables. The coding of these parameters is a contrast of the level of interest with the highest coded level of the independent variable. The function number shown in (k3) is a contrast of the level of the dependent variable against the highest coded level of the dependent variable. Note that a categorical variable of k classes is represented by k–1 functions. In column (k4), we obtain the *p*-values of the significance of the

TABLE 5.5

Artificial Data for Candidates Running for President

Y Party	X₁ Gender	X₂ Ethnicity	X₃ Age	X₄ Education Level
1	1	3	41	3
1	1	4	25	2
1	1	4	56	3
1	1	3	45	3
1	1	4	35	2
1	1	4	21	3
1	0	2	54	1
1	0	2	49	3
1	1	4	34	3
1	1	1	47	2
1	1	3	23	3
1	1	3	67	3
2	0	4	45	1
2	1	4	30	1
2	0	1	28	1
2	0	2	34	1
2	0	2	49	3
2	0	4	44	2
2	0	4	37	1
2	0	3	53	1
2	1	3	62	1
2	1	2	71	1
2	0	2	80	1
2	0	4	42	1
2	0	2	78	1
2	0	2	76	1
2	0	4	51	1
2	0	2	36	1
2	0	2	46	1
2	0	4	43	1
2	0	2	48	1
3	0	4	65	3
3	0	1	55	2
3	0	1	37	1
3	0	2	51	1
3	0	2	41	1
3	0	4	39	3
3	0	4	27	2
3	0	3	29	1
3	1	3	57	2

level given in column (k2) of the explanatory variable in the prediction of the level indicated in column (k3). Consider the *p*-value of 0.0114 shown in column (k4) in the line of (k2) = 0 and (k3) = 1 for the parameter X_1. This *p*-value indicates that for $X_1 = 0$ (males versus females) is significant in predicting the voting pattern for Democrats versus Independents. Note that the highest coded level of the dependent variable Y is that the candidate is Independent and the function number 1 is that the candidate is Democrat. Consider the *p*-value of 0.0228 given in column (k4) in the line of (k2) = 1 and (k3) = 2 for the parameter X_4. This *p*-value indicates that for $X_4 = 1$ (high school education versus graduate or professional education) is significant in predicting the voting pattern for Republican and Independents. Consider the *p*-value of 0.4478 given in column (k4) in the line of (k2) = 3 and (k3) = 2 for the parameter X_2. This *p*-value indicates that for $X_2 = 3$ (Hispanic versus Others) is not significant in predicting the voting pattern of Republicans and Independents.

5.6.3 Cumulative Logistic Model

When the response is an ordered categorical variable, the *cumulative logistic model* (McCullagh, 1980) is used to explain the role of the explanatory variables. One should note that a large sample size will be needed to consider this model. One can use any number of categories for this model; however, it should be noted that with increased number of categories ordinary least squares is a better alternative procedure.

Suppose a loan officer categorizes his clients into three categories of the dependent variable Y: low risk = 1, moderate risk = 2, or high risk = 3. The explanatory variables for classifying the risk are annual income, X_1: (1 = low income, 2 = medium income, 3 = high income), and credit scores, X_2: (1 =< 500, 2 = [500 to 650], 3 = >650). The frequency of the number of clients falling into these categories along with their explanatory variables is given in Table 5.6.

We can dichotomize the response variable by combining the classes of response. By doing this we obtain different regression coefficients for the explanatory variables. For three levels of response, two logit models are

TABLE 5.6

Artificial Data on the Client's Risk Level

	Low Risk			Moderate Risk			High Risk		
	Credit Scores Category			Credit Scores Category			Credit Scores Category		
	1	2	3	1	2	3	1	2	3
Low income	20	20	20	20	23	10	50	25	33
Average income	20	20	20	23	34	24	56	12	15
High income	20	20	65	15	35	40	32	35	40

computed as the log odds of low risk versus moderate and high risk; low and moderate risk versus high risk. Both the odds focus on more to less favorable response. To avoid this situation, the cumulative logistic model is used. This gives k–1 intercept parameters for k classes of response variables and 1 regression coefficient for each explanatory variable. The regression coefficients reasonably explain the role of the explanatory variables. One can use dummy variables for the levels of the explanatory variable if the responses are not equally spread out over the levels. For simplicity of illustration, we will not use dummy variables in this example. The programming lines corresponding to the dichotomous logistic regression provide the cumulative logistic model when the categorical response variable has more than two classes; see below:

```
data a;
input y x1 x2 freq@@;cards;
1 1 1 20 1 1 2 20 1 1 3 20 1 2 1 20 1 2 2 20 1 2 3 20 1 3 1 20
  1 3 2 20
1 3 3 65 2 1 1 20 2 1 2 23 2 1 3 10 2 2 1 23 2 2 2 34 2 2 3 24
  2 3 1 15
2 3 2 35 2 3 3 40 3 1 1 50 3 1 2 25 3 1 3 33 3 2 1 56 3 2 2 12
  3 2 3 15
3 3 1 32 3 3 2 35 3 3 3 40
;
proc logistic descending;
freq freq; model y=x1 x2; run;
```

***

Model Convergence Status
Convergence criterion (GCONV = 1E-8) satisfied.
Score Test for the Proportional Odds Assumption

Chi-Square	DF	Pr > ChiSq
1.1604	2	0.5598 (11)

***

The LOGISTIC Procedure
Testing Global Null Hypothesis: BETA = 0

Test	Chi-Square	DF	Pr > ChiSq
Likelihood ratio	30.7138	2	<0.0001 (12)
Score	29.5551	2	<0.0001 (13)
Wald	30.7362	2	<0.0001 (14)

Analysis of Maximum Likelihood Estimates

Parameter	DF	Estimate	Std Error	Wald Chi-Square	Pr > ChiSq
Intercept 3	1	0.7246	0.2310	9.8404	0.0017 (17)
Intercept 2	1	2.0188	0.2417	69.7445	<0.0001 (18)
x1	1	−0.1626	0.0838	3.7690	0.0522 (15)
x2	1	−0.3980	0.0838	22.5825	<0.0001 (16)

```
                        Odds Ratio Estimates
    Effect      Point Estimate      95% Wald Confidence    Limits
                    (l9)                    (l10)           (l11)
    x1              0.850                   0.721           1.002
    x2              0.672                   0.570           0.791
                                 ****
```

By retaining the *proportional odds assumption*, the cumulative logistic model can be used to interpret the data. In this case, the regression lines for cumulative logits are parallel for each dependent variable category and they differ only by the intercept parameter. The *p*-value of the Score test for the proportional odds assumption is 0.5598 given at (l1) and hence the proportional odds assumption is not rejected. This tests whether the parameters are all the same versus whether they are different for the groups of dependent variables. If this null hypothesis is rejected, then one needs to use generalized logits (Stokes et al., 1995), or other models. The global hypothesis test is used to test the null hypothesis that all regression coefficients of the explanatory variables are zero against the alternative that at least one regression coefficient is not zero. We can use any of the *p*-values of the three tests (l2), (l3), or (l4), to test the global hypotheses of all the regression coefficients being 0. In our problem, all these tests indicate rejection of the null hypothesis that all regression coefficients are 0. The individual significance of the parameters can be observed by looking at the *p*-values (l5) and (l6). The *p*-value for X_2 is significant, while the *p*-value for the X_1 variable is a borderline case and is not significant. The *i*th intercept corresponds to the *i*th or higher category of the response versus the categories less than *i* (because of the DESCENDING option in PROC LOGISTIC), and the *p*-value corresponding to the intercept *i* can be used to test its significance. In our problem, the *p*-value corresponding to (l8) is significant indicating that the intercept term corresponding to the second and third categories versus the first category is significant. Similarly, the *p*-value (l7) is also significant showing that the intercept corresponding to the third category versus the first and second category is significant. The odds ratio estimates given in column (l9) indicate the odds of classifying the response in a higher category against the lower category, in whichever way we dichotomize the ordered response variable. The CIs for the odds ratio estimates are given in columns (l10) and (l11). For example, the value 0.850 in column (l9) against X_1, indicates that with increased income level, the odds of the individual belonging to the higher category decrease.

5.7 Poisson Regression

The *Poisson regression* model is used when the response variable takes nonnegative integer values corresponding to some rare events. Examples of this

TABLE 5.7

Artificial Data of the Number of Grass Cuttings in a Month

Number of Cuttings	Fertilizer	Rainfall	Time Interval (Months)	Number of Cuttings	Fertilizer	Rainfall	Time Interval (Months)
3	0	3	1	8	1	6	2
6	1	1	3	5	0	4	2
6	0	4	5	4	1	3	4
3	0	0.1	7	3	1	4	5
8	1	5	5	5	1	5	6

include the number of grass cuttings in a month, the number of times one catches a cold during the winter months, and so on. In some cases, the response variable data may be collected during different time intervals. In that case we need to get the number of events for a specified time interval and the appropriate adjustments need to be made in the program.

Let us consider the number of grass cuttings in a month at 10 different cities in a country. The explanatory variables in this case are the average rainfall (in inches) in a month and whether fertilizer (treatment) is used (0 = no, 1 = yes). The data are given in Table 5.7.

First we will not consider the time interval for the cuttings and assume that all the cuttings are for a one-month period. The following programming lines provide the necessary output. In the model statement the Poisson distribution is indicated as *P* because the responses are assumed to follow a Poisson distribution.

```
Data grasscut; input cut treat rainfall @@; Cards;
3 0 3 6 1 1 6 0 4 3 0 .1 8 1 5
8 1 6 5 0 4 4 1 3 3 1 4 5 1 5
;
proc genmod; model cut = treat rainfall/dist = p;run;
```

```
            Criteria for Assessing Goodness of Fit
   Criterion                  DF           Value        Value/DF
   Deviance                 7 (m2)       4.1053 (m1)     0.5865
   Scaled deviance            7          4.1053          0.5865
   Pearson chi-square         7          3.9739          0.5677
   Scaled Pearson X2          7          3.9739          0.5677
   Log likelihood                       33.2466

                    Algorithm converged.
             Analysis of Parameter Estimates
 Parameter  DF Estimate   Std       Wald 95%       Chi-  Pr > ChiSq
                          Error    Confidence     Square
                                     Limits
               (m3)                (m4)   (m5)                (m6)
 Intercept  1   1.1420   0.3713   0.4143 1.8696   9.46    0.0021
```

treat	1	0.1581	0.3187	−0.4665	0.7828	0.25	0.6198
rainfall	1	0.1051	0.0930	−0.0773	0.2874	1.28	0.2587
Scale	0	1.0000	0.0000	1.0000	1.0000		

Note: The scale parameter was held fixed.

If the deviance value/df is close to 1, then the model fits the data. If it is much greater than 1 then overdispersion is indicated. However, one may use the following programming lines to obtain the p-values to test the goodness of fit using the deviance.

```
data a; deviance = 4.1053; *given in (m1); df = 7; *given in (m2);
pvalue = 1 − probchi(deviance,df); keep pvalue; proc print;run;
```

```
   Pvalue
   0.76757 (m7)
```

In our problem value/df for deviance does not indicate overdispersion. The p-value for assessing goodness of fit given at (m7) is 0.76757, indicating that the model is a good fit. The estimates of the parameters are given in column (m3) and their lower and upper confidence limits are given in columns (m4) and (m5). By taking $e^{estimate}$, we obtain the odds ratio, where the estimate is given by (m3). The p-value for testing the significance of the parameters is given in column (m6). None of the p-values corresponding to the explanatory variables indicate significance.

Sometimes the data may have larger variation than predicted by the sampling model and in that case we say that the data show overdispersion. Poisson regression is one where overdispersion normally occurs. In the case of Poisson, the mean and variance are the same and the usual analysis does not account for this in the estimates. To correct the situation we need to use the scale option after the model statement. We use scale=d or scale=p depending upon using deviance or the Pearson Chi-Square statistic. The output by this option provides the same estimates of the regression coefficients as before. However, the standard error and the p-value for testing the coefficients may not be the same as before. For further details, refer to Allison (1999).

```
proc genmod; model cut = treat rainfall/dist = p scale = p;run;
```

Algorithm converged.
Analysis Of Parameter Estimates

Parameter	DF	Estimate (m8)	Std Error	Wald 95% Confidence Limits		Chi-Square	Pr > ChiSq (m9)
Intercept	1	1.1420	0.2797	0.5937	1.6902	16.67	<0.0001
treat	1	0.1581	0.2401	−0.3125	0.6288	0.43	0.5102
rainfall	1	0.1051	0.0701	−0.0323	0.2425	2.25	0.1339
Scale	0	0.7535	0.0000	0.7535	0.7535		

Note: The scale parameter was estimated by the square root of Pearson's Chi-Square/DOF.

Note that the values in columns (m3) and (m8) are the same. The values in columns (m6) and (m9) are different because of the change in the standard errors. We can interpret the results in the same way as before.

Considering the time intervals given in Table 5.7, interpret the number of cuttings given in the specified time interval. To consider time for the Poisson model, the model statement in the program has to be modified considering the log of the time interval as an explanatory variable and keep the estimated coefficient of the log of the time interval that we need to *offset*. The following programming lines produce the necessary output.

```
Data grasscut; Input cut treat rainfall time @@; Cards;
3 0 3 1 6 1 1 3 6 0 4 5 3 0 .1 7 8 1 5 5
8 1 6 2 5 0 4 2 4 1 3 4 3 1 4 5 5 1 5 6
;
data grasscut; set grasscut; logtime = log(time);
proc genmod; model cut = treat rainfall/dist = p
  offset = logtime;run;
```

The output can be interpreted as before.

***

```
           Criteria For Assessing Goodness Of Fit
       Criterion              DF     Value    Value/DF
       Deviance               7     16.9714   2.4245
       Scaled deviance        7     16.9714   2.4245
       Pearson chi-square     7     19.9754   2.8536
       Scaled Pearson X2      7     19.9754   2.8536
       Log likelihood               26.8136

                    Algorithm converged.
```

```
                Analysis of Parameter Estimates
                        Std         Wald 95%          Chi-
Parameter DF Estimate  Error  Confidence Limits  Square Pr > ChiSq

Intercept  1  -0.3245 0.3622 -1.0343   0.3854    0.80   0.3703
treat      1  -0.1521 0.3386 -0.8158   0.5116    0.20   0.6532
rainfall   1   0.1846 0.0980 -0.0076   0.3767    3.54   0.0598
Scale      0   1.0000 0.0000  1.0000   1.0000
```

Note: The scale parameter was held fixed.

When the response variable has few very large values, then *Gamma regression* is used and can be programmed similarly by using the following option after the model statement:

```
dist = g link = log.
```

5.8 Robust Regression

In real-life data there may be outliers influencing the parameter estimates. However, discarding these outliers may not be desirable. Sometimes these outliers may be an indication that the data are not normally distributed or the model is inappropriate. In the presence of outliers, *Robust Regression* is used to limit their influence on the estimated parameters.

Depending on the distribution of the errors, by giving different weights to the residuals, the robust estimators (*M*-estimators) as discussed in Section 6.4 are obtained. It should be noted that *M*-estimators are not useful in the presence of influential observations. The SAS Manual provides different weight functions and the default weight function is a *bisquare weight function* defined by

$$
W(x,c) = \begin{cases} \left(1 - \left(\dfrac{x}{c}\right)^2\right)^2 & \text{if } |x| < c, \\ 0 & \text{otherwise.} \end{cases}
$$

Usually different cs in the weight function gives different estimators and a choice of a reasonable c is needed. For further details, refer to Huber (1981).

Consider the data given in Table 5.4. We will now analyze the data by the Robust Regression method. The following program provides the required output with a bisquare weight function as discussed earlier:

```
data a;
/***input data***/
input x1 x2 x3 x4 x5 y @@; cards;
35 1 2 9 50 60 40 1 3 15 85 89 25 1 3 13 69 70 30 0 2.9 12 73
70 42 0 2.7 15 76 80 29 0 3.5 16 80 85 33 1 3 9 59 57 39 1 3.5
12 92 95 45 1 2.8 17 70 79 51 1 3.5 12 73 79 22 0 2.9 15 75 70
49 0 3.7 16 95 99 45 1 3.6 18 80 85 40 1 3.4 10 85 85 35 1 3.2
18 85 77 23 1 2.9 12 59 63 42 1 2.5 15 75 70 27 0 3 15 80 85
;
/***end of input data***/
proc robustreg method = m (wf = bisquare (c = 5.0));* method = m
   indicates M- estimates; model y = x1 x2 x3 x4 x5;test
   x1-x5;;*the test statement can be modified as needed
   depending on which variables one wants to test; run;
```

★★★

Parameter Estimates

Parameter	DF	Estimate	Std Error	95% Confidence Limits		Chi-Square	Pr > ChiSq
		(n1)		(n5)	(n6)		(n4)
Intercept	1	4.2403	10.9162	−17.1552	25.6357	0.15	0.6977
x1	1	0.2812	0.1714	−0.0548	0.6172	2.69	0.1009

```
x2          1  -1.9163   3.0719  -7.9371   4.1045   0.39   0.5327
x3          1   2.5128   4.3535  -6.0199  11.0456   0.33   0.5638
x4          1   0.0607   0.5471  -1.0116   1.1331   0.01   0.9116
x5          1   0.7415   0.1926   0.3641   1.1189  14.83   0.0001
Scale       1   5.8706
```

***

Robust Linear Tests
Test

Test	Test Statistic	Lambda	DF	Chi-Square	Pr > ChiSq
Rho	7.7447	0.8157	5	9.49	0.0909 (n2)
Rn2	69.2531		5	69.25	<0.0001 (n3)

The estimated regression equation by using the M-estimators is

$$\hat{Y} = 4.24 + 0.2812X_1 + (-1.9163)X_2 + 2.5128X_3 + 0.0607X_4 + 0.7415X_5.$$

The coefficients in the above equation are taken from column (n1). To test whether all regression coefficients are 0, we have two methods (the ρ and the R_n^2) and the p-value for both the methods are given in (n2) and (n3). The value in (n3) is significant, whereas the value in (n2) is not significant. It may be noted that the rho test is analogus to the F-test discussed for multiple regression. The significance of each of the regression coefficients can be tested by looking at the p-values given in column (n4). These p-values in column (n4) are obtained for testing each coefficient by the R_n^2 method. Looking at column (n4), the only significant explanatory variable is (X_5). The 95% confidence limits for the parameters are given in columns (n5) and (n6).

The estimates and the 95% CIs are given in Table 5.8 for comparing GLM and robust regression methods.

For these data, the estimates and the CIs are almost the same.

TABLE 5.8

Robust and GLM Estimates

	Robust			GLM		
		95% CI			95% CI	
Parameter	Estimate	Upper	Lower	Estimate	Upper	Lower
Intercept	4.2403	−17.1552	25.6357	4.414405711	−18.17084607	26.999657487
X_1	0.2812	−0.0548	0.6172	0.285550596	−0.069140443	0.640241635
X_2	−1.9163	−7.9371	4.1045	−2.109134262	−8.464730085	4.246461561
X_3	2.5128	−6.0199	11.0456	2.603644079	−6.403620665	11.610908824
X_4	0.0607	−1.0116	1.1331	0.038383421	−1.093605876	1.170372719
X_5	0.7415	0.3641	1.1189	0.738172710	0.339744953	1.136600468

5.9 Nonlinear Regression

Sometimes the dependent variable Y and the independent variable(s) used to predict Y may not have a linear relationship. This is especially true in dose–response curves. The fitting of the nonlinear equation is much harder than the fitting of linear equations. There are many types of nonlinear regression forms that are meaningful in different settings. We will only consider three parameter models with only one independent variable and a four-parameter model with two independent variables. In obtaining the equations it is very important that we specify initial values for the parameters. If the parameters specified do not provide the convergence for the estimates, we may have to modify the initial values to get convergence as the estimation is iterative. One way to give the initial values is to use the values based on previous studies. For more details to find the initial values, refer to Draper and Smith (1981).

Let us consider the following model to fit the data given in Table 5.9:

$$Y = \theta_1 + \theta_2(\theta_3)^{X1} + \varepsilon.$$

The following program gives the necessary estimates of the three-parameter model with one independent variable:

```
data a;
input y x1 @@; cards;
600 .5 675 .5 750 .5 680 1 635 1 655 1
700 1.5 675 1.5 650 1.5 725 2 730 2 685 2
;
proc nlin method = gauss; parms theta1 = 500 theta2 = 100
   theta3 = 1.5;
model y = theta1 + theta2*(theta3**x1); run;
                            ***
```

Note: Convergence criterion met.

```
                            ***
                    Estimation Summary
                        ***
```

Parameter	Estimate (o1)	Approx Std Error	***
theta1	666.5	19.9747	
theta2	0.0139	0.2924	
theta3	58.0844	602.3	

```
                        ***
```

Using the estimates given in column (o1), we have the nonlinear regression equation using the three parameters:

TABLE 5.9

Artificial Data on Dose–Response

Dose (X_1)	Method of Administration (X_2)	Response (AUC) (Y)	Dose (X_1)	Method of Administration (X_2)	Response (AUC) (Y)
0.5	1	600	1.5	1	700
0.5	2	675	1.5	2	675
0.5	3	750	1.5	3	650
1	1	680	2	1	725
1	2	635	2	2	730
1	3	655	2	3	685

Note: X_2 is 1 = oral, 2 = IV, 3 = rectal.

$$\hat{Y} = 666.5 + 0.0139(58.08)^{X_1}$$

For the data given in Table 5.9 we fit a four-parameter model with two independent variables as given below:

$$Y = \theta_1 + \theta_2(1 - e^{(\theta_3 X_1 + \theta_4 X_2)}) + \varepsilon.$$

The following program provides the necessary output:

```
data a; input y x1 x2@@; cards;
600 .5 1 675 .5 2 750 .5 3 680 1 1 635 1 2 655 1 3
700 1.5 1 675 1.5 2 650 1.5 3 725 2 1 730 2 2 685 2 3
;
proc nlin method = gauss; parms theta1 = 600 theta2 = 200
  theta3 =-8 theta4 =-5;
model y = theta1 + theta2* (1 - exp (theta3*x1 + theta4*x2)); run;
                                  ***
```

Note: Convergence criterion met.

```
                               ***
                      The NLIN Procedure
          Parameter        Estimate (o2)        Approx      ***
                                                Std Error
          theta1              664.1             20.8776
          theta2             -0.3772             3.9656
          theta3              2.8357             5.2580
          theta4             -0.4262             0.7047
```

Using the estimates given in column (o2), we have the nonlinear regression equation using four parameters:

$$\hat{Y} = 664.1 + (-0.377)(1 - e^{(2.8 X_1 + (-0.43) X_2)}).$$

For a patient treated with a dose of $X_1 = 1.25$ and $X_2 = 2$, the three-parameter model with one independent variable X_1 estimates Y as

$$\hat{Y} = 666.5 + 0.0139(58.08)^{1.25} = 668.729$$

and with the four-parameter model, using two independent variables X_1 and X_2, the estimate is

$$\hat{Y} = 664.1 + (-0.377)(1 - e^{((2.8)(1.25)+(-0.43)(2))}) = 669.006.$$

Note that the two estimates are close to one another for this data set.

5.10 Piecewise Regression

In some cases throughout the entire domain of the independent variable we may not get one regression equation to predict Y. It is possible that the predicted equation of Y may be different over the domain of the X values. For example, consider (X) as the number of hours a student studies for a test and (Y) as the test score for the course. It is obvious that with the initial increase in the X values, the Y values may increase at a faster rate and finally it may taper off as X is increased further. In Table 5.10, the artificial data are given for the number of hours studied and the test score.

The investigator believes that the change in the regression equations occurs at about 7.5 h, after studying for the test. The regression equation is expected to be quadratic up to $X < 7.5$ and will be linear for $X \geq 7.5$. The necessary program for the equation is given below:

TABLE 5.10

Artificial Data on the Number of
Hours Studied and the Test Score

X	Y	X	Y
2	45	7	90
3	55	8	92
4	60	9	95
5	80	10	97
6	85		

```
data a; input x y @@; cards;
2 45 3 55 4 60 5 80 6 85 7 90 8 92 9 95 10 97
;
data a1; set a; x1 = (x < 7.5)*x; x2 = (x < 7.5)*(x*x);
  x3 = (x >= 7.5)*x;
```

```
proc glm; model y = x1 x2 x3;run;
                              ***
```

```
                    The GLM Procedure
                  Dependent Variable: y
Source       DF Sum of Squares Mean Square   F Value    Pr > F
Model         3   2865.981650   955.327217    40.47  0.0006 (p2)
Error         5    118.018350    23.603670
Corrected     8   2984.000000
  total
```

```
      R-Square          Coeff. Var    Root MSE      y Mean
      0.960450 (p1)       6.255400    4.858361     77.66667
```

```
    Parameter      Estimate     Std Error   t Value  Pr > |t|
                    (p4)                               (p3)
    Intercept    28.40145120   13.41305261    2.12    0.0878
    x1            8.83508184    6.58102490    1.34    0.2372
    x2            0.05119341    0.72862574    0.07    0.9467
    x3            7.32310538    1.51040966    4.85    0.0047
```

We note that the R^2 value of 96.0% given at (p1) is high and the model fits the data very well. This is also supported by the p-value of 0.0006 given at (p2) for testing the global hypothesis that all regression coefficients are zero. Column (p3) gives the p-values for testing the parameters, and the p-value corresponding to the linear component for $X \geq 7.5$ is significant. Using the estimates given in column (p4) we obtain the predicted score

$$\hat{Y} = 28.40 + 8.84X + 0.05X^2, \quad \text{if } X < 7.5$$
$$= 28.40 + 7.32X, \quad \text{if } X \geq 7.5.$$

If one wants the linear component to be the same for $X < 7.5$ and $X \geq 7.5$, this could have been attained by placing $X_1 = X$, $X_2 = (X < 7.5)*(X*X)$ and the

$$\text{model } Y = X_1 \, X_2$$

in the programming lines.

In the piecewise exponential model described in Allison (1995), the time-scale is divided into intervals, where in each interval the hazard is considered to be constant, but the hazards vary across the intervals. The necessary programming details are provided in his book *Survival Analysis Using the SAS System: A Practical Guide*.

5.11 Accelerated Failure Time (AFT) Model

Three commonly used SAS procedures are PROC LIFETEST, PROC LIFEREG, and PROC PHREG for analyzing censored survival data. In Section 4.7, we used PROC LIFETEST to construct the KM survival function and to compare two or more survival curves. In LIFETEST we cannot obtain any parameter estimates. PROC LIFEREG and PROC PHREG are used to estimate the hazard function and the regression coefficients attached to the covariates in the hazard function. PROC LIFEREG is not usable to deal with time-dependent covariates. It provides the estimates of the regression parameters for the covariates in the survival function. We need to specify the error distribution to derive the estimates by using LIFEREG. PROC PHREG provides the survival function with regression coefficients in a broad generality. It also allows the estimation of regression coefficients for time-dependent covariates. The PROC PHREG procedure is less restrictive than the PROC LIFEREG procedure. In this section we will discuss the PROC LIFEREG procedure used for the AFT model and will discuss the PROC PHREG procedure in Section 5.12, which is used for the proportional hazards model.

In the presence of the censored data (see Chapter 4), two popular models used are the AFT model and the Cox proportional hazards model. In the AFT model, the relationship of the survival functions for two individuals i and j, is assumed to be

$$S_i(t) = S_j(\phi_{ij}t), \quad \text{for all } t,$$

where ϕ_{ij} is a constant that is specific to the pair (i, j).

The response variable is assumed to be a linear combination of the covariates $X_1, X_2, \ldots, X_k$ and a random disturbance term. The model takes the form

$$Y_i = \log (T_i) = \beta_0 + \beta_1 X_{i1} + \cdots + \beta_k X_{ik} + \sigma\varepsilon,$$

where the response variable is the log of the failure times, σ is an unknown *scale parameter*, and ε is a random error from a distribution that may depend on additional *shape parameters*. Usually, the variance of ε is taken to be 1. The distributions of ε are usually extreme value distributions with 1 or 2 parameters such as log-gamma, logistic, or normal. Consequently, the distributions of T_i are exponential, Weibull, gamma, log-logistic, or log-normal. One of the AFT models is lognormal because the T has a lognormal distribution when $\log(T)$ has a normal distribution.

Let us consider the time for relief of the headache after taking one of the two medications. If there is no relief of the headache within 2 h, we consider that observation to be censored. Let us consider gender and age to be the covariates for the headache relief.

The data are given in Table 5.11.

The following program provides estimates using the exponential model for the distribution of the time variable, followed by the output:

```
data a;
input drug headache time gender age@@;
cards;
```

```
1 1 3 1 35 1 1 6 1 45 1 1 8 1 55 1 1 4 1 36 1 1 1 0 43 1 1 8 0
67 1 1 5 0 56 1 1 3 0 67 1 0 5 1 25 1 0 1 0 34 1 0 5 1 44 1 0
1 0 26 1 0 3 1 51 1 0 7 0 43 1 0 2 1 25 1 0 2 0 35 0 1 1 1 34
0 1 6 1 35 0 1 4 1 50 0 1 4 1 36 0 1 4 0 41 0 1 6 1 61 0 1 5 0
51 0 1 1 0 71 0 0 5 1 50 1 0 2 0 49 0 0 5 1 44 0 1 1 0 50 0 1
3 1 76 0 0 7 1 73 0 1 5 1 65 0 1 4 0 55 0 0 4 1 87 0 0 3 1 77
0 0 1 1 34 0 1 4 0 27
;
data a1;set a;
if time > 2 and headache = 1 then do; time = 2;headache = 0; end;
if time > 2 and headache = 0 then time = 2;
proc lifereg; model time*headache(0) = drug age gender/
   dist = exponential;
run;
```

***
Algorithm converged.
***

Analysis of Parameter Estimates

Parameter	DF	Estimate	Std Error	95% Confidence Limits		Chi-Square	Pr > ChiSq
		(q3)		(q4)	(q5)		(q2)
Intercept	1	1.5802	1.8035	-1.9546	5.1151	0.77	0.3809
drug	1	1.3316	1.1664	-0.9544	3.6177	1.30	0.2536
age	1	-0.0009	0.0349	-0.0693	0.0675	0.00	0.9795
gender	1	1.8090	1.1917	-0.5266	4.1446	2.30	0.1290
Scale	0	1.0000	0.0000	1.0000	1.0000		
Weibull shape	0	1.0000	0.0000	1.0000	1.0000		

Lagrange Multiplier Statistics

Parameter	Chi-Square	Pr > ChiSq
Scale	3.2849	0.0699 (q1)

The exponential model specifies the distribution of T to be exponential and ε has a standard extreme-value distribution with one parameter and constrains $\sigma = 1$. The p-value given at (q1) is used to test the null hypothesis that $\sigma = 1$. If the hypothesis is not rejected, then the hypothesis $\sigma = 1$ is retained and there is a constant hazard over time. If the hypothesis is rejected, then the hazard is not constant with time, and one should consider other distributions for the ε parameter. In our example the null hypothesis is retained indicating that the hazard function is constant over time. In column (q2), the p-values are given for testing each of the parameters to be zero. In our example none of the parameters corresponding to the three variables drug, age, and gender are significant. The estimates given in column (q3) can be used to obtain the hazard ratios. The exponent of the estimate provides the odds ratio. For gender, the estimate given in column (q3) is 1.809 and hence exp(1.809) = 6.104 is the odds

TABLE 5.11

Artificial Data on Relief of Headache

Drug (0 = Placebo, 1 = Active Drug)	Headache (1 = Relief, 0 = No Relief)	Time (h)	Gender (1 = Female, 0 = Male)	Age (Years)
1	1	3	1	35
1	1	6	1	45
1	1	8	1	55
1	1	4	1	36
1	1	1	0	43
1	1	8	0	67
1	1	5	0	56
1	1	3	0	67
1	0	5	1	25
1	0	1	0	34
1	0	5	1	44
1	0	1	0	26
1	0	3	1	51
1	0	7	0	43
1	0	2	1	25
1	0	2	0	35
0	1	1	1	34
0	1	6	1	35
0	1	4	1	50
0	1	4	1	36
0	1	4	0	41
0	1	6	1	61
0	1	5	0	51
0	1	1	0	71
0	0	5	1	50
1	0	2	0	49
0	0	5	1	44
0	1	1	0	50
0	1	3	1	76
0	0	7	1	73
0	1	5	1	65
0	1	4	0	55
0	0	4	1	87
0	0	3	1	77
0	0	1	1	34
0	1	4	0	27

ratio. This implies that the odds of getting relief for females are more than the odds for getting relief for males. The estimated parameter for age is −0.0009 and exp(−.0009) = 0.999 and we infer that with every 1 year increase in age the odds of getting relief are decreased. The CIs for the parameters are given in (q4) and (q5) and the CI for the odds ratio can be obtained from them.

By replacing *dist* = *exponential* with *dist* = *weibull*, we obtain the following output:

***

Analysis of Parameter Estimates

Parameter	DF	Estimate	Std Error	95% Confidence Limits		Chi-Square	Pr > ChiSq
Intercept	1	1.2175	1.1346	−1.0062	3.4413	1.15	0.2832
drug	1	0.8197	0.8088	−0.7655	2.4050	1.03	0.3108
age	1	−0.0011	0.0217	−0.0437	0.0414	0.00	0.9583
gender	1	1.1432	0.8909	−0.6030	2.8894	1.65	0.1994
Scale	1	0.6123 (q6)	0.2882	0.2434	1.5403		
Weibull shape	1	1.6331 (q7)	0.7686	0.6492	4.1078		

We note that the scale parameter σ at (q6) is 0.6123. When $\sigma > 1$, the hazard decreases with time; when $0.5 < \sigma < 1$, the hazard increases at a decreasing rate; when $0 < \sigma < 0.5$, the hazard increases at an increasing rate. It goes through the origin when $\sigma = 0.5$.

If the shape parameter for the Weibull distribution given at (q7) is 1, then the assumption of Weibull distribution is valid. When the estimated shape parameter is zero, the distribution is log normal and when the shape and scale parameters are equal we obtain the gamma distribution; particularly, when both the shape and the scale parameter equals 1, we obtain the exponential distribution. We can make similar interpretations of the p-values and parameter estimates as shown for the exponential distribution. By changing the distribution we can obtain other specified models that are provided in SAS.

Further details on the AFT model are given in Allison (1995).

5.12 Cox Regression

5.12.1 Proportional Hazards Model

The Cox proportional hazards model is widely used in estimating the hazard function for survival data and is semiparametric. This model assumes that the hazards are constant over time between two individuals, implying that the hazards for the two individuals are parallel and is also known as a *proportional hazards model.* Thus, initially if the risk for individual A is twice as likely as individual B, then throughout the latter time points, A's risk will be twice as that of B. The *hazard function* is positive and is modeled as follows:

$$h(t) = h_0(t) \exp(\Sigma \beta_i X_i).$$

If A has the covariate values X_{iA} and B has covariate values X_{iB}, then their hazards will be

$$h_A(t) = h_0(t) \exp(\Sigma \beta_i X_{iA}),$$

$$h_B(t) = h_0(t) \exp(\Sigma \beta_i X_{iB}).$$

The ratio of the hazards is then

$$\frac{h_A(t)}{h_B(t)} = \exp(\Sigma \beta_i (X_{iA} - X_{iB})),$$

and is independent of time implying that the hazards are proportional. The covariates X_is may be categorical or continuous variables, and may even depend on time. We first consider the case where X_is are independent of time and in Section 5.12.4 we consider time-dependent covariates. In the problems discussed in this section, it is necessary to check for the proportional hazards assumption as discussed in Section 5.12.2. Some of the covariates considered are gender, race, and so on, which are not time dependent. The covariates such as height and weight for a child are time dependent.

The baseline hazard function $h_0(t)$ involves t but does not involve X. The *Cox model* reduces to the baseline hazard model when all of the Xs are equal to 0. The $h_0(t)$ has no specified function attached to it and there are parameter coefficients of the covariates. Hence, we have a semiparametric situation in this model. Clearly, the hazard $h(t)$ and the baseline hazard $h_0(t)$ are nonnegative. In some settings the Cox model will almost give similar estimated parameters as the AFT model. Note that the Cox model is more general than the AFT model in estimating the hazard functions.

In the Cox model, the parameters are estimated using the maximum likelihood method considering the hazards excluding the baseline hazard. Since a part of the hazard function is considered in estimating the parameters, the method of estimation used here is known as *partial likelihood*. In this case, we also obtain the hazard ratios of two individuals belonging to different dichotomous categorical covariates, and also differing by 1 unit in case of continuous covariates. The CIs for the hazard ratios are also provided in the computer output. It may be noted that the covariates can be selected by forward, backward, or stepwise methods as discussed in the multiple regression setting.

Consider the laid off time for workers till they are reemployed. Some workers may leave the area and go elsewhere or may get trained for a different kind of employment. These workers are censored for this analysis. The covariates considered are age, gender (1 = Female, 0 = Male), race (1 = White, 2 = African American, 3 = Hispanic, 4 = Other), education (1 = High School, 2 = Undergraduate or technical school, 3 = Other) (Table 5.12).

Since education and race have more than two categorical responses, we use dummy variables as follows:

Education	Race	ed1	ed2	race1	race2	race3
1		0	0			
2		1	0			
3		0	1			
	1			0	0	0
	2			1	0	0
	3			0	1	0
	4			0	0	1

TABLE 5.12

Artificial Data on Time (in days) until Reemployment

Days	Censor	Education	Age	Gender	Race
120	1	2	45	1	3
88	1	3	50	1	2
260	1	3	55	0	3
94	0	2	24	1	2
80	0	2	18	0	4
29	0	3	47	1	4
90	0	2	35	1	3
82	0	3	55	0	4
77	1	3	19	0	3
23	1	2	27	0	1
90	1	3	45	1	4
75	1	2	19	1	1
16	1	1	33	1	1
24	1	2	20	1	4
100	1	2	47	0	3
139	1	1	45	0	3
36	1	2	53	0	1
90	1	3	34	0	4
49	1	1	25	1	1
33	0	2	39	0	1
68	0	2	21	1	2

The following program gives the necessary output:

```
data a;
input censor education days age gender race@@;
datalines;
1 2 120 45 1 3 1 3 88 50 1 2 1 3 260 55 0 3 0 2 94 24 1 2 0 2
80 18 0 4 0 3 29 47 1 4 0 2 90 35 1 3 0 3 82 55 0 4 1 3 77 19
0 3 1 2 23 27 0 1 1 3 90 45 1 4 1 2 75 19 1 1 1 1 16 33 1 1 1
2 24 20 1 4 1 2 100 47 0 3 1 1 139 45 0 3 1 2 36 53 0 1 1 3 90
34 0 4 1 1 49 25 1 1 0 2 33 39 0 1 0 2 68 21 1 2
;
data b;set a;
if education = 1 then do; ed1 = 0;ed2 = 0;end;
else if education = 2 then do; ed1 = 1;ed2 = 0;end;
else if education = 3 then do; ed1 = 0;ed2 = 1;end;
if race = 1 then do; race1 = 0;race2 = 0;race3 = 0;end;
else if race = 2 then do;race1 = 1;race2 = 0;race3 = 0;end;
else if race = 3 then do race1 = 0;race2 = 1;race3 = 0;end;
else if race = 4 then do race1 = 0;race2 = 0;race3 = 1;end;
proc phreg;
model days*censor(0) = ed1 ed2 age gender race1 race2 race3/
  risklimits;
run;
```

Convergence Status

Convergence criterion (GCONV = 1E-8) satisfied.

***

Testing Global Null Hypothesis: BETA = 0

Test	Chi-Square	DF	Pr > ChiSq (r1)
Likelihood ratio	15.6419	7	0.0286
Score	19.5926	7	0.0065
Wald	10.1304	7	0.1813

The PHREG Procedure

Analysis of Maximum Likelihood Estimates

Variable	DF	Parameter Estimate (r2)	Std Error	Chi-Square	Pr > ChiSq (r3)	Hazard Ratio (r4)	95% Hazard Ratio Confidence Limits (r5)	(r6)
ed1	1	-0.13364	0.77196	0.0300	0.8626	0.875	0.193	3.972
ed2	1	0.00959	1.11771	0.0001	0.9932	1.010	0.113	9.027
Age	1	-0.02059	0.03696	0.3104	0.5774	0.980	0.911	1.053
Gender	1	0.10093	0.70075	0.0207	0.8855	1.106	0.280	4.368
race1	1	-3.13993	1.44813	4.7014	0.0301	0.043	0.003	0.740
race2	1	-4.05441	1.55080	6.8351	0.0089	0.017	0.001	0.362
race3	1	-2.42600	1.34418	3.2574	0.0711	0.088	0.006	1.232

The p-values for the Global Null Hypothesis for testing all regression coefficients, β_is, are zero and are given in column (r1) corresponding to three different test statistics. These test statistics for large sample size are asymptotically equivalent. Note that the p-values corresponding to the likelihood ratio and the score test in our problem are significant indicating that at least one β is not zero. The p-values corresponding to different covariates are given in column (r3) with the parameter estimates given in column (r2). Of the p-values given in column (r3), race1 and race2 are significant. This implies that there is a significant difference between whites and African Americans, and between whites and Hispanics for their reemployment.

The hazard ratios are given in column (r4) with their 95% confidence limits given in columns (r5) and (r6). Consider the hazard ratio 1.106 for gender. This implies that the hazard rate for females is 1.106 times that of the males. The CI for this hazard ratio is (0.280, 4.368) and it can be interpreted as before. Consider the hazard ratio of 0.980 for age. Hence, for every year increase in age, the hazard rate is 0.98 from the previous age. Thus, with increased age of one year, the hazard decreases by 2% [(1 – 0.098)*100]. The CI for this hazard ratio is (0.911, 1.053) and can be interpreted as before.

The failure time ties are handled using Breslow (1974) and is the default in SAS.

The variables can be selected by forward and backward selection similar to the method described in Section 5.3.4. Diagnostics can be checked as described by Lawless (1982) and Allison (1995).

5.12.2 Proportional Hazard Assumption

For the data considered in Section 5.12.1, we add the following programming lines after the model statement, to check for the proportional hazards model assumption for the covariate of interest:

```
assess var = (race1 race2 race3 ed1 ed2 gender age) ph/resample;
  *the variables in parenthesis are checked for the
  proportional hazard assumption;
```

The following is the necessary output:

***

	Supremum Test for Proportionals Hazards Assumption			
	Maximum Absolute			
Variable	Value	Replications	Seed	Pr > MaxAbsVal (r7)
ed1	1.0239	1000	488875001	0.3650
ed2	0.9240	1000	488875001	0.3690
Age	0.9246	1000	488875001	0.2860
Gender	0.4275	1000	488875001	0.8730
race1	0.5633	1000	488875001	0.5540
race2	1.0559	1000	488875001	0.2460
race3	1.1298	1000	488875001	0.2790

The *p*-values for testing the proportional hazards assumption for different covariates are given in column (r7). If any of the *p*-values is less than 0.05, then the proportional hazards model assumption is not valid for the corresponding covariate. For all covariates in this problem, the proportional hazards assumption is valid.

5.12.3 Stratified Cox Model

Sometimes we may stratify some of the covariates and discuss the Cox model over those strata. In those cases their regression coefficients β_is are assumed to be the same over all the strata. The hazard functions differ only on the baseline hazard functions.

In Section 5.12.1, we considered the baseline hazards to be constant over time for all the subjects. In this section we will consider that certain groups have different baseline hazards. We consider the groups as strata and use the stratified Cox model for the analysis. The strata variable used is not of interest for the interpretation of the data (no estimates in the output will be provided) and is usually categorical.

Consider the example of Section 5.12.1 and assume the baseline hazard to be different for the two genders. We apply the stratified Cox model for the factor gender at the two levels. The strata statement in the model makes the difference for the *stratified Cox model*.

```
proc phreg;
model days*censor(0) = ed1 ed2 age race1 race2 race3/
  risklimits; strata gender; run;
```

* * *

Testing Global Null Hypothesis: BETA = 0

Test	Chi-Square	DF	Pr > ChiSq
Likelihood ratio	14.6250	6	0.0234
Score	16.0427	6	0.0135
Wald	7.9946	6	0.2385

The PHREG Procedure

Analysis of Maximum Likelihood Estimates

Variable	DF	Parameter Estimate	Std Error	Chi-Square	Pr > ChiSq (s1)	Hazard Ratio	95% Hazard Ratio Confidence Limits	
ed1	1	−0.68458	0.95006	0.5192	0.4712	0.504	0.078	3.246
ed2	1	0.14636	1.11194	0.0173	0.8953	1.158	0.131	10.234
age	1	−0.03997	0.03763	1.1278	0.2882	0.961	0.893	1.034
race1	1	−3.11587	1.63119	3.6488	0.0561	0.044	0.002	1.085
race2	1	−4.02888	1.56262	6.6476	0.0099	0.018	0.001	0.381
race3	1	−2.73894	1.49185	3.3707	0.0664	0.065	0.003	1.203

The significance of the parameters can be tested using the *p*-values given in column (s1). The parameter estimates and hazard ratios can be interpreted

as in the previous sections. Note that the parameter for gender is not estimated. The estimates of the other variables may be seen to be different for
those given in Section 5.12.1 with no stratification. The estimates given here
are averaged over gender, whereas the estimates of Section 5.12.1 separate
out gender.

5.12.4 Time-Varying Covariates

Sometimes the covariates may affect the response depending on the times
that the covariates are considered. In that case the Cox model handles the
time-varying covariates. These covariates' values may change during the
time of the study and are called *time-dependent covariates*. In the example
discussed in Section 5.12.1 the age of the subject for reemployment may
affect the chance of reemployment. For example, when age <25, the chance
of reemployment is less; when the age is ≥25 and <50 the chance of reemployment is high; and the chance of reemployment is less when age ≥50. We
consider the reemployment within 30 days or at least 30 days for the person
to be reemployed. In this case, the age covariate is separated into three covariates as follows:

$$Age1 = 1, \quad \text{if age} <25 \text{ and days} >30$$
$$= 0, \quad \text{otherwise}$$

$$Age2 = 1, \quad \text{if age} >= 25 \text{ and age} <50 \text{ and day} <= 30$$
$$= 0, \quad \text{otherwise}$$

$$Age3 = 1, \quad \text{if age} >= 50 \text{ and days} >30$$
$$= 0, \quad \text{otherwise.}$$

We modify the program by adding the following lines after the model
statement;

```
proc phreg;
model days*censor(0) = ed1 ed2 age1 age2 age3 gender race1
  race2 race3/risklimits;
if age <25 and days >30 then age1 = 1;else age1 = 0;
if age >=25 and age <50 and days <= 30 then age2 = 1;else
  age2 = 0;
if age >=50 and days >30 then age3 = 1;else age3 = 0;      run;
```

The output is given below:

```
          Testing Global Null Hypothesis: BETA = 0
Test                    Chi-Square      DF        Pr > ChiSq
Likelihood ratio          15.7317        9          0.0727
Score                     18.8159        9          0.0268
Wald                       9.5835        9          0.3852
```

```
                          The PHREG Procedure
                 Analysis of Maximum Likelihood Estimates


              Parameter   Std    Chi-  Pr > ChiSq Hazard 95% Hazard Ratio
Variable  DF  Estimate   Error  Square   (s2)      Ratio Confidence Limits
ed1       1    0.09952 0.91989 0.0117  0.9138     1.105   0.182     6.702
ed2       1   -0.58939 1.58336 0.1386  0.7097     0.555   0.025    12.354
age1      1   -0.60023 1.31497 0.2084  0.6481     0.549   0.042     7.222
age2      1    0.51343 1.31449 0.1526  0.6961     1.671   0.127    21.972
age3      1    0.32296 1.41873 0.0518  0.8199     1.381   0.086    22.278
gender    1    0.27353 0.70327 0.1513  0.6973     1.315   0.331     5.217
race1     1   -3.03197 1.53355 3.9089  0.0480     0.048   0.002     0.974
race2     1   -4.51370 1.61017 7.8582  0.0051     0.011   0.000     0.257
race3     1   -2.17559 1.61544 1.8137  0.1781     0.114   0.005     2.693
```

The significance of the parameters of covariates and hazard ratios can be interpreted as before. In the (s2) column, if any *p*-value corresponding to a time-dependent covariate is significant, we interpret that part of the covariate affects the response. Had the *p*-value of age1 been significant we could have inferred that the time for reemployment for the cohort of workers under the age 25 and not reemployed for 30 days is significantly different from other unemployed workers.

5.12.5 Competing Risks

Sometimes the events considered in a problem may be of different types. A death may be due to heart attack, cancer, stroke, motor accident, or other types. The covariates considered for death in survival distribution models may not be the same for each of these types of death. When a person dies of a heart attack, the person cannot die afterward from any other type of death, and the study involving several events and the risk factors is known as *competing risk* (see Kalbfleisch and Prentice, 2002; Lee and Wang, 2003). Once the time of event of a given type is known, that subject is censored for any other type of event and will be considered as censored for other types. In this case, we run different models for each of the type of events and test the effect of covariates on any two types of events of interest.

In Table 5.13, we consider three types of death and give three covariates. The three types of death considered result from heart attack, stroke, and others and the covariates are cholesterol level, A1C (sugar levels), and exercise at least thrice a week (Yes or No).

```
data a;
/***input data***/
input ha hacensor stroke strokecensor other othercensor
  cholesterol a1c
exercise @@; cards;
```

```
55 1 55 0 55 0 250 10 0 55 1 55 0 55 0 200 11 0 50 0 50 1 50 0
275 11 0 75 0 75 0 75 1 250 9 0 72 1 72 0 72 0 200 10 1 79 0
79 0 79 1 150 8 1 68 1 68 0 68 0 225 9.5 1 63 1 63 0 63 0 200
10 0 58 0 58 1 58 0 275 8 1 59 0 59 1 59 0 250 6.5 0 72 0 72 0
72 1 200 7 1 75 1 75 0 75 0 210 8 0 80 1 80 0 80 0 200 7 0 77
0 77 1 77 0 175 7 1 60 0 60 0 60 1 200 9 1
;* for each individual, the time is given forall the types of
  death giving 1 for the actual type of death and 0 for other
  types death;
/***end of input data***/
data a1;set a;
proc phreg;model ha*hacensor(0)=cholesterol a1c exercise; run;
data a1;set a;
proc phreg;model stroke*strokecensor(0)=cholesterol a1c
  exercise; run;
data a1;set a;
proc phreg;model other*othercensor(0)=cholesterol a1c
  exercise; run;
```

TABLE 5.13

Artificial Data on Different Causes of Death

Cause of Death	Time (Age)	Cholesterol	A1C	Exercise (0 = No, 1 = Yes)
Heart attack	55	250	10	0
Heart attack	55	200	11	0
Stroke	50	275	11	0
Others	75	250	9	0
Heart attack	72	200	10	1
Others	79	150	8	1
Heart attack	68	225	9.5	1
Heart attack	63	200	10	0
Stroke	58	275	8	1
Stroke	59	250	6.5	0
Others	72	200	7	1
Heart attack	75	210	8	0
Heart attack	80	200	7	0
Stroke	77	175	7	1
Others	60	200	9	1

```
                    The PHREG Procedure
                    Model Information
             Data set               WORK.A1
             Dependent variable     ha
             Censoring variable     hacensor
             Censoring value(s)     0
             Ties handling          BRESLOW
```

***
The PHREG Procedure
Analysis of Maximum Likelihood Estimates

Variable	DF	Parameter Estimate	Std Error	Chi-Square	Pr > ChiSq	Hazard Ratio
cholesterol	1	−0.00137	0.02111	0.0042	0.9484	0.999
a1c	1	1.58413 (t1)	0.64661 (t2)	6.0021	0.0143	4.875
exercise	1	−0.84737	1.20415	0.4952	0.4816	0.429

The PHREG Procedure
Model Information

Data set	WORK.A1
Dependent variable	stroke
Censoring variable	stroke censor
Censoring value(s)	0
Ties handling	BRESLOW

***
The PHREG Procedure
Analysis of Maximum Likelihood Estimates

Variable	DF	Parameter Estimate	Std Error	Chi-Square	Pr > ChiSq	Hazard Ratio
cholesterol	1	0.07969	0.04141	3.7040	0.0543	1.083
a1c	1	0.15569 (t3)	0.54027 (t4)	0.0830	0.7732	1.168
exercise	1	0.96257	1.32417	0.5284	0.4673	2.618

Data set	WORK.A1
Dependent variable	other
Censoring variable	other censor
Censoring value(s)	0
Ties handling	BRESLOW

***
The PHREG Procedure
Analysis of Maximum Likelihood Estimates

Variable	DF	Parameter Estimate	Std Error	Chi-Square	Pr > ChiSq	Hazard Ratio
cholesterol	1	0.08212	0.05412	2.3022	0.1292	1.086
a1c	1	−0.22386	0.59945	0.1395	0.7088	0.799
exercise	1	5.32019	3.33466	2.5454	0.1106	204.422

From the outputs looking at the *p*-values for the parameters we note that A1C is significant for heart attack (*p*-value = 0.0143). Cholesterol is a borderline case for stroke. Suppose we want to test that A1C hazard is/is not the same for heart attack and stroke. We test the null hypothesis that the beta coefficients for A1C are the same for heart attack and stroke. The two estimated parameters (t1) and (t3) and their standard errors (t2) and (t4) from the above output are, respectively,

```
Estimate      Std error
1.58413        0.64661
0.15569        0.54027
```

The *p*-value for the test, assuming that the two estimates are independent, will be given by using the following programming lines:

```
data a;
/***input the data***/
estimate1 = 1.58413;*heart attack estimate;
se1 = 0.64661;*heart attack se;
estimate2 = 0.15569; *stroke estimate;
se2 = 0.54027;*stroke se;
/***end of input data***/
z = (estimate1 - estimate2)/(sqrt((se1**2) + (se2**2)));
pvalue = 2* (1 - probnorm(abs(z))); proc print;var pvalue;run;
```

Output:

```
              pvalue
            0.090028
```

Since this *p*-value is greater than 0.05, we conclude that the hazard due to A1C is the same for heart attack and stroke. Similarly, other hazard rates of the covariates on the types of death can be tested.

5.13 Parallelism of Regression Equations

Suppose we know that the dependent variable Y can be expressed as a linear combination of p independent variables $X_1, X_2, ..., X_p$ and that the regression coefficients $\beta_1, \beta_2, ..., \beta_p$ are the same or different for k different populations (groups). When the regression coefficients are the same for k populations with different constant terms, the regression equations are parallel implying that the rate of changes in the Y variable for the k populations is the same for a unit change of each of the independent variables with no change in other independent variables. Let us consider the data given in Table 5.4. We are interested in testing whether the regression equations are parallel for men and women if we fit a multiple regression equation of Y (final grade) on X_1 (age), X_3 (GPA), X_4 (number of credit hours), and X_5 (midterm score).

To run the SAS program, for each independent variable X_i, we create k independent variables $X_{i1}, X_{i2}, ..., X_{ik}$, where X_{ij} are values of X_i for the jth group and zero for other $k-1$ groups $X_{i1}, X_{i2}, ..., X_{i,j-1}, X_{i,j+1}, ..., X_{ik}$. We introduce k columns corresponding to the k groups where the ith column has 1s corresponding to the ith group and 0s elsewhere. We run two regression equations without intercept where the full model equation regresses Y on the columns corresponding to the groups and the covariates X_{ij}s, and the reduced model equation regresses Y on the columns corresponding to the groups and the covariates X_is. Based on the two residual mean squares, we test the parallelism of the regression equations.

The following program provides the necessary output to compare the parallelism of the regression equations for the two genders.

```
data a;
/***input data***/
input x1 x2 x3 x4 x5 y @@;
cards;
35 1 2 9 50 60 40 1 3 15 85 89 25 1 3 13 69 70 30 0 2.9 12 73
70 42 0 2.7 15 76 80 29 0 3.5 16 80 85 33 1 3 9 59 57 39 1 3.5
12 92 95 45 1 2.8 17 70 79 51 1 3.5 12 73 79 22 0 2.9 15 75 70
49 0 3.7 16 95 99 45 1 3.6 18 80 85 40 1 3.4 10 85 85 35 1 3.2
18 85 77 23 1 2.9 12 59 63 42 1 2.5 15 75 70 27 0 3 15 80 85
;
/***end of input data***/
data a;set a;
if x2 = 0 then x2male = 1; else x2male = 0;
if x2 = 1 then x2female = 1; else x2female = 0;
*reduced model; *Data given for the k independent variables;
proc reg; model y = x1 x2male x2female x3 x4 x5/noint;run;
```

***

Analysis of Variance

Source	DF	Sum of Squares	Mean Square	F Value	Pr > F
Model	6	110566	18428	712.41	<0.0001
Error	12 (u2)	310.40067 (u1)	25.86672		
Uncorrected total	18	110876			

***

```
data a2;set a;
*In our example k = 2 and hence we create 2 independent
  variables for each of the original independent variable,
  except for the grouping variable. These independent variables
  will contain 0s for other groups than the group they are
  representing. In our example gender is the grouping variable
  and Xinew contains the data corresponding to the data for
  females and 0s for males, whereas the original X variable
  will contain the data for males and 0s for the females.;
x1new = x1; x3new = x3; x4new = x4; x5new = x5;
if x2 = 1 then do;
```

```
x1new = 0;  x3new = 0;  x4new = 0;  x5new = 0;  end;
if x2 = 0 then do;  x1 = 0;  x3 = 0;  x4 = 0;  x5 = 0;  end;
proc reg; model y = x1 x2male x2female x1new x3 x3new x4 x4new
  x5 x5new/noint; run;
```

```
                            * * *
                   Analysis of Variance
                                    Mean
Source          DF      Sum of Squares    Square    F Value    Pr > F
Model           10         110603         11060      324.60   <0.0001
Error           8 (u4)    272.58610 (u3)   34.07326
Uncorrected     18        110876
  total
                            * * *
```

```
data a3;
rssfull = 272.58610 ;*full model residual SS (u3);
rssdffull = 8;* full model error df (u4);
rssreduced = 310.40067 ;*reduced model residual SS (u1);
rssdfred = 12;*reduced model error df (u2);
f = ((rssreduced - rssfull)/(rssdfred - rssdffull))/(rssfull/
  rssdffull);
pvalue = 1 - probf(f, rssdfred - rssdffull, rssdffull);
keep pvalue; proc print;run;
```

```
                        pvalue
                        0.88455 (u5)
```

Since the *p*-value at (u5) is at least 0.05, we conclude that the regression equations are parallel for both genders.

5.14 Variance-Stabilizing Transformations

When the variable Y has got the variance σ^2 and mean μ and if the variance is not the same for all observed Y values, we may perform weighted least squares as discussed before, or we may use a variance stabilizing transformation to get the same variance for all observations as needed by the least-squares method. The commonly used transformations are *arcsine, square root, logarithmic*, or any of the *power transformations*. Table 5.14 indicates the necessary transformation depending on the relationship of the variance σ^2 and the mean μ.

The regression equations will be obtained on these transformed dependent variables.

The square root transformation to the dependent variables is carried out when the dependent variables follow a Poisson distribution. In this case, the responses will have smaller values. If the value is 0, it is customary to use 0.5 in place of 0.

TABLE 5.14

Transformation Depending on the Relationship of Variance and Mean

Relation of σ to μ	Transformation
$\sigma \propto \mu^{1/2}(1-\mu)^{1/2}$	$\sin^{-1}\left(\sqrt{Y/n}\right)$
$\sigma \propto \mu$	$Ln(Y)$
$\sigma \propto \mu^{1/2}$	$sqrt(Y)$
$\sigma \propto \mu^{k}$	Y^{1-k}

When the dependent variable Y is integral and has a binomial distribution based on n independent trials, each trial with two outcomes yes (= 1), no (= 0), the arcsine transformation $\sin^{-1}\left(\sqrt{Y/n}\right)$ is used. If the number of trials are different for each response, arcsine transformation will not stabilize the variance. If Y is 0 or n, it is customary to replace $0/n$ by $1/n$ and if it is n, then n/n is replaced by $(1 - 1/n)$.

When a dependent variable follows an exponential distribution, the dependent variable takes large positive values and in that case the ln transformation is used.

5.15 Ridge Regression

Sometimes we come across ill-conditioned data for obtaining the multiple regression equation. This is the case when there is *multicollinearity* of the independent variables. One method is to regress the dependent variable on some independent variables, ignoring other independent variables. This means that we retain independent variables that are of interest and ignore the other variables that may depend on these variables. When the independent variables are random, another method is to consider principal components of the independent variables with their associated variances and apply the weighted multiple regression equation.

An alternative way of solving this problem is given by Hoerl and Kennard (1970) and is widely known as *ridge regression*. In this case, a constant k is added to the sums of squares of the independent variables and regression analysis is carried out. The choice of the constant k is important and in our program we first find the constant as given by Draper and Smith (1981, p. 317) and use it to obtain the estimated parameters by using the ridge regression.

Let us consider the data given in Table 5.4 and find the ridge regression estimators. The necessary program is given below:

```
data a;
/***input data***/
```

```
input x1 x2 x3 x4 x5 y @@; cards;
35 1 2 9 50 60 40 1 3 15 85 89 25 1 3 13 69 70 30 0 2.9 12 73
70 42 0 2.7 15 76 80 29 0 3.5 16 80 85 33 1 3 9 59 57 39 1 3.5
12 92 95 45 1 2.8 17 70 79 51 1 3.5 12 73 79 22 0 2.9 15 75 70
49 0 3.7 16 95 99 45 1 3.6 18 80 85 40 1 3.4 10 85 85 35 1 3.2
18 85 77 23 1 2.9 12 59 63 42 1 2.5 15 75 70 27 0 3 15 80 85
;
/***end of input data***/
data a1;set a;
proc reg outest = b tableout; model y = x1 x2 x3 x4 x5; run;
data parms;set b;
if _type_ = 'PARMS'; s = _rmse_ ;s2 = s*s;
/***input data***/
numberparms = 5;
/***end of input data***/
a = 1; proc sort;by a;
proc print;run; data stderr;set b; if _type_ ='STDERR'; a = 1;
x1stderr = x1; x2stderr = x2; x3stderr = x3; x4stderr = x4;
x5stderr = x5; *number of independent variables;
drop x1 x2 x3 x4 x5; keep x1stderr x2stderr x3stderr x4stderr
  x5stderr a; a = 1;
proc sort;by a;
data final;merge parms stderr; by a;
sum = ((x1*x1stderr)**2) + ((x2*x2stderr)**2) +
      ((x3*x3stderr)**2) +  ((x4*x4stderr)**2) +
      ((x5*x5stderr)**2);*modify based on the number of
      independent variables;
optimal = (numberparms*s2)/sum; keep optimal; proc print;run;
```

$$\text{optimal}$$
$$0.84133$$

Using the optimal k from the output, one performs ridge regression by the ridge regression program using this optimal k.

```
data final1;set a;
proc reg outest = c ridge = .84133; *input optimal theta for
  ridge;
model y = x1 x2 x3 x4 x5; run;
data c; set c; regression = _type_;
proc print; var regression intercept x1 x2 x3 x4 x5; run;
```

Output:

Regression	Intercept	x1	x2	x3	x4	x5
PARMS		4.4144	0.28555	−2.10913	2.60364	0.03838	0.73817
RIDGE (v1)	22.5931	0.22103	−1.88961	5.27302	0.43445	0.34619

In the output, the last line corresponds to the ridge regression estimates and the PARMS line provides the standard regression estimates. The ridge regression equation, using the coefficients given in the row (v1), is

$$\hat{Y} = 22.59 + 0.22X_1 + (-1.89)X_2 + 5.27X_3 + 0.43X_4 + 0.35X_5.$$

5.16 Local Regression (LOESS)

Many types of regression models can be handled using REG, NLIN, and GLM; however, in certain situations the parametric regression model is not adequate. The *LOESS model* is used when we want a robust model or when the parametric model is unknown. The response variable Y is formed using a smoothing function $g(x)$ and the random error with a mean of 0 and a constant variance as

$$Y_i = g(x_i) + \varepsilon.$$

For each observation at x, a polynomial is estimated using a smoothing parameter and the second parameter indicating the degree of the fitted polynomial. The choice of these two parameters is up to the researcher and for full details the interested reader is referred to the SAS Manual or Der and Everitt (2006, p. 228).

5.17 Response Surface Methodology: Quadratic Model

Experimenters will be interested to find the optimal levels of factors in a factorial experiment to maximize or minimize the response. For this purpose, initially we fit the first-order model to identify the factors of interest and move the center of the factors by a method known as steepest ascent to reach a center from where they can determine the optimal levels of the factors. The experiment conducted at the center may enable the experimenter to fit a *quadratic regression equation* and determine the optimal levels of the factors.

The commonly used design to fit a quadratic polynomial is *central composite design*. In this design there are three types of points where the data are collected. Using the coded levels one set of points is the center points $(0, 0, ..., 0)$ enabling the researcher to see whether the model fits the data. In addition there will be factorial points $(\pm1, \pm1, ..., \pm1)$ and a set of axial points $(\pm a, 0, ..., 0)$, $(0, \pm a, ..., 0)$, ..., $(0, 0, ..., \pm a)$ on each axis. The points are selected so that the design is rotatable in the sense that the points at the same distance from the center provide equal variance to the estimated response. We will give an experimental

TABLE 5.15

Artificial Data to Determine Stability

Coded			Actual			Expiration
X_1	X_2	X_3	X_1	X_2	X_3	Y (Months)
1	1	1	25	275	2750	25
1	1	-1	25	275	2250	20
1	-1	1	25	225	2750	24
1	-1	-1	25	225	2250	20
-1	1	1	15	275	2750	20
-1	1	-1	15	275	2250	22
-1	-1	1	15	225	2750	24
-1	-1	-1	15	225	2250	22
-2	0	0	10	250	2500	26
2	0	0	30	250	2500	22
0	-2	0	20	200	2500	20
0	2	0	20	300	2500	18
0	0	-2	20	250	2000	18
0	0	2	20	250	3000	24
0	0	0	20	250	2500	24
0	0	-2	20	250	2000	28
0	0	2	20	250	3000	22
0	0	0	20	250	2500	30

setting in this section with $a = 2$, which is not a rotatable design. For further details the interested reader is referred to Myers and Montgomery (1995).

Suppose we are experimenting with three factors: the time taken to grind the compound (X_1), the temperature at grinding (X_2), and the speed (X_3) at which the grinder is operated for the stability (Y) of the tablets manufactured. Suppose the minimum and maximum time for grinding is 10–30 min, the temperatures at 200°–300°F and the speed of grinding is 2000–3000 rpm. In Table 5.15, we provide artificial data for the coded and the actual levels of the factors for determining the stability of the product. While center points are repeated to get pure error, one may repeat axial points to get pure error as we had done in Table 5.15.

Note that in Table 5.15, for each factor, the minimum and maximum levels are identified with the coded -2 and 2 levels and the other coded levels are used to determine the actual levels.

```
data a;
input codedx1 codedx2 codedx3 actualx1 actualx2 actualx3
  expiration @@;
cards;
                1       1     1    25     275     2750    25
                1       1    -1    25     275     2250    20
                1      -1     1    25     225     2750    24
```

```
        1    -1   -1   25   225   2250   20
       -1     1    1   15   275   2750   20
       -1     1   -1   15   275   2250   22
       -1    -1    1   15   225   2750   24
       -1    -1   -1   15   225   2250   22
       -2     0    0   10   250   2500   26
        2     0    0   30   250   2500   22
        0    -2    0   20   200   2500   20
        0     2    0   20   300   2500   18
        0     0   -2   20   250   2000   18
        0     0    2   20   250   3000   24
        0     0    0   20   250   2500   24
        0     0   -2   20   250   2000   28
        0     0    2   20   250   3000   22
        0     0    0   20   250   2500   30
;
data a1;set a;
proc rsreg;model expiration = actualx1 actualx2 actualx3/
  lackfit; *one may replace actual Xi by coded Xi in the
  model, get the output and transform the coded values to
  actual values to get the stationary point; run;
```

The following is the necessary output:

★★★

Residual	DF	Sum of Squares	Mean Square	F Value	Pr > F
Lack of fit	5	20.400000	4.080000	0.17	0.9549 (w1)
Pure error	3	70.000000	23.333333		
Total error	8	90.400000	11.300000		

Parameter	DF	Estimate (w3)	Std Error	t Value	Pr > |t| (w2)	★★★
Intercept	1	-243.225000	199.831191	-1.22	0.2582	
actualx1	1	-2.387500	3.624397	-0.66	0.5286	
actualx2	1	1.632500	0.845748	1.93	0.0897	
actualx3	1	0.072500	0.077096	0.94	0.3745	
actualx1* actualx1	1	-0.030000	0.033615	-0.89	0.3982	
actualx2* actualx1	1	0.005000	0.009508	0.53	0.6132	
actualx2* actualx2	1	-0.003200	0.001345	-2.38	0.0446	
actualx3* actualx1	1	0.000900	0.000951	0.95	0.3716	
actualx3* actualx2	1	-0.000060000	0.000190	-0.32	0.7604	
actualx3* actualx3	1	-0.000014800	0.000011515	-1.29	0.2346	

```
                        The RSREG Procedure
      Canonical Analysis of Response Surface Based on Coded Data
                          Critical Value
           Factor                 Coded                   Uncoded
                                                           (w5)
        actualx1              - 0.168493               18.315067
        actualx2              - 0.082478              245.876110
        actualx3                0.015608             2507.803829
        Predicted value at stationary point:  26.515653  (w4)
                                 ★★★
                Stationary point is a maximum.  (w6)
```

From (w1) the p-value for testing the lack of fit of the quadratic model is 0.9549 and is not significant indicating that the quadratic model fits the data. From column (w2) the p-value for the X_2^2 term is 0.0446 and is significant and other linear, quadratic, and cross-product terms are not significant. Column (w3) provides the estimated parameters and from them we have the following predicting equation:

$$\hat{Y} = -243.23 + (-2.39)X_1 + (1.63)X_2 + (0.073)X_3 + (-0.03)X_1^2 + 0.005X_1X_2$$
$$+ (-0.0032)X_2^2 + 0.001X_1X_3 + 0X_2X_3 + 0X_3^2.$$

The stationary point provides the maximum for the equation and this can be seen from (w6). The optimum values for X_1, X_2, and X_3 are given in column (w5) and the values at the levels of the three factors providing local maxima for the response are

$$X_1 = 18.32, \quad X_2 = 245.88, \quad X_3 = 2507.80.$$

The maximum response at the above levels of the three factors is given in (w4) and is 26.52.

5.18 Mixture Designs and Their Analysis

We consider the factorial experiments in k factors and the sum of the levels of all the factors is 1. For example, consider a tour package costing $800. The tour package consists of lodging, food, and entertainment expenses.

Suppose the package consists of 0.5 for lodging, 0.3 for food, and 0.2 for entertainment resulting in the cost of $0.5 \times 800 = \$400$ for lodging, $0.3 \times 800 = \$240$ for food, and $0.2 \times 800 = \$160$ for entertainment. Here the levels of the three factors are 0.5, 0.3, and 0.2 and the sum of the levels is 1.

TABLE 5.16

Artificial Data of the Choice in a 10-Point Mixture Design

	Levels		Rating
X_1	X_2	X_3	Y
1	0	0	2
0	1	0	3
0	0	1	3
0.33	0.67	0	4
0.67	0.33	0	5
0.33	0	0.67	4
0.67	0	0.33	6
0	0.33	0.67	5
0	0.67	0.33	7
0.33	0.33	0.33	6

The provider of the package wants to determine the optimal levels of these three factors so that the package is attractive to the customers. For this purpose, we prepare mixture designs and analyze them to determine the preferred levels of the factor. The designs commonly used in this context are *simplex lattice designs* {k, m}. In these designs there are k factors, and the number of equally spaced levels for each of the factors are $m + 1$, denoted by 0, $1/m$, $2/m$, ..., $m/m = 1$. If $k = 3$ and $m = 3$, we consider equally spaced levels for each factor as 1, $1/3$, $2/3$, $3/3 = 1$. We form triplets because we have $k = 3$ factors consisting of these levels where in each triplet the sum of all the three levels is 1. The required design in this case consists of 10 points (runs, profiles, and treatment combinations):

```
(1, 0, 0), (0, 1, 0), (0, 0, 1), (1/3, 2/3, 0), (2/3, 1/3, 0),
(1/3, 0, 2/3), (2/3, 0, 1/3), (0, 1/3, 2/3), (0, 2/3, 1/3),
(1/3, 1/3, 1/3).
```

Each of these 10 profiles will be presented to a panel of prospective customers and each customer will rate one of the 10 profiles on a Lickert scale of seven points. We present the artificial data in Table 5.16.

The necessary program to obtain the optimal combination of levels is given below:

```
data a;
/***input data***/
input x1 x2 x3 y @@;
cards;
1 0 0 2 0 1 0 3 0 0 1 3 .33 .67 0 4 .67 .33 0 5 .33 0 .67
4 .67 0 .33 6 0 .33 .67 5 0 .67 .33 7 .33 .33 .33 6
;
```

```
/***end of input data***/
data a2; set a;
/***input data***/
k = 3;*the number of factors;
/***end of input data***/
x1star = x1 - x3;*x3 is the highest level;
x2star = x2 - x3;* continue for Xistar = Xi - Xk, for i = 1,2,..., k◻1;
proc rsreg;model y = x1star x2star;*use k - 1 xistar terms;run;
```

Parameter	***	Estimate (y4)	***
Intercept		6.297466	
x1star		-1.289215	
x2star		0.356874	
x1star*x1star		-2.424767	
x2star*x1star		1.124909	
x2star*x2star		-3.508388	

The RSREG Procedure

Canonical Analysis of Response Surface Based on Coded Data

Critical Value

Factor	***	Uncoded (y1)
x1star		-0.263858
x2star		0.008559

Predicted value at stationary point: 6.469078 (y2)

***

Stationary point is a maximum. (y3)

```
data b;
/***input data***/
k = 3;
x1star = -0.263858;*take from column (y1);
x2star = 0.008559; *take from column (y1) upto xk - 1star;
x3 = (1 - x1star - x2star)/k;*x3 = xk, up to xk - 1star in the
  numerator;
x1 = x1star + x3;*xistar + xk, for i = 1 to k - 1;
x2 = x2star + x3;
/***end of input data***/
proc print; var x1 x2 x3;* all the k variables; run;
```

X1	X2	X3
0.15458 (y5)	0.42699 (y6)	0.41843 (y7)

From (y3), we note that at the optimal levels of the three factors, the response is maximum. The levels of the three factors where the response is maximized are given at (y5), (y6), and (y7). This means that the tour package must consist of a proportion of $X_1 = 0.15$, $X_2 = 0.43$, and $X_3 = 0.42$ and thus the

$800 tour package must assign 0.15*800 = $120 for lodging, 0.43*800 = $344 for food, and 0.42*800 = $336 for entertainment. From (y2) we note that the maximum response is 6.47. Column (y4) provides the required estimates to form the predicting equation for the response Y as given below:

$$\hat{Y} = 6.30 - 1.29(X_1 - X_3) + 0.36(X_2 - X_3) - 2.42(X_1 - X_3)^2$$
$$+ 1.12(X_1 - X_3)(X_2 - X_3) - 3.51(X_2 - X_3)^2.$$

The above model can be expressed in its Canonical form

$$\hat{Y} = b_1 X_1 + b_2 X_2 + b_3 X_3 + b_{12} X_1 X_2 + b_{13} X_1 X_3 + b_{23} X_2 X_3$$

by noting that $X_1 + X_2 + X_3 = 1$, $X_1^2 = X_1(1 - X_2 - X_3)$, and so on.

This equation can be used to see the responses at any level of the three factors especially near the optimal response to see how the change in the levels for the optimal response affects the predicted response. This example is similar to the one discussed by Raghavarao and Wiley (2009) who also discussed mixture-amount designs, to determine the preferred cost of the package and its assignment, for the customers.

5.19 Analysis of Longitudinal Data: Mixed Models

Suppose we take a random sample of n patients who have diabetes and are treated with oral medication. The A1C levels are noted at the baseline and every 3 months for 1 year. The response on the ith subject at the jth period is given by the following equation:

$$Y_{ij} = \mu + u_i + \beta_j + u_{ij} + e_{ij},$$

where β_j is the period effect, u_i is the subject effect, u_{ij} is the jth period effect on the ith subject, and e_{ij} are random errors, $i = 1, 2, ..., n; j = 0, 1, ..., p$. In our example, $p = 4$. The β_j is considered to be a fixed effect, u_i, u_{ij}, and e_{ij} are independent random effects with mean $= 0$. The variances of u_i, u_{ij}, and e_{ij} are assumed to be σ_1^2, σ_2^2, and σ^2. Further u_i and e_{ij} are assumed to be uncorrelated as well as u_{ij} and e_{ij}. In addition, u_i and u_{ij} are correlated with covariance σ_{12}. Consider the artificial data given in Table 5.17.

The following program provides the required output:

```
data a;
input subject a1c0 a1c1 a1c2 a1c3 a1c4@@;
y = a1c0; period = 0; output;   y = a1c1; period = 1; output;
y = a1c2; period = 2; output;   y = a1c3; period = 3; output;
```

```
y = a1c4;period = 4;output; drop a1c0 a1c1 a1c2 a1c3 a1c4;cards;
1 9.8 8.0 8.0 7.9 7.8
2 9.3 8.9 8.7 8.5 7.7
3 8.0 7.9 7.4 7.0 6.9
4 9.0 8.7 8.4 8.0 7.9
5 8.0 7.8 7.6 7.1 6.8
6 7.9 7.5 7.4 7.1 7.0
7 8.2 8.0 7.8 7.5 7.1
8 8.5 8.2 8.2 7.9 7.8
9 8.9 8.4 8.3 8.4 8.0
10 8.6 8.4 10.2 10.3 7.5
;
data a1;set a;
proc mixed covtest; class subject;
model y = period /s;
random Int period / sub = subject type = un cl; run;
```

TABLE 5.17

A1C Levels of Patients with Diabetes Treated with Oral Medication

Subject	Period				
	0	1	2	3	4
1	9.8	8.0	8.0	7.9	7.8
2	9.3	8.9	8.7	8.5	7.7
3	8.0	7.9	7.4	7.0	6.9
4	9.0	8.7	8.4	8.0	7.9
5	8.0	7.8	7.6	7.1	6.8
6	7.9	7.5	7.4	7.1	7.0
7	8.2	8.0	7.8	7.5	7.1
8	8.5	8.2	8.2	7.9	7.8
9	8.9	8.4	8.3	8.4	8.0
10	8.6	8.4	10.2	10.3	7.5

Output:

```
                              ***
                   Convergence criteria met.
                              ***
                       The Mixed Procedure
                  Covariance Parameter Estimates
```

Cov Parm	Subject	Estimate (z1)	Std Error	Z Value	Pr Z (z2)
UN(1,1)	subject	0.1485	0.1355	1.10	0.1366
UN(2,1)	subject	0.03708	0.03601	1.03	0.3031
UN(2,2)	subject	2.9E−18	.	.	.
Residual		0.2178	0.04932	4.42	<0.0001

```
                              ***
```

Solution for Random Effects

Effect	subject	Estimate	Std Error Pred	DF	t Value	Pr > |t| (z4)
Intercept	1	0.01225	0.09526	30	0.13	0.8985
period	1	0.06418	0	30	Infty	<0.0001
Intercept	2	0.2325	0.09526	30	2.44	0.0208
period	2	0.09559	0	30	Infty	<0.0001
Intercept	3	-0.4103	0.09526	30	-4.31	0.0002
period	3	-0.07360	0	30	-Infty	<0.0001
Intercept	4	0.1565	0.09526	30	1.64	0.1108
period	4	0.05023	0	30	Infty	<0.0001
Intercept	5	-0.3988	0.09526	30	-4.19	0.0002
period	5	-0.07093	0	30	-Infty	<0.0001
Intercept	6	-0.3798	0.09526	30	-3.99	0.0004
period	6	-0.1021	0	30	-Infty	<0.0001
Intercept	7	-0.2203	0.09526	30	-2.31	0.0278
period	7	-0.04526	0	30	-Infty	<0.0001
Intercept	8	0.08216	0.09526	30	0.86	0.3953
period	8	-0.01454	0	30	-Infty	<0.0001
Intercept	9	0.2361	0.09526	30	2.48	0.0191
period	9	0.02518	0	30	Infty	<0.0001
Intercept	10	0.6897	0.09526	30	7.24	<0.0001
period	10	0.07127	0	30	Infty	<0.0001

Type 3 Tests of Fixed Effects

Effect	Num DF	Den DF	F Value	Pr > F
period	1	9	29.86	0.0004 (z3)

In column (z1), the estimated variances and covariances are given for the terms indicated in the first column. In our example, 0.1485 is the estimated variance σ_1^2, 0.03708 is the estimated covariance σ_{12}, 2.9E–18 is the estimated variance σ_2^2, and 0.2178 is the estimated σ^2. In column (z2), we have the p-values to test the significance of these variances and covariances. In the example, the residual variance of 0.2178 is significant. If σ_2^2, comes to be significant, then the slopes for the time periods on the subjects are not the same. At (z3) we have the p-value to test the fixed period effects and in this example it is significant. This implies that the A1C level for different periods is not the same, and there is slope of the A1C levels over the periods. In column (z4), the p-values are given for testing the significance of the slopes and intercepts across each subject as indicated in the row corresponding to periods and intercepts. For example, the intercept and period for subject 2 are significant.

For further details see Diggle et al. (1994).

6

Miscellaneous Topics

6.1 Missing Data

Missing data may occur in surveys, clinical trials, and even in planned experiments using appropriate design. Initially this was realized in experimental designs and Yates (1933) and Bartlett (1937a) provided methods for analyzing the data. In these problems the analysis is carried out using only the available data. Missing values result in having nonorthogonal setting and the analysis can easily be made using computer programs. Before computers were introduced, Yates had substituted estimates for missing data which made the residuals small. Bartlett provided covariance analysis by using covariates for the missing observations where the ith covariate takes 0 values for all responses except for the ith missing response and 1 or –1 was given for the ith missing observation. These methods allowed the researcher to get the analysis on the observed responses only using the available statistical methods.

In longitudinal data, when the missing observation arises at a given time point, no more future observations are available on that unit and such missing value pattern is called monotone missing data pattern.

A very simple way of dealing with this issue is to perform the analysis based on the available complete observations. In this scenario, information on the incomplete data is not used; thus, the analysis only uses the information that is based on subjects remaining in the trial, and may lead to biased inferences. One should also note that statistical power may be lost due to the missing data. Another commonly used methodology in clinical trial is to use the last available observation for the future responses. This method assumes that the patients' condition stays the same from the time the responses are not available. The treatment effect may be conservative by this method. One should be cautious when using this method if there are early dropouts, or if the rates of dropouts are different. A worst-case scenario imputes the worst-observed response value for the active treatment group and the best-observed response value among the placebo group (Myers, 2000). This is usually done as a sensitivity analysis so as to assess the robustness of the endpoint. Nonparametric methods are also available to handle the missing data problems.

Single imputations for the missing value can be obtained; however, this does not account for the variability that is present in the data. One way of doing this is by taking the mean across all the subjects and this value is then imputed for the missing value. This should be done separately for the treatment groups and the placebo group. This method biases the treatment group downward and the placebo group upward.

With the growing need of handling the missing data, Rubin (1987) developed *multiple imputation methods* for the missing data and SAS uses these methods. *Missing at random (MAR)* and *missing completely at random (MCAR)* are two commonly used missing data mechanisms. Little and Rubin (2002) consider the MCAR mechanism assumed that the missing data are a simple random sample of all possible data and the missing data pattern does not depend on observed or missing patterns. In MAR assumption, missing data can depend on previously observed measures or baseline covariates for an individual.

Multiple imputations can be used for longitudinal measurements or single responses. By using multiple imputation, a set of values are obtained by drawing random samples from the distribution for the missing value. Usually, about 3–5 imputations are enough. Each data set is analyzed separately using standard methods such as regression and GLM. The estimates are then combined so that one can draw inferences. However, one should note that these estimates will not produce unique solutions.

By looking at the pattern of the missing data, one selects the method for the multiple imputation such as regression, *MCMC (Markov Chain Monte Carlo)*, or *propensity score*. For instance, if the data set has a monotone missing pattern, one can use regression or MCMC for a parametric or the propensity score method for nonparametric cases. When data are missing, *monotone missing data pattern* is the missing observations from a given time point and onward for an individual. These methods rely on the MAR assumption. When data are missing on a variable it is not necessary that the missing values occur because of that variable; it may be based on other variables in the study. For the regression method, a regression model is fitted for each variable with missing values using previous variables as covariates, and estimates the regression coefficients and the residuals variance. Next, a new model is then fitted and used to impute the missing data for the variables. This process is repeated sequentially for the monotone missing pattern. The previous variables are used as covariates. The MCMC method is used for a monotone or a nonmonotone arbitrary missing data pattern. In MCMC the current variable distribution is based on the previous distribution. The data are assumed to follow a multivariate normal distribution. Simulations using Bayesian prediction from normal data are used for the imputation. For the propensity score method, the observations are grouped based on the propensity scores. For each group an approximate *Bayesian bootstrap* is applied.

In SAS, the procedure PROC MI is used to create multiply imputed data sets and PROC MIANALYZE is used to generate valid statistical inferences by combining the data sets and drawing inferences about the parameters.

As an example, let us consider a fitness center interested in surveying 20 individuals for their loss of weight in 6 months and regress the loss on the daily caloric intake and the initial and 3 months loss of weight. They recorded the weight at the start of the program and at 3 months into the program. They also recorded the food intake in caloric value. Due to several reasons the data on all items from all individuals are not available. The artificial data are given in Table 6.1. From these data we see that the missing pattern is not monotonic and is arbitrary and hence we will use MCMC as an imputation technique. The *chain = multiple* tells the procedure to use multiple chains with a default of 200 burn iterations so that the iterations converge to a stationary distribution, before imputation. The initial estimate(s) is(are) *EM posterior* mode(s) with Jeffreys prior. Other initial estimates can be specified, including bootstrap (see SAS manual for further details). The number of imputations is 5 by default and can be changed by using *nimpute* in the PROC MI statement (refer to the SAS manual for further details).

The following program provides multiple imputation results and the final analysis by using PROC MI and PROC MIANALYZE.

TABLE 6.1

Weight Loss in 6 Months

Lbs Lost[a]	Calories/ Day	Initial Body Weight	Weight Loss after Three Months	Lbs Lost[a]	Calories/ Day	Initial Body Weight	Weight Loss after Three Months
40	1200	163	12	5	.	.	1
33	1800	200	.	30	1400	186	7
27	1850	195	10	20	1700	195	10
15	.	179	5	43	.	.	20
8	2200	.	2	.	1800	160	1
11	1575	176	.	15	1900	180	7
.	2200	205	.	4	1250	208	1
17	.	185	.	2	1000	.	.
32	1300	174	15	44	2200	.	20
25	1860	170	15	8	.	168	.

[a] Total pounds lost in 6 months is final weight minus initial weight.

```
data a; input lbslost calories initialwgt threemonth@@; cards;
40  1200  163  12  33  1800  200  .  27 1850  195  10  15  .  179  5
8  2200  .  2  11  1575  176  .  .  2200  205  .  17  .  185  .
32  1300  174  15  25  1860  170  15  5  .  .  1  30  1400  186  7
20  1700  195  10  43  .  .  20  .  1800  160  1  15  1900  180  7
4  1250  208  1  2  1000  .  .  44  2000  .  20  8  .  168  .
;
```

```
data a1;set a; proc mi out=a2;mcmc displayinit chain=multiple;
var lbslost calories initialwgt threemonth;run;
proc reg data=a2 outest=a3 covout noprint; model
  lbslost=calories initialwgt threemonth; by
  _imputation_;run;
proc mianalyze data=a3 edf=16 theta0= 0 0 0 0;*edf is the
  number of observations minus the number of independent
  variables including intercept;
*theta0 is the hypothesized values for the intercept and the
  slopes of the independent variables;
modeleffects intercept calories initialwgt threemonth;run;
```

The MI Procedure
Model Information

Data set	WORK.A1
Method	MCMC
Multiple imputation chain	Multiple chains
Initial estimates for MCMC	EM Posterior Mode
Start	Starting Value
Prior	Jeffreys
Number of imputations	5
Number of burn-in iterations	200
Seed for random number generator	95375001

Missing Data Patterns (a1)

Group	lbslost	calories	initialwgt	threemonth	Freq	Percent
1	X	X	X	X	8	40.00
2	X	X	X	.	2	10.00
3	X	X	.	X	2	10.00
4	X	X	.	.	1	5.00
5	X	.	X	X	1	5.00
6	X	.	X	.	2	10.00
7	X	.	.	X	2	10.00
8	.	X	X	X	1	5.00
9	.	X	X	.	1	5.00

The MIANALYZE Procedure
★★★
Multiple Imputation Parameter Estimates

Parameter	Estimate (a2)	Std Error (a3)	95% Confidence Limits (a4)	(a5)	DF
intercept	22.214457	25.642931	−46.8716	91.30047	4.3336
calories	−0.005543	0.004084	−0.0148	0.00375	8.6736
initialwgt	−0.043383	0.141989	−0.4396	0.35285	3.9493
threemonth	1.924011	0.255000	1.3218	2.52619	7.0462

```
                Multiple Imputation Parameter Estimates
                                       t for H0:
Parameter  Minimum    Maximum     Theta0 Parameter = Theta0  Pr > |t|
                                                                (a6)
intercept    1.123850 46.274536      0            0.87        0.4317
calories    -0.007915 -0.003132      0           -1.36        0.2089
initialwgt -0.183824   0.071588      0           -0.31        0.7754
threemonth   1.760372  2.055628      0            7.55        0.0001
```

At (a1), one can see the distinct missing patterns. The multiple imputation parameter estimates are displayed in (a2). The standard error of these estimates is shown in (a3). The 95% CI is given at [(a4), (a5)]. The p-values at (a6) are used to test that the parameters (intercept and slopes) are hypothesized as θ_0 vector specified by the *theta0* option in the program. The estimates in the output change with each run of the program due to the change in the imputed data, and the imputed estimates are not unique.

6.2 Diagnostic Errors and Human Behavior

6.2.1 Introduction

Diagnostic tests, such as blood and urine analysis, are used to assess whether an individual has a particular disease or not. These tests are not always 100% accurate. If the test shows a positive result, the patient may or may not have the corresponding disease. Similarly, if the test shows a negative result, the patient may not be disease free.

As discussed in Chapter 1, two types of *misclassification errors* can occur: a *false-positive error* with probability ℓ_1 and a *false-negative error* with probability ℓ_2. The later misclassification error is usually considered to be more serious of the two errors.

These misclassification error rates can be estimated directly if the test can be applied to individuals whose true disease statuses are known, but it is usually difficult or not feasible. The misclassification errors on these diagnostic tests are shown in Table 6.2, assuming π to be the true prevalence rate of the disease. Let p be the prevelance rate estimated in the presence of misclassification errors.

In the following sections we will calculate the sample sizes and power for testing the hypothesis in the presence of misclassification errors.

TABLE 6.2

Misclassification Error Rates

Actual Disease Status	Test Result		
	Positive	Negative	Total
Positive	$(1-\ell_2)\pi$	$\ell_2\pi$	π
Negative	$\ell_1(1-\pi)$	$(1-\ell_1)(1-\pi)$	$(1-\pi)$
Total	P	$(1-p)$	

6.2.2 Independent Samples

6.2.2.1 Two Independent Samples

Let us consider the two-sample case in the presence of misclassification errors. Let a health scientist be interested in drawing inference in the prevalence rate of a disease. The prevalence rates will be determined based on a diagnostic test which is not free of false-positive (negative) errors. The scientist wants to determine the sample sizes of the male and female populations to test the null hypothesis $\pi_1 \le \pi_2$ against the alternative $\pi_1 > \pi_2$ using an α-level test, where π_1 and π_2 are the incidence rates in the male and female populations, and wants to get a power of $1 - \beta = 0.80$ for the test when $\pi_1 - \pi_2 = \delta = 0.05$. It is assumed that $\ell_1 = \ell_2 = 0.01$ and $n_1 = f\, n_2$, where $f = 1$. The following program provides the sample sizes n_1, n_2 as output for the test based on arcsine transformation of the proportions given in Lakshmi (1995).

```
Data a;
/**input data ***/
alpha = 0.05; Power = 0.8; d = .05; f = 1; l1 = .01; l2 = .01;
/**end of input data**/
z2side = probit(1 - alpha/2); z1side = probit(1 - alpha);
  zbeta = probit(power);
delta = arsin(sqrt(((1 + l1 - l2) + d*(1 - l1 - l2))/2)) -
      arsin(sqrt(((1 + l1 - l2)-d*(1 - l1 - l2))/2));
n21side = floor((((z1side + zbeta)/delta)**2)*
        ((1/(4*f)) + 1/4)) + 1;
n22side = floor((((z2side + zbeta)/delta)**2)*
        ((1/(4*f)) + 1/4)) + 1;
n11side = n21side*f; n12side = n22side*f; keep n11side n12side
  n21side n22side; proc print;var n11side n21side n12side
  n22side;run;
```

The sample sizes are on the generous side in the sense that they may be more than needed to test the hypothesis and are given in the following output:

N11SIDE	N21SIDE	N12SIDE	N22SIDE
1287	1287	1634	1634

Without the false-positive and false-negative error rates the sample sizes would be

N11SIDE	N21SIDE	N12SIDE	N22SIDE
1236	1236	1569	1569

Now, suppose the samples of sizes $n_1 = 1634$, $n_2 = 1634$ are taken independently of the two populations for a two-sided test. Let the number of "Yes" responses in the two samples be 500 and 400, respectively, as shown in Table 6.3.

The following program, using normal approximation, provides the p-values at (b1) and (b2) of the output.

```
data a;
/***input data***/
yes1 = 500; yes2 = 400; *number of yes answers for groups 1 and
  2;
n1 = 1634;*sample size for group 1;
n2 = 1634;*sample size for group 2;
l1 = .01; l2 = .01;
/***end of input data**/

p1hat = yes1/n1; p2hat = yes2/n2;pcomb = (yes1 + yes2)/(n1 + n2);
theta1 = l1 + p1hat*(1 - l1 - l2); theta2 = l1 + p2hat*(1 - l1 - l2);
z = (arsin(theta1) - arsin(theta2))/(sqrt((1/(4*n1))+
   (1/(4*n2)))));
zabs = abs(z); PVALUE1 = (1 - probnorm(Z));
PVALUE2 = 2*(1 - probnorm(zabs));
keep pvalue1 pvalue2; proc print; run;
```

We obtain the following output:

PVALUE1	PVALUE2
0.000177096 (b1)	0.000354193 (b2)

From (b2), the p-value is less than 0.05 for a two-sided test. Hence, we conclude that the proportions of males and females affected by the disease are different based on a 0.05-level test.

TABLE 6.3

Incidence Rates of the Disease in Females and Males with Misclassification Errors

	Gender		
Outcome	Female	Male	Total
No Disease	1134(69.4%)	1234(75.5%)	2368
Disease	500(30.6%)	400(24.5%)	900
Total	1634	1634	3268

Let us suppose that the scientist can only recruit 1000 subjects in each of the two groups. The power is then given in the output of the following program:

```
Data a;
/**input data ***/
alpha = 0.05; d = .05; n1 = 1000; n2 = 1000; l1 = .01; l2 = .01;
/**end of input data**/
z2side = probit(1 - alpha/2); z1side = probit(1 - alpha);
delta = arsin (sqrt(((1 + l1 - l2) + d* (1 - l1 - l2))/2)) -
      arsin(sqrt(((1 + l1 - l2) - d* (1 - l1 - l2))/2));
POWER1 = 1 - probnorm(z1side - (delta/(sqrt((1/(4*n1)) +
      (1/(4*n2))))));
POWER2 = 1 - probnorm(z2side - (delta/(sqrt((1/(4*n1)) +
      (1/(4*n2))))));
proc print;var power1 power2; run;
```

```
        POWER1      POWER2
        0.70794     0.59183
```

From the above output one can see that the power for detecting a difference of 0.05 between the prevalence rates with 1000 subjects in each of the groups using a two-sided test is 0.59, and using a one-sided test is 0.71.

6.2.2.2 k Independent Samples

Let us now consider the k sample case. Continuing our example from Section 6.2.2.1, suppose now the scientist is interested in testing the equality of the prevalance rates of the disease for three races: African Americans, whites, and others. Let p_1, p_2, and p_3 be the incidence rates of the disease in whites, African Americans, and other populations. She needs to determine the common sample size needed to test this. She expects that $\ell_1 = \ell_2 = 0.01$. The maximum difference between the proportions, $d = 0.05$, has to be detected with power 0.80 using a level of significance, $\alpha = 0.05$. The following program provides the common sample size n as in the output.

```
data a;
/***input the data ***/
alpha = .05; groups = 3; *number of groups;
power = .8; l1 = 0.01; l2 = 0.01; mdelta = .05; *maximum difference;
/** end of data ***/
y = quantile('CHISQ', .95, groups - 1,); nc = cnonct
    (y, groups - 1, 1 - power);
N = floor((nc* (1 - l1 + l2) * (1 + l1 - l2))/(2* (mdelta**2) *
    (1 - l1 - l2) **2)) + 1;
keep n; proc print; run;
```

The output is as follows:

```
N
2007
```

If there were no misclassification errors, then the common sample size for the three groups would have been 1927. She takes a random sample of size 2007 from each of the three races independently and determines the number of whites, African Americans, and others having the disease. The artificial data are provided in Table 6.4.

The following program, using normal approximation, provides the *p*-value in the output.

```
data a;
/***input data***/
yes1 = 300; yes2 = 350; yes3 = 325;
 *number of yes answers for groups 1, 2 and 3;
n = 2007;*sample size for each group;  l1 = .01; l2 = .01;
 groups = 3;
/***end of input data**/
p1hat = yes1/n; p2hat = yes2/n; p3hat = yes3/n;
theta1hat = l1 + p1hat*(1 - l1 - l2); theta2hat = l1 + p2hat*(1 - l1 - l2);
theta3hat = l1 + p3hat*(1 - l1 - l2);
ph1 = arsin(sqrt(theta1hat)); ph2 = arsin(sqrt(theta2hat));
ph3 = arsin(sqrt(theta3hat)); mean = mean(ph1,ph2,ph3);
T = 4*n*(((ph1 - mean)**2) + ((ph2 - mean)**2) + ((ph3 - mean)**2));
PVALUE = 1 - probchi(t,groups - 1); keep pvalue; proc print; run;
```

We obtain the following output:

```
PVALUE
0.11820
```

The *p*-value of the output is used to test the null hypothesis of equal incidence rate in all groups against the alternative that at least one incidence rate is different from the others. For our data, the *p*-value of 0.11820 is greater

TABLE 6.4

Incidence of Disease for Three Races with Misclassification Errors

		Race		
Outcome	Whites	African Americans	Other	Total
No disease	1707 (85.1%)	1657 (82.6%)	1682 (83.8%)	5046
Disease	300 (14.9%)	350 (17.4%)	325 (16.2%)	975
Total	2007	2007	2007	6021

than 0.05 and hence we do not reject the null hypothesis of equal incidence rates in the three groups.

6.2.3 Two Dependent Samples

Let us now consider the problem of testing the equality of the proportions in dependent samples. Let n pairs of siblings be classified to have a disease (1) or no disease (0). Let π_{ij} be the probability that the two siblings are classified as i and j, respectively, where $i, j = 0, 1$. The null hypothesis, H_0, of interest is $H_0: \pi_{01} + \pi_{11} = \pi_{10} + \pi_{11}$ against the alternative $H_A: \pi_{01} + \pi_{11} \neq \pi_{10} + \pi_{11}$. Testing this null hypothesis reduces to comparing the two off-diagonal entries (discordant responses) in the 2×2 table of Table 6.5; that is, $H_0: \pi_{01} = \pi_{10}$ against $H_A: \pi_{01} \neq \pi_{10}$ and this test is known as McNemar test and is discussed in Section 2.3.1 for data without any misclassification errors. We will now discuss these results in the presence of false-positive (negative) error rates, with $\ell_1 = \ell_2$ as given by Lakshmi (1995).

Let $\psi = \pi_{01} + \pi_{10}$ be the probability of discordant responses of the siblings and the researcher should have a guess value of this ψ and let $\psi = 0.2$. Let $\ell_1 = 0.01 = \ell_2$. The researcher wants the test to have a power of $1 - \beta = 0.8$ when the difference $\pi_{01} - \pi_{10} = \delta = 0.1$. The level of significance of the test is $\alpha = 0.05$. The following program provides the number of siblings required.

```
data a;
/***input the data***/
sigh = .2;*expected pi01 + pi10; alpha = .05; beta = .2;
l = .01;*both false positive(negative) error rates;
delta = .1;*difference between pi01 and pi10;
/***end of input data***/
sighstar = 2*l*(1 - l) + sigh*(2*l - 1)**2;
deltastar = delta*(1 - 2*l);
z2side = probit(1 - alpha/2); zpower = probit(1 - beta);
N = floor((sighstar*((z2side + zpower)**2))/(deltastar**2) +
  (1/sighstar)) + 1;
keep n;proc print;run;

  N
 178
```

TABLE 6.5

Paired Data Analysis in the Presence of Misclassification Errors

	Sibling 1		
Sibling 2	Disease	No Disease	Total
Disease	25(55.6%)	15(11.3%)	40
No disease	20(45.4%)	118(88.7%)	138
Total	45	133	178

On the basis of the output, the researcher should collect data on 178 siblings with misclassification errors. The research needs data on 162 siblings without misclassification errors. In Table 6.5, the artificial data for the first and second sibling disease status are given.

The inference for testing the null hypothesis $\pi_{10} = \pi_{01}$ can be tested by using the McNemar test given in Section 2.3.1 and the p-value for our data is 0.3980 which is greater than 0.05 and hence is not significant. We conclude that the incidence rates of the disease are the same for both siblings.

6.2.4 Finding the Threshold for a Screening Variable

When a physician conducts procedures on a subject, they can be very expensive and time consuming. Instead, *screening variables* can be used to classify an experimental unit into either normal (N) or abnormal ($\overline{N}$) categories. Collecting data on these screening variables tends to be cheaper and faster with a price of increasing false-positive (negative) error rates.

Let us consider catheterization, an invasive procedure, which cardiologists perform only if they are pretty certain that the patient has arteriosclerosis. A *screening variable X*, where X is the number of minutes a patient can walk on the treadmill, may be used to determine whether a patient has arteriosclerosis. For example, if $X > u$ minutes, then the cardiologist may determine that the patient is okay and there is no need to do the catheterization. On the other hand, if $X \leq u$ minutes, the cardiologist may conclude that the patient has some blocked artery and will need a catheterization. The determination of "u" is important to minimize the misclassification error rates.

In banks the credit worthiness of a client is determined from the threshold "u" of the credit score and it is important that the threshold "u" be determined to minimize the misclassification error rates.

Given the screening variable we decide the threshold "u" by maximizing the correlation between the predicted response from the screening variable and the actual status. If ℓ_1 and ℓ_2 indicate the false-positive and false-negative error rates, the correlation between the classification based on the screening variable and the actual status is known to be

$$r = \frac{\left(1 - \ell_1 - \ell_2\right)^2}{1 - \left(\ell_1 - \ell_2\right)^2}.$$

Damaraju (2009) showed that the correlation given above is also the *asymptotic relative efficiency* for testing the equality of the two proportions based on the sample size with and without false-positive (negative) errors.

Let us consider the historical data on patients who had or had not undergone catheterization and the amount of time they walked on the treadmill is given in Table 6.6. We assume that the catheterization is positive (1) if catheterization was performed on the subject and negative (0), otherwise.

TABLE 6.6

Treadmill Time and Catheterization Status

Subject No.	Catheterization ($Y=1, N=0$)	Treadmill (min)	Subject No.	Catheterization ($Y=1, N=0$)	Treadmill (min)
1	0	10	21	1	10
2	0	25	22	0	20
3	1	5	23	0	5
4	0	20	24	0	13
5	1	10	25	1	5
6	0	22	26	1	19
7	1	6	27	1	6
8	1	24	28	0	12
9	1	17	29	1	4
10	0	20	30	1	17
11	1	6	31	1	2
12	0	30	32	0	20
13	1	12	33	0	5
14	0	22	34	0	12
15	1	7	35	1	6
16	0	17	36	0	25
17	1	4	37	0	9
18	0	25	38	0	16
19	1	2	39	1	12
20	0	19	40	0	14

We choose a range on the screening variable in which the threshold belongs and we plot the correlation against these thresholds. The maximum of the graph is at the *threshold* value of "*u*." It is possible that there may not be a maximum in the range selected by the researcher. The mathematics of finding this threshold when the screening variable has normal and exponential distributions for each of the normal and abnormal disease status are given by Lakshmi (1995) and Damaraju (2009).

The program and output are given below.

```
data a;
/***input data***/
input cath treadmill @@; cards;
0 10 0 25 1 5 0 20 1 10 0 22 1 6 1 24 1 17 0 20 1 6 0 30 1 12
   0 22 1 7 0 17 1 4 0 25 1 2 0 19 1 10 0 20 0 5 0 13 1 5 1 19
   1 6 0 12 1 4 1 17 1 2 0 20 0 5 0 12 1 6 0 25 0 9 0 16 1 12 0
   14
;
/***end of input data***/
data b;
%macro threshold(u,in);*input threshold value u and
   dataset name;
```

```
data &in;set a; retain fpcount 0 fncount 0; n=40;*total
  number of subjects; u=&u;
if cath=0 and treadmill <=&u then fpcount+1; if cath=1 and
  treadmill > &u then fncount+1; data &in;set &in;
  falsepositive=fpcount/n; falsenegative=fncount/n;
if _n_=n; keep u falsepositive falsenegative;   run; %mend
  threshold;
*sall the macro for the possible threshold u values;
%threshold(4,in1); * choose the threshold u for possible
  values;
%threshold(5,in2);
%threshold(6,in3);
%threshold(7,in4); %threshold(8,in5); %threshold(9,in6);
%threshold(10,in7); %threshold(11,in8); %threshold(12,in9);
%threshold(13,in10); %threshold(14,in11); %threshold(15,in12);
data final; set in1 in2 in3 in4 in5 in6 in7 in8 in9 in10
  in11 in12;
*all datasets of interest need to be included;
r=((1-falsepositive-falsenegative)**2)/(1-((falsepositive-
  falsenegative)**2));
proc print;run;
```

u	falsepositive	falsenegative	r
4	0.000	0.375	0.45455
5	0.050	0.325	0.42258
6	0.050	0.225	0.54223
7	0.050	0.200	0.57545
8	0.050	0.200	0.57545
9	0.075	0.200	0.53397
10	0.100	0.150	0.56391
11	0.100	0.150	0.56391
12	0.150	0.100	0.56391
13	0.175	0.100	0.52860
14	0.200	0.100	0.49495
15	0.200	0.100	0.49495

From the graph (Figure 6.1) and the above output we note that the maximum correlation occurs when u is in the interval [7,8].

6.2.5 Analyzing Response Data with Errors

Double-blind studies in clinical trials are designed to mask the treatment assignment from investigators and patients. Even if double-blind studies are planned, the investigators and patients may identify the treatment assignment due to the side effects and the expectations of the affects of the active drug. This problem is prevalent in trials involving psychotropic drugs and extends to many other areas as well. Basoglu et al. (1997) and Brownwell and Stunkard (1982) report that about 70–80% of the investigators and patients correctly identify the treatment assignment.

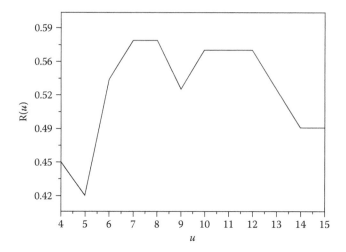

FIGURE 6.1
Determination of the threshold.

DeLucca et al. (1999) and DeLucca and Raghavarao (2000) studied the effect of the treatment assignment perception and the bias in response due to the treatment supposed to be received, on the commonly used Z test and Wilcoxon test for the ordered categorical responses.

The response biases may also be prevalent in open-label studies and other surveys where subjective responses are elicited. In the quality-of-life studies, most of the patients usually indicate their true status. However, a small fraction of respondents who have positive enthusiastic attitudes toward life overevaluate their true status. Similarly, those who have negative pessimistic attitudes underrate their status. In a survey aimed at comparing the amount of time spent on daily exercise, some people overestimate or underestimate the true time for daily exercise.

The proportion of people who overstate (or understate) the responses and the extent of overstatement or understatement differs from population to population. While instruments are available to determine whether a person is a pessimist or an optimist, the author is not aware of the percentage of people who are pessimists or optimists in the general population. For illustration purposes, we will study the effect when 10–25% of people overstate their response and a similar percentage of people understate their response and the absolute value of the overevaluation (or underevaluation) of the response is about 0.3–0.7 standard deviation units. Damaraju and Raghavarao (2005) considered the effect of such overstatements and understatements by the respondents on the commonly used Z, F in ANOVA, and chi-square distributions. The conclusions of these papers are that the tests have got higher level of significance and power increases in these settings. In a study, if the norms mentioned in the paper by Damaraju and Raghavarao are not applicable, the investigators may use the appropriate norms and draw conclusions similar to the ones obtained in their paper.

One may wonder whether these results are similar to the results in *measurement errors* on response variables. When measurement errors occur on response variables, in the context of testing hypotheses problems, the power of the test is noted to decrease (see Carroll, 1998), while in our setting we observe that the power increases. Carroll considers that this is due to measurement errors on response variables that favor the null hypotheses while increasing the variability in the data, whereas in our context, the biases favor the alternative hypotheses without increasing the variability too much.

The suggestion made with these misclassification errors is to use smaller significance level in these tests instead of using the usual 0.05 level of significance. The interested readers may consult the references to see the effect of the misspecifications on these tests.

6.2.6 Responders' Anonymity

When one conducts surveys, the respondents may view certain questions as sensitive in nature and may not want to divulge their personal information to strangers. To rectify this situation, Warner (1965) suggested two statements:

1. I belong to the sensitive category.
2. I do not belong to the sensitive category.

The responders are provided with a random mechanism to select statement 1 or 2 with probability p or $1 - p$ and they are asked to answer the selected statement with a "Yes" or "No" answer without divulging which statement they are responding. One should select p close to 1/2, but not 1/2 to draw the inferences and maintain anonymity to the maximum extent. By doing this the respondents' anonymity is maintained. A random sample of n respondents are taken without replacement and using the proportion of subjects who answered "Yes," the proportion of people belonging to the *sensitive category* is estimated. There are several modifications for this technique and the interested reader is referred to the monograph by Chaudhuri and Mukerjee (1988).

Even with this device, still some people may not truthfully answer the statement they had selected. Inferences on the probability that the respondents are lying and the extent of the proportion of people lying were considered by Krishnamoorthy and Raghavarao (1991) and Lakshmi and Raghavarao (1992) assuming that the proportion giving untruthful answers is the same in both sensitive and nonsensitive categories. Their methods involve asking the sensitive question twice with different or same selection probabilities of statements 1 and 2.

6.3 Density Estimation

Sometimes we may have data from an unknown distribution and we would like to see the data distribution from the given data. *Density estimation* provides a mechanism to find an approximate density form such as skewness, symmetry, modality, and so on from a given data set. This can be done by parametric or nonparametric methods. In parametric density estimation, the density form is assumed from a known family of distributions and estimating the parameters of the model that fit the data. In nonparametric methods no functional form for the density function is assumed and the density estimates are driven entirely by the observed data. In this form the *kernels* and *bandwidth* are needed. The kernel type can be normal, triangular, or rectangular and it determines the shape of the peaks in the data. The bandwidth is the smoothing parameter. We will provide a brief discussion of these results in this section.

6.3.1 Parametric Density Estimation

Let us consider the systolic blood pressure of randomly selected 50 subjects as given below.

110	120	130	115	125	135	150	140	148	137
120	139	147	143	127	126	145	150	139	130
130	140	132	153	145	120	150	128	140	128
140	138	135	129	143	120	140	130	145	150
150	140	139	145	150	120	110	119	140	127

For testing the data to follow a normal distribution, we gave the Shapiro–Wilk test in Chapter 1. Instead of the test we want to have a probability plot of the data for a normal distribution or any other distribution. We can plot the curves by the following program. In this program we show the plot for a normal and exponential distribution. The researcher can use either of the two distributions or any other distribution by specifying the distribution in the probplot programming statement. The *probplot* should be at a 45° angle to the *x*-axis for the data to follow the specified distribution indicated in the program.

```
data a; input sysbp@@; cards;
110 120 130 115 125 135 150 140 148 137 120 139 147 143 127
  126 145 150 139 130 130 140 132 153 145 120 150 128 140 128
  140 138 135 129 143 120 140 130 145 150 150 140 139 145 150
  120 110 119 140 127
;
```

```
data a1;set a; proc univariate; var sysbp; histogram sysbp/
  normal;probplot sysbp/normal;  histogram sysbp/exp
  (theta = 100);
*specify the location parameter theta as less than or equal to
  the minimum data point;probplot sysbp/exp (theta = 100);run;
```

Of the two graphs given in Figures 6.3 and 6.5, the normal probability plot is closer to a 45° angle and we assume that the data are normally distributed based on the two graphs. Further comparing Figures 6.2 and 6.4, we note that the normal plot given in Figure 6.2 closely agrees with the histogram of the data.

6.3.2 Nonparametric Univariate Density Estimation

The histogram is the frequently encountered nonparametric density estimator. It depends on the width and end points of the bars. By shifting the width and the origin of the histogram we obtain a different view of the data. By using the kernel density estimator we smooth out the data. The researcher must specify the *kernel* type to smooth the data to follow a specific distribution and the *bandwidth* corresponding to the width of the histograms used in forming the frequency tables of the data. Often one uses normal kernel by specifying in the program $(k = n)$. The bandwidth is set by the standard parameter c which by default is 1. If the bandwidth is too small, the estimated density is undersmoothed and introduces unnecessary detail. If the bandwidth is too large, the density is oversmoothed and hides some important details. The *mean integrated squared error (MISE)* and *asymptotic mean integrated squared error (AMISE)* are commonly used to determine the appropriate bandwidth. For further details, see Silverman (1986). For the data given in

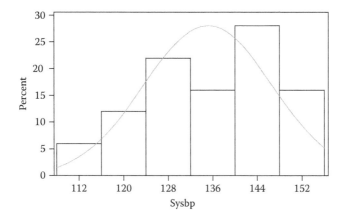

FIGURE 6.2
Histogram and fitted normal density.

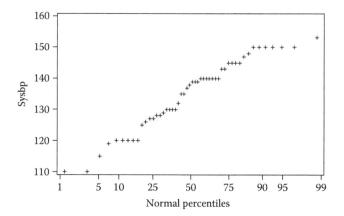

FIGURE 6.3
Normal probability plot.

Section 6.3.1 we will use the following program to get the nonparametric density estimate.

```
/***Data from previous section***/
data a1;set a; proc univariate; var sysbp;
  histogram sysbp/kernel (k=n c=1);
* If one uses the option C=MISE, the bandwidth that minimizes
  AMISE is obtained; run;
```

We can change c to 2 or 3 to make the curve in Figure 6.6 to become wider. We can see that this curve is similar to that in Figure 6.2. If we change $c = 1$ to c = MISE in our program, the graph is still similar to Figures 6.6 and 6.2.

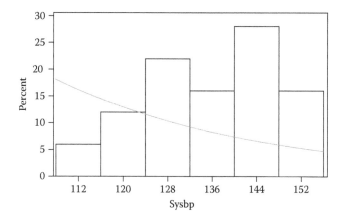

FIGURE 6.4
Histogram and fitted exponential density.

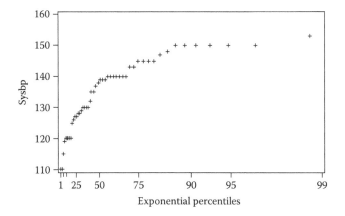

FIGURE 6.5
Exponential probability plot.

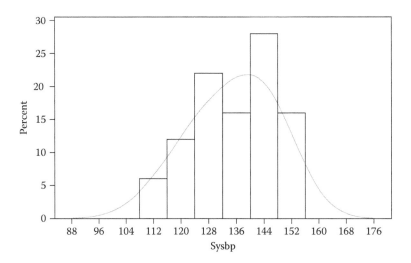

FIGURE 6.6
Histogram with a *normal kernel* density estimate.

6.3.3 Bivariate Kernel Estimator

We will now consider a bivariate kernel density estimator. We need to specify the kernel type and the bandwidth for each of the two variables. Let us take the systolic blood pressure data given in Section 6.3.1 and for those subjects let the following be the diastolic blood pressure measurements.

60	61	95	69	80	70	90	65	75	90
69	68	88	79	90	60	80	59	65	80

```
70  71  80  76  85  82  79  90  68  85
75  79  75  85  75  89  88  85  92  88
90  85  84  85  80  90  90  78  76  87
```

The following programming lines provide the bivariate density estimate:

```
data a; input sysbp@@; cards;
110   120   130   115   125   135   150   140   148   137   120   139   147
143   127   126   145   150   139   130   130   140   132   153   145   120
150   128   140   128   140   138   135   129   143   120   140   130   145
150   150   140   139   145   150   120   110   119   140   127
;
data a;set a; subject = _n_; proc sort;by subject; run;
data b; input diasbp@@; cards;
60   61   95   69   80   70   90   65   75   90   69   68   88   79   90   60   80
59   65   80   70   71   80   76   85   82   79   90   68   85   75   79   75   85
75   89   88   85   92   88   90   85   84   85   80   90   90   78   76   87
;
data b;set b; subject = _n_; proc sort;by subject; run;
data final;merge a b;by subject;
data anno;retain ysys xsys '2' function 'SYMBOL' test 'CIRCLE';
y = sysbp; x = diasbp;run; proc kde data = final; bivar sysbp
  diasbp/bivstats levels percentiles unistats; run;
proc kde data = final out = final1; var sysbp diasbp;run;
proc gcontour data = final1;plot sysbp*diasbp = density/
  nlevels = 5 nolegend annotate = anno; * by removing no legend
  from the programming line provides the density along the
  contours; run;
```

Univariate Statistics

	sysbp	diasbp
Mean	135	79.10
Variance	129	92.30
Std deviation	11.37	9.61
Range	43.00	36.00
Interquartile range	18.00	17.00
Bandwidth	5.92	5.01

Bivariate Statistics

Covariance	9.87
Correlation	0.090

Percentiles

	sysbp	diasbp
0.5	110	59.00
1.0	110	59.00
2.5	110	60.00
5.0	115	60.00
10.0	120	65.00

```
              25.0        127       71.00
              50.0        139       80.00
              75.0        145       88.00
              90.0        150       90.00
              95.0        150       90.00
              97.5        150       92.00
              99.0        153       95.00
              99.5        153       95.00
```

		Levels			
Percent	Density	Lower for sysbp	Upper for sysbp	Lower for diasbp	Upper for diasbp
1	0.000140	110	153	59.00	95.00
5	0.000171	110	153	59.00	95.00
10	0.000257	113	153	60.22	95.00
50	0.000756	122	151	67.54	90.73
90	0.001008	137	146	74.25	85.85
95	0.001019	138	146	74.86	85.85
99	0.001059	140	144	77.31	82.19
100	0.001065	142	142	79.75	79.75

The output shows the summary statistics for each of the two variables and also the correlation between the variables. The percentage of observations beyond the levels of each variable are also provided. Figure 6.7 shows the bivariate distribution for the systolic and diastolic blood pressure variables. Points on the same contour provide the same probability of having systolic and diastolic blood pressures.

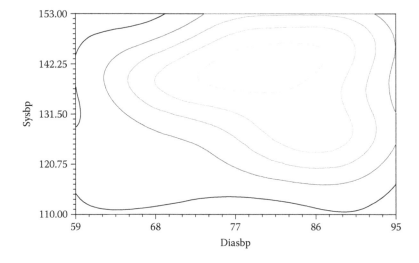

FIGURE 6.7
Estimated bivariate density for systolic and diastolic blood pressures.

6.4 Robust Estimators

When the data contain outliers (very large or very small observations compared to the observations of the main body of the data), the estimators discussed in Chapter 1 do not represent the parameters they are estimating. In that case we use robust estimators that are not affected by the outliers. Some of the commonly used robust estimators are M-, L-, and R-estimators using the ranked observations or the ranks of the observations. Discussion of these estimators is beyond the scope of this book and readers with very strong mathematical background can refer to Huber (1981).

In this section we discuss some robust estimators of location and scale. Consider a random sample of 10 employees in a job with ages

   35, 40, 37, 42, 36, 38, 39, 65, 40, 38

The PROC UNIVARIATE of Chapter 1 gives the estimate of the mean as 41 and the standard deviation as 8.68. Looking at the data one can easily note that 8.68 is not representing the variability of the data because the data contain the outlier age 65. If 65 is removed from the data, the standard deviation is clearly much less than 8.68. In this case, we need to get robust estimators of location and scale. The following program provides the required robust estimators as output.

```
Data a;
/***Input data***/
Input Age @@; Cards;
35  36  37  38  38  39  40  40  42  65
;
/***end of input data***/
proc univariate trimmed = 2 winsorized = .2 robustscale; var
  age;run;
```

```
Basic Statistical Measures
        Location                              Variability
Mean              41.00000        Std deviation              8.67948
Median            38.50000 (c1)   Variance                  75.33333
Mode              38.00000        Range                     30.00000
                                  Interquartile range        3.00000
```

Note: The mode displayed is the smallest of two modes with a count of 2.
                                      ★★★

		Trimmed Means		
Percent	Number		Std error	
Trimmed	Trimmed	Trimmed	Trimmed	
in Tail	in Tail	Mean	Mean	95% Confidence Limits
20.00	2 (c3)	38.66667 (c2)	0.739369	36.76606 (c4) 40.56728 (c5)

```
                        Winsorized Means

Percent        Number                    Std error
Winsorized  Winsorized Winsorized Winsorized   95% Confidence
in Tail      in Tail     Mean       Mean           Limits
20.00          2(c7)    38.60000   0.768375   36.62483   40.57517
                        (c6)                   (c8)       (c9)

                    The UNIVARIATE Procedure

                        Variable: Age
                  Robust Measures of Scale
Measure                          Value      Estimate of Sigma(c13)
Interquartile range          3.000000(c10)         2.223903
Gini's mean difference       7.422222(c11)         6.577773
MAD                          1.500000(c12)         2.223900
```

The median 38.5 given at (c1) is a robust estimator of location and was discussed in Chapter 1. The *trimmed mean* 38.7 given at (c2) is a robust estimator of location and is the mean computed after the two smallest observations and two largest observations are deleted. The program lines *trimmed* = 2 indicate that two observations are deleted at each tail of the data and this number of trimmed observations in each tail is shown at (c3) of the output. The trimmed mean 38.7 is slightly smaller than the mean of 41. Approximately 95% CI for the population mean is given in [(c4), (c5)], using the trimmed mean as a robust estimator of the population mean.

The *winsorized mean* 38.6 given at (c6) is also a robust estimator of location and is the mean computed after replacing the k smallest observations with the $(k + 1)$th smallest observation and the k largest observations with the $(k + 1)$th largest observations. In this program we indicate this by showing *wisorized* = 0.2, indicating that $k = 0.2 * 10 = 2$ observations are winsorized at each tail. This is shown at (c7) of the output. The 95% CI for the population mean is given at [(c8), (c9)], based on the winsorized mean as a robust estimator of the population mean.

For symmetric distributions the trimmed means and winsorized means are unbiased estimators of the population mean. However, the sampling distribution of these two means even for large samples is not normal.

The robust estimator for scale is given at (c10), (c11), and (c12). The interquartile range 3.0 given at (c10) is the difference between the third and first quartiles of the data as discussed in Chapter 1. The *Gini's measure* 7.4 given at (c11) is the mean of the absolute difference of every distinct pair of observations. The median absolute deviation from the median (MAD) is 1.5 given at (c12) is the median of all the absolute values of the deviations of the observations from its median. For normal data, these robust estimators provide an estimate for the population standard deviation and these are given in column (c13).

6.5 Jackknife Estimators

In some problems we use biased estimators in the sense that the average value of the estimator in repeated sampling does not equal the parameter estimated. The difference in the average value of the estimator and the parameter is called the bias of the estimator and Tukey provided *Jackknife estimators* to reduce this bias.

Suppose we want to estimate the proportion of people attending a college for at least 1 year in a community. A simple random sample of households will be taken, and in those households the number of people in the house-hold who attended at least 1 year of college is recorded. The ratio of the num-ber of people attending college and the total number of people in the households is used to estimate the necessary proportion. This estimator is called the ratio estimator and is biased. To minimize this bias we use the Jackknife estimator. We illustrate this by providing artificial data in Table 6.7.

```
data a;
input household numpeople college@@; cards;
1  4  2  2  1  1  3  5  3  4  3  1  5  2  2
;
data a1;set a; obs = _n_; *n pairs of observations;
data jackknife;
%macro jackknife(n); data in;set a1;
if obs = &n then delete; proc univariate noprint;var numpeople
   college;
output out = stats&n sum = sumnumpeople sumcollege n = n; run;
%mend jackkinfe;
data call;
%jackknife(0); %jackknife(1); %jackknife(2);
%jackknife(3); %jackknife(4); %jackknife(5);
*Do until the nth paired observation;
*One subject is dropped each time;
data final;set stats0 stats1 stats2 stats3 stats4 stats5;
*update according to the maximum number of paired
   observations;
r = sumcollege/sumnumpeople;obs = _n_;
data finalone;set final; if _n_ = 1; a = 1; keep n r a;
   proc sort;by a;
```

TABLE 6.7

Number of People in the Household Attending College

Household	1	2	3	4	5
Number of people	4	1	5	3	2
Number of people attending college for at least 1 year	2	1	3	1	2

```
data final2;set final; if obs = 1 then delete;
proc univariate noprint;var r;output out = final3 mean = meanrj;
data final6;set final3;  a = 1; proc sort;by a;
data final0;merge finalone final6;by a;
rjackknife = r*n- (n-1) *meanrj; keep r rjackknife;
  proc print;run;
```

```
  R        RJackknife
  0.6      0.58966
```

We note that the standard estimator is $R = 0.6$ and the bias reducing jack-knife estimator is Rjackknife = 0.58966.

6.6 Bootstrap Method

For some of the estimators we use, the standard error may not be in a nice neat mathematical expression and we need to find the standard error of such estimators. For this purpose, the *bootstrap method* developed by Efron (1979) is very useful. There are parametric and nonparametric bootstrap methods and we will briefly describe the nonparametric method. We take repeated samples from the original sample of the same size with replacement and the variance of these estimators is the necessary variance of the original estimator.

Returning to the example of Section 6.5, the variance of the ratio estimator is not in a compact form and the following program provides the standard error of the ratio estimator R by using the Bootstrap method with 200 repeated samples. Usually, 200 repeated samples are taken to obtain the bootstrap estimator.

```
data a;
%let replicate = 200;*replicate = 200, the number of repeated
  samples;
%let unit = 5;*unit = the number of original sample size (number
  of house holds);
proc plan seed = 100;
factors replicate = &replicate ordered unit = &unit t = 1 of
  &unit/noprint;
output out = a; run; end; data a;set a;
do j = 1 to &unit;*number of different observations;
output;end; keep replicate t unit j;
data a1;set a; drop unit; proc sort;by replicate j;
data a2;set a;
keep replicate j unit; proc sort;by replicate j unit;
data a;merge a1 a2;by replicate j;  proc sort;by replicate j;
  data b;
/***input data***/
```

```
input household numpeople college@@; cards;
1  4  2  2  1  1  3  5  3  4  3  1  5  2  2
;
/***end of input data***/
data b;set b; do i = 1 to &replicate; replicate = i; output;
  end;
data b;set b; keep numpeople college replicate household j;
do j = 1 to &unit; output; end; proc sort; by replicate j;
  data final; merge a b;
by replicate j;  proc sort;by replicate j; data final1;
  set final;
if j = unit;  tkeep = t; keep replicate j tkeep; proc sort;
  by replicate j;
data final2;merge final final1;by replicate j; if
  tkeep = household; proc sort;
by replicate; proc univariate noprint;var numpeople college;
output out = stats sum = sumnumpeople sumcollege n = n;
  by replicate;
data stats;set stats; r = sumcollege/sumnumpeople;
proc univariate noprint;var r; output out = stats1 n = n
  mean = meanr std = std; run;
data stats1;set stats1; proc print;run;
```

The output is

```
    n     meanr      Std
   200   0.61076   0.096866
```

From the above output, we note that the standard deviation of the ratio estimate is 0.096866. The mean*r* is the mean of the 200 sample means using simple random samples with replacement, from a finite population with mean 0.6.

6.7 Propensity Scores

Given a set of covariates for two groups of individuals the *propensity score* gives the conditional probability that an individual with given covariates belongs to a specific group. Let us consider the two groups as treatment and control groups. From the logistic regression model with the covariates as independent variables and the treatment group as a dependent variable, the predicted probability that the unit with the specified covariates belongs to the treatment group is the propensity score. This score is useful in three settings such as matching, forming subclassification, and regression adjustment.

Let us consider a study with a treatment and control arm. We recognize that the subjects may have different baseline covariates such as age, smoking history, hypertension, high cholesterol, A1C, and so on. The comparison of the treatment and control groups needs to balance over the covariates. In Table 6.8, we give the artificial data of the covariates and treatment group.

The following program provides the necessary output for classifying the units into five groups using quantile partitioning.

```
data a;input subject treatment age smoker hypertension
  cholesterol A1c@@; cards;
1  1  60  1  1  1  7  2  1  55  1  0  1  7.5  3  1  81  0  1  1  7  4
1  63  0  0  1  10  5  1  50  0  1  0  8  6  1  69  1  0  0  7  7  1
71  0  1  1  10  8  1  59  1  0  1  9  9  1  45  1  1  1  9  10  1
60  0  1  1  10  11  1  58  0  0  1  11  12  1  62  1  0  0  7  13
1  55  1  0  1  7  14  1  68  1  0  0  8  15  1  59  0  1  1  6.5
16  1  71  0  1  0  7.5  17  1  78  0  1  1  6.5  18  1  45  1  0  1
7  19  1  71  0  1  1  7.5  20  1  65  1  1  0  8  21  0  75  1  0
0  7.5  22  0  40  0  1  0  6.5  23  0  64  1  0  1  7.5  24  0  56
1  0  1  6.5  25  0  66  0  0  1  7  26  0  39  1  1  1  7.5  27  0
75  1  1  0  7  28  0  46  1  1  0  11  29  0  70  1  0  1  8.5  30
0  78  0  0  0  8  31  0  65  1  0  0  9  32  0  35  0  0  0  6.5
33  0  59  1  1  1  7  34  0  49  1  1  0  7  35  0  71  1  0  1  10
36  0  47  1  0  1  7.5  37  0  39  0  0  0  10  38  0  35  1  0  1
11  39  0  64  0  1  1  11  40  0  55  0  0  1  7
;
data a;set a; proc logistic descending noprint;
model treatment = age smoker hypertension cholesterol a1c;
  output out = a2 pred = pred; proc rank groups = 5
out = score; ranks blocks; var pred;
data block;set score; keep blocks subject; proc sort;by blocks
  subject;
proc transpose out = block1;by blocks; data block1;set block1;
rename col1-col8= subject1-subject8; drop _name_;
  proc print;run;
```

The following is the output indicating the five groups of patients in the five lines.

				blocks				
0	12	18	28	31	32	36	37	38
1	2	6	8	13	14	21	22	34
2	5	9	11	20	23	24	26	40
3	1	4	25	27	29	30	33	35
4	3	7	10	15	16	17	19	39

We will now use the above five blocks corresponding to the quantile partitioning of the propensity scores. The response data on the treatments and control will now be analyzed from these five blocks formed by the propensity scores, using the CMH method or GLM or any other method. It may be noted that any number of blocks can be formed using propensity scores. For further details, refer D'Agostino (1998).

TABLE 6.8

Baseline Covariates

Subject	Treatment (1 = Drug, 0 = Control)	Age (Years)	Smoker (1 = Yes, 0 = No)	Hypertension (1 = Yes, 0 = No)	High Cholesterol (1 = Yes, 0 = No)	A1C
1	1	60	1	1	1	7
2	1	55	1	0	1	7.5
3	1	81	0	1	1	7
4	1	63	0	0	1	10
5	1	50	0	1	0	8
6	1	69	1	0	0	7
7	1	71	0	1	1	10
8	1	59	1	0	1	9
9	1	45	1	1	1	9
10	1	60	0	1	1	10
11	1	58	0	0	1	11
12	1	62	1	0	0	7
13	1	55	1	0	1	7
14	1	68	1	0	0	8
15	1	59	0	1	1	6.5
16	1	71	0	1	0	7.5
17	1	78	0	1	1	6.5
18	1	45	1	0	1	7
19	1	71	0	1	1	7.5
20	1	65	1	1	0	8
21	0	75	1	0	0	7.5
22	0	40	0	1	0	6.5
23	0	64	1	0	1	7.5
24	0	56	1	0	1	6.5
25	0	66	0	0	1	7
26	0	39	1	1	1	7.5
27	0	75	1	1	0	7
28	0	46	1	1	0	11
29	0	70	1	0	1	8.5
30	0	78	0	0	0	8
31	0	65	1	0	0	9
32	0	35	0	0	0	6.5
33	0	59	1	1	1	7
34	0	49	1	1	0	7
35	0	71	1	0	1	10
36	0	47	1	0	1	7.5
37	0	39	0	0	0	10
38	0	35	1	0	1	11
39	0	64	0	1	1	11
40	0	55	0	0	1	7

6.8 Interim Analysis and Stopping Rules

Usually many clinical trials take a long time to complete. To obtain a quick decision whether the trial is going to be successful or not, analyses are performed several times before the trial is completed. The analysis performed during a trial is called *interim analysis*.

Let us consider a trial with m interim analyses, where the final analysis is based on the entire data. The total number of subjects for the trial is n. Let the ith interim analysis be based on n_i subjects and let $t_i = n_i/n$ for $i = 1, 2, ..., m$. The symbol t_i is known as the time information factor. Let Z_i be the standardized normal distribution statistic used to test the hypothesis at the ith interim analysis. The significance level, α, now satisfies for all the m interim analyses

$$\Pr(Z_1 \geq c_1, \text{ or } Z_2 \geq c_2, \text{ or } ..., Z_m \geq c_m \,|\, H_0) = \alpha.$$

This equation is equivalent to

$$\sum_{i=1}^{m} \Pr\left\{ Z_i \geq c; Z_j < c, j \leq i-1 \,|\, H_0 \right\} = \alpha.$$

Here

$$c_i = \left(\frac{c}{\sqrt{t_i}} \right), \quad i = 1, 2, ..., m.$$

The statistical problem of interest is to determine the c_is and c, and will be discussed in Section 6.8.1.

6.8.1 Stopping Rules

Letting $\Pr(Z_1 \geq c_1, \text{ or } Z_2 \geq c_2, \text{ or } ..., Z_i \geq c_i \,|\, H_0) = \alpha(t_i)$, we have $\Pr(Z_1 < c_1, \text{ or } Z_2 < c_2, \text{ or } ..., Z_{i-1} < c_{i-1}, Z_i \geq c_i \,|\, H_0) = \alpha(t_i) - \alpha(t_{i-1})$. This problem of finding the boundaries was considered by Pocock (1977), O'Brien and Fleming (1979), Lan and DeMets (1983), and others. Lan and DeMets introduced the idea of *alpha spending function* and many of these boundaries are particular cases of that spending function. The boundaries c_i obtained by Pocock satisfy

$$\alpha_i = \alpha(t_i) = \alpha \ln(1 + (e-1)t_i), \quad i = 1, 2, ..., m,$$

and the boundaries obtained by O'Brien and Fleming satisfy

$$\alpha_i = \alpha(t_i) = 2 - 2\Phi\left(\frac{Z_{\alpha/2}}{\sqrt{t_i}} \right), \quad i = 1, 2, ..., m.$$

The boundaries of Pocock are all the same, whereas the boundaries given by O'Brien and Fleming are not all the same. When using *Pocock boundaries*, if the trial does not stop early, this boundary pays a high penalty for the final analysis. *O'Brien and Fleming's bounds* have smaller α_i in the early stages and large α_i at the later stages. Since this method pays a high penalty in the beginning of the study, it may be difficult to stop the trial early. However, at the final analysis, little penalty is paid. The critical values c_i have to be found by numerical integration of the density functions. Geller and Pocock (1987) gave the spending function of α_i for level of significance of 0.05 and 0.1, and the critical values of c_i for different stopping rules for 2–5 stages in their Table 1a and b.

According to them for $\alpha = 0.05$, Pocock's boundaries and spending function

for $m = 2$ are $\alpha_1 = 029$, $c_1 = 2.178$; $\alpha_2 = 0.029$, $c_2 = 2.178$, and

for $m = 3$ are $\alpha_1 = 0.022$, $c_1 = 2.289$; $\alpha_2 = 0.022$, $c_2 = 2.289$, $\alpha_3 = 0.022$, $c_3 = 2.289$.

For $\alpha = 0.05$, O'Brien and Flemming's boundaries and spending function

for $m = 2$ are $\alpha_1 = 0.005$, $c_1 = 2.797$; $\alpha_2 = 0.048$, $c_2 = 1.977$, and

for $m = 3$ are $\alpha_1 = 0.0005$, $c_1 = 3.471$; $\alpha_2 = 0.014$, $c_2 = 2.454$, $\alpha_3 = 0.045$, $c_3 = 2.004$.

To use these boundaries, the t_is must be equally spaced. For further details, refer to Jennison and Turnbull (2000).

6.8.2 Conditional Power

Conditional power is the probability that the study will be successful at the final analysis based on data observed in the first part of the study. This approach was described by Lan and Wittes (1988).

Let us consider N subjects for a clinical study comparing a drug to placebo. Suppose we are having an interim analysis with n subjects. Then $t = n/N$ be the amount of information. Of the n subjects, let approximately $n/2$ belong to the drug and placebo groups. Let $\bar{X}$ and $\bar{Y}$ be the means for the drug and placebo at the time of the interim analysis.

Let μ_1 and μ_2 be the effects of the drug and placebo, respectively. Let $\delta = (\mu_1 - \mu_2)/\sigma$. We are testing the null hypothesis that $\mu_1 = \mu_2$. At the end of the trial, we expect to have $N/2$ subjects to the treatment and placebo groups and the test statistic for the final analysis is a two-sample Z test.

By using the information available at the interim analysis the conditional power is calculated to determine if the trial is a success by assuming the two alternatives:

1. The current observed trend should be assumed for the remaining part of the study or
2. The alternative hypothesis in the originally outlined expected rates, in the remaining part of the study.

Let us assume that we are starting our study with a drug and placebo to test that the effects are the same for diastolic blood pressure. The sample sizes are determined by assuming under the alternative that $\mu_1 = 87$ and $\mu_2 = 80$ where μ_1 and μ_2 are the means for the placebo and drug. Let the standard deviation of the blood pressure of both the groups be 15. Let us assume that we are using a 0.05-level test and expect the power of 0.8. The sample sizes in both groups are assumed to be equal. The program in Section 3.2.1.1 gives $N/2 = 73$. Suppose an interim analysis is planned with 74 subjects, 37 in each of the two groups. Let $\bar{X} = 100$ and $\bar{Y} = 95$. We would like to calculate the conditional power under the two types of alternatives as mentioned earlier. The following program provides this output:

```
data a;
/***input data***/
*input information for interim analysis;
mu1 = 87;*hypothesized mean for placebo; mu2 = 80;*hypothesized
  mean for drug;
xmean = 100;*sample mean for placebo; ymean = 95;*sample mean
  for drug;
sigma = 15; alpha = .05;*final alpha value;
n1 = 37;* sample size at interim analysis for placebo;
n2 = 37;*sample size at interim analysis for drug;
totaln = 146;*total sample size for trial;
/***end of input data***/

n = n1 + n2; t = n/totaln; estimated_delta = (xmean-ymean)/sigma;
delta = (mu1 - mu2)/sigma; theta = (delta*sqrt(totaln))/2;
z_n = ((xmean - ymean)*(sqrt(n)))/(2*sigma);
b_t = z_n*sqrt(t); zalpha = probit(1 - alpha/2);
current_trend = 1 - probnorm((zalpha-b_t/t)/(sqrt(1-t)));
alt_hyp = 1 - probnorm( (zalpha - b_t -((1-t)*theta))/(sqrt(1-t)));
proc print;var current_trend alt_hyp; run;
```

current_trend	alt_hyp
0.53058	0.73970

On the basis of the above output, the conditional power from the current trend and postulated alternative hypothesis are 0.53 and 0.74, respectively, and the completed study is expected to be a success. Generally, a conditional power of 10–20% or less assuming current trend and 50% or less assuming alternative hypothesis indicate futility, and the study may be terminated at the interim analysis stage.

6.9 Microarrays and Multiple Testing

6.9.1 Microarrays

Currently, researchers are interested in identifying the genes between the normal subjects and people with some disease. For this purpose, the genes of normal people and people with a disease will be put on Affymetrix gene chips and using two colors of dye to determine the gene expressions. On these chips several thousands of genes can be compared for the expressions. There is a lot of noise in these expressions and the researchers have to normalize the data to remove the nonbiological variation and provide the required gene expression.

When several gene expressions are available for a particular gene between the normal subjects and people with a disease, the standard *t*-test or Wilcoxon rank-sum test are performed to determine the genes with different expressions between normal subjects and people with a disease. In this process we need to perform several tests of significance, and controlling *family-wise error rate (FWER)* or test-wise error rate will not adequately protect the level of significance for the overall significance of the genes. At present, *multiple testing procedures* are developing and they protect the level of significance for testing all the genes. We will discuss one of these methods in Section 6.9.2. It may be noted that if multiple observations are not available (i.e., sample size 1) because the disease is a rare disease, Ding and Raghavarao (2008) developed a method for testing the significance of the genes where only one replicate is available for people with the disease.

6.9.2 Multiple Testing

In Section 3.3.1, we considered FWER in multiple comparisons setting. We come across testing several null hypotheses, and in that case, FWER will not adequately protect the level of significance. To this end, several multiple testing procedures have been developed in the last decade and we will discuss the Benjamini and Hochberg (1995) method of controlling *False Discovery Rate (FDR)*. FDR is the fraction of false rejections of the null hypotheses in the set of rejected null hypotheses. To control this, Benjamini and Hochberg gave a step-down method of sequentially testing the null hypotheses and drawing conclusions for independent *p*-values. Suppose we have m null hypotheses and let $p_1, p_2, ..., p_m$ be the *p*-values for the m tests. The ordered *p*-values are $p_{(1)} \leq p_{(2)} \leq ... \leq p_{(m)}$. The null hypotheses corresponding to the ordered *p*-values are $H_{0(1)}, H_{0(2)}, ..., H_{0(m)}$. The null hypotheses $H_{0(1)}, H_{0(2)}, ..., H_{0(i)}, i \leq m$ are rejected if i is maximum satisfying

$$p_{(i)} \leq \frac{i\alpha}{m},$$

where α is the overall level of significance. To achieve this, first $p_{(m)}$ will be compared with α and if $p_{(m)}$ is less than or equal to α, all m hypotheses are rejected. If not, $p_{(m-1)}$ will be compared with $(m-1)\alpha/m$ and if it is less than or equal to α, then $H_{0(1)}, H_{0(2)}, ..., H_{0(m-1)}$ are rejected; otherwise, $p_{(m-2)}$ will be compared with $(m-2)\alpha/m$, and so on. This is a step-down procedure of testing the null hypotheses. Under very general conditions this method controls

FDR at the α level, whatever be the truth or false of the null hypotheses $H_{0(1)}$, $H_{0(2)}$, ..., $H_{0(m)}$.

Consider the 20 p-values given below:

0.0910,	0.6912,	0.0017,	0.0340,	0.4984,	0.0245,
0.3456,	0.0950,	0.0278,	0.5123,	0.0763,	0.0043,
0.0023,	0.0204,	0.0982,	0.0901,	0.0117,	0.0690,
0.0142,	0.0005				

We will now give the program and output for rejecting the null hypotheses.

```
data a; input Raw_p @@; cards;
0.0910 0.6912 0.0017 0.0340 0.4984 0.0245 0.3456 0.0950 0.0278 0.5123
0.0763 0.0043 0.0023 0.0204 0.0982 0.0901 0.0117 0.0690 0.0142 0.0005
;
data a1;set a; proc sort;by raw_p; proc multtest pdata=a1 fdr; run;
```

The output is

The Multitest Procedure

p-Values

Test	Raw	False Discovery Rate
1	0.0005	0.0100
2	0.0017	0.0153
3	0.0023	0.0153
4	0.0043	0.0215
5	0.0117	0.0468
6	0.0142 (d2)	0.0473 (d1)
7	0.0204	0.0583
8	0.0245	0.0613
9	0.0278	0.0618
10	0.0340	0.0680
11	0.0690	0.1227
12	0.0763	0.1227
13	0.0901	0.1227
14	0.0910	0.1227
15	0.0950	0.1227
16	0.0982	0.1227
17	0.3456	0.4066
18	0.4984	0.5393
19	0.5123	0.5393
20	0.6912	0.6912

The FDR is bounded above by $np_{(i)}/i$ and hence looking at the column for FDR in the output we reject all the null hypotheses before the FDR reaches the α-value 0.05 and it is not less than 0.05 afterward. It should be noted that an FDR may be less than 0.05 for one test and the next may be more than 0.05 and less than 0.05 for another test. In our example, the FDR is less than 0.05 that occurs at (d1) and it is not less than 0.05 afterward. Thus, we reject all the null hypotheses with p-values ≤ 0.0142 corresponding to the FDR 0.0473. The value 0.0142 is given at (d2), in the same row as (d1).

6.10 Stability of Products

We observe that every drug manufactured and all perishable products we eat carry an expiration date. We will now discuss how the expiration date is calculated for the drugs to meet the requirements of the FDA. FDA recommends that under all storage conditions the product's potency is determined over a period of time and for the degradation curves 95% confidence lower bounds are calculated. The expiration date is the acceptable limit of the potency on the confidence bound. FDA put forth guidelines for the stability studies. It is required that three batches of the product under different conditions should be tested for potency in 3-month interval for the first year, 6-month interval for the second year, annually for the third year, and onward. The slopes for the degradation curves are determined for each of the three batches and if the slopes are not significant, the three batches will be combined and the expiration date is calculated. If the slopes for the three batches are different, the expiration date is determined for each batch and the smallest limit is the expiration date. Inclusion of all factors that affect the potency of the drug will involve substantial cost both in terms of direct product costs and experimental assay costs. To reduce these costs and time, matrixing and bracketing is allowed by the FDA. In *matrix designs* a fraction of all possible factor combinations are tested at a given sampling time. All chosen factor combinations are tested initially and at the end of long-term testing. With *bracketing*, the extreme levels for each factor are tested instead of testing at all the levels of the factor. The design issues and details are briefly discussed by DeWoody and Altan (2001).

6.11 Group Testing

When the blood tests are carried out providing a positive or negative test result, we can save time and money by pooling some samples and testing the pooled blood sample for positive or negative results. If the pooled blood sample gives a negative result, each of the blood samples included in the pool provides negative results. If the pooled blood sample gives a positive result, at least one of the blood samples in that pool gives a positive test result. This idea was first used by Dorfman (1943) in testing the military recruits for syphilis in the World War II.

The *group testing* can be done *sequentially* and *nonsequentially*. In the sequential group testing procedure, the tests are performed one after another using the information provided by the preceding test on the succeeding test. Professor Milton Sobel is a pioneer in developing the group testing procedures. The main theme here is to test all the samples first and if the first test result is positive, then split the samples into two equal groups and test again until the split samples test result is negative.

This procedure, at the end, will identify every blood sample included in the test to be either positive or negative.

The nonsequential procedure is also called a *nonadaptive group testing procedure*. In this, different groups of samples are made and tested simultaneously to identify the positive or negative result on each sample. If one knows the number of positive samples before starting the testing procedure, the procedure is called *hypergeometric nonadaptive group testing procedure*. If the number of positive samples is unknown, the procedure is called *binomial nonadaptive group testing procedure*. Du and Hwang (1993) extensively discussed this topic, and Raghavarao and Padgett (2005) discussed these results in the context of block designs.

We will provide an illustration of this procedure and the interested reader may look at the above books for further details.

Consider six samples $S_1, S_2, \ldots, S_6$ and let us consider the tests based on test1 $= (S_1, S_2, S_3)$; test2 $= (S_1, S_4, S_5)$; test3 $= (S_2, S_4, S_6)$; test4 $= (S_3, S_5, S_6)$. Assume that one of the six samples is positive. Table 6.9 provides the outcomes.

If it is known that only one sample gives a negative result, among the six samples, without testing all the six samples separately, the results provided in the four tests can be used to identify the negative sample by using the information provided in Table 6.9. It may be noted that the procedure given above will not give only one positive and three negative test results. This method uses only four tests for testing six samples and cuts the cost and time of experimentation.

6.12 Correspondence Analysis

Correspondence analysis is similar to the principal component analysis and factor analysis. This is primarily used for contingency tables to find the clustering of the rows (columns) having similar profiles across the columns

TABLE 6.9

Identifying Positive Test Sample

Positive Sample	Positive Tests	Negative Tests
S_1	test1,test2	test3, test4
S_2	test1,test3	test2,test4
S_3	test1,test4	test2,test3
S_4	test2,test3	test1,test4
S_5	test2,test4	test1,test3
S_6	test3,test4	test1,test2

(rows). This is a graphic representation and is visually examined to identify the association between the rows and columns. It should be noted that this does not involve any hypothesis testing.

Consider a market research situation in which four brands of refrigerators A, B, C, and D with colors maroon, black, white, gray, and gold are sold per year from a large store. The data are given in Table 6.10.

The following program provides the necessary output as a graph.

```
data brand;
input maroon black white grey gold brand $ @@;
cards;
100  60  150  50  90  a  50  30  105  40  10  b
125  45  140  60  80  c  55  35  80   45  55  d
;
proc corresp data = brand out = outdata short;
var maroon black white grey gold;
id brand;run;
%plotit (data = outdata,  datatype = corresp,  plotvars = Dim1
  Dim2);run;
```

From the graph (Figure 6.8), brands A and D seem to have a similar color for the brand profile as indicated by the closeness of their points. Brand B has an entirely different profile compared to the other three brands. White and gray have similar profiles of brands. Gold has an entirely different brand

TABLE 6.10

Sales Data for Brand and Colors of Refrigerators

Brand	Maroon	Black	White	Gray	Gold
A	100	60	150	50	90
B	50	30	105	40	10
C	125	45	140	60	80
D	55	35	80	45	55

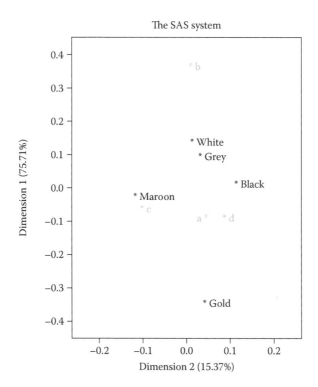

FIGURE 6.8
Graph of brands and colors.

profile compared to the other four colors. Brand C seems to be exclusively associated with the color maroon. The percentages shown on the x and y axis are the percentages of the χ^2 test of goodness of fit.

For further details, refer to Greenacre (1984) and Van der Heijden and de Leeuw (1985).

6.13 Classification Regression Trees

To make a prediction on a response variable using 1 or more predictor variables, classification and regression trees (CARTs) (Brieman et al., 1984) are used. The popularity of using this method for data mining arises due to its simple interpretation of the results based on a decision tree. When distributional assumptions are used, the predictions can be made by discriminant analysis, logistic regression, or multiple regression. However, CART achieves this prediction by graphical representation without any distributional assumptions. The advantage of using CART is that outliers are not affected. Transformations made to these data will not change the tree structure. A disadvantage of this method is that the tree shape can change based on the sample size selected (instability of the tree).

If the response variable is categorical, then we get classification trees, and when it is continuous, we get regression trees. One first uses historical data (learning sample) to construct the decision trees. These decision trees are based on rules that split the data based on predictor variables. The tree starts from the root and branches are created based on the split. Many branches can be used, but most researchers prefer to use two branches. The leaves of the tree are the terminal nodes (nodes that will not be split). These split nodes have the maximum homogeneity among all the possible variables based on impurity functions. The impurity function finds a split at each node that generates the greatest improvement in predictive accuracy. This process is then repeated. Gini's function is the commonly used impurity function for classification trees, and for the regression tree, the split uses the squared residuals minimization algorithm which is similar to the Gini method. The size of the tree is very critical. If one keeps splitting the tree, one will obtain the maximum tree; however, one should note that by splitting the tree into many levels one may be overfitting the tree. This tree can be very complex and may not be the optimal tree. If the tree is small, then you may not be able to make good classifications since the data may not fit well.

One approach so as not to create over-fitted trees is to create stopping rules. This may include creating any new splits if the overall prediction is improved minimally, or if the researcher feels that the impurity is low enough. One should note that by using the stopping rules the optimal tree may not be obtained. There is a trade-off between the impurity measure and the number of levels of a tree. As the impurity measure increases, the terminal nodes decrease, and with a maximum tree the impurity measure is 0 with a maximum number of nodes.

As an alternative to stopping rules, some researchers create a larger tree and then prune the tree back to create a simpler, more optimal tree. This tree can be pruned by withholding some of the learning sample data. The tree can be pruned by using cross-validation. In cross-validation one also has another independent set of observations different from the learning sample, and if the prediction for this sample is good then one can infer that the selected tree is making satisfactory predictions.

Suppose we are interested to predict whether the second-year undergraduate students will graduate at the end of the fourth year of the program. Let I and II denote their completion or noncompletion of the degree requirements at the end of the fourth year. We use the predictor variables A: SAT score >1000, B: at least 20 h per week on a job, C: GPA at the end of the second year is > 2.7, D: Age at the admission is <20 years. The form of the decision tree is shown in Figure 6.9.

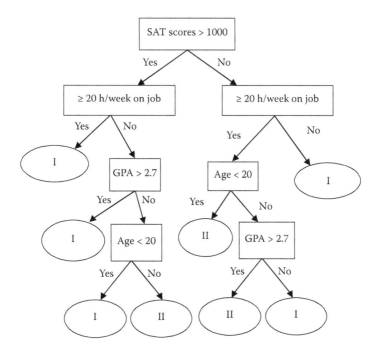

FIGURE 6.9
Decision tree for Completion I and Noncompletion II of degree requirements.

This tree has eight leaves and five levels and can be converted to a set of rules. For example,

If the SAT scores <1000 and work <20 h, then the students graduate.

If the SAT scores >1000 and work at least 20 h, then the students graduate.

If the SAT scores ≤1000 and work ≥20 h with age <20 years, then the student does not graduate.

Other methods have also been developed (Loh and Shih, 1997) like QUEST (Quick Unbiased Efficient Statistical Tree). An extension of the CART is known as random forest. Here many classification trees are grown using a probabilistic scheme where each tree gives a classification (Brieman, 2001).

6.14 Multidimensional Scaling

Multidimensional scaling (MDS) is used in marketing, psychology, sociology, and other areas to group similar objects based on distance or *similarity*

(*dissimilarity*) measure. It is similar to principal components, factor, and cluster analysis. This technique involves visual representation of the data so that the clustering of the objects can be identified. The data are usually represented in a *two-dimensional grid* which can be orientated in any way, to make meaningful interpretation. One can increase the number of dimensions, but it should be noted that with more dimensions the graph becomes more complicated to comprehend. However, in certain situations the extra dimensions are needed as there may be a lack of fit in the two dimensions. In this grid, objects that seem similar (dissimilar) are placed near (far away) each other. It should be noted that this method does not involve any hypothesis testing.

A *similarity matrix* is the similarity (distance) between the (i, j) objects. One can also use the distances between the objects in the similarity matrix. The diagonal element of the similarity matrix is 1 when similarity measures are used and 0 when the distance is used. Instead of a similarity matrix a dissimilarity matrix can also be used to plot the data. Similarities of qualitative (quantitative) data are referred to as *nonmetric* (*metric*) MDS.

The *stress function* is a measure of goodness of fit and is an indicator of how well the graph fits the data. It ranges from 0 to 1. A large positive stress implies insufficient dimensionality in the fit. As the number of dimensions increase, the stress will not increase, and using $n-1$ dimensions with n objects the stress function will be 0. Usually the stress should be under 0.15, and if it is less than 0.1, then the graphical fit is considered excellent for the data. In SAS, the stress is the "*badness-of-fit criteria*" and is analogous to residual sums of square in a regression context. For further details, refer to Kruskal and Wish (1978) and the SAS programming details in the SAS manual.

Suppose there are six auto body shops and a researcher is interested in grouping the body shops based on their repair costs. A damaged car was taken to each of the six body shops and the quoted repair costs for the same repair are given below:

$3000; \quad $4000; \quad $2500; \quad $3750; \quad $3500; \quad $2800

The absolute value of the difference in the repair costs are shown in the following similarity matrix.

$$
\begin{bmatrix}
0 & 1000 & 500 & 750 & 500 & 200 \\
1000 & 0 & 1500 & 250 & 500 & 1200 \\
500 & 1500 & 0 & 1750 & 1000 & 300 \\
750 & 250 & 1750 & 0 & 250 & 950 \\
500 & 500 & 1000 & 250 & 0 & 700 \\
200 & 1200 & 300 & 950 & 700 & 0
\end{bmatrix}
$$

The following program provides the visual pattern as the output:

```
data bodyshop;
input (shop_A shop_B shop_C shop_D shop_E shop_F)(5.)
@59 bodyshop $15.; Cards;
0                                    shop_A
1000  0                               shop_B
500   1500  0                          shop_C
750   250   1750  0                     shop_D
500   500   1000  250  0                 shop_E
200   1200  300   950  700  0             shop_F
;
proc mds data = bodyshop level = absolute out = out;
id bodyshop; run;
%plotit(data = out, datatype = mds, labelvar = bodyshop,
vtoh = 1.75, labfont = swissb); run;
```

```
        Multidimensional Scaling: Data = WORK.BODYSHOP.DATA
          Shape = TRIANGLE Condition = MATRIX Level = ABSOLUTE
              Coef = IDENTITY Dimension = 2 Formula = 1 Fit = 1
          Gconverge = 0.01 Maxiter = 100 Over = 1 Ridge = 0.0001
```

Iteration	Type	Badness-of-Fit Criterion	Change in Criterion	Convergence Measure
0	Initial	0.2373	.	0.8685
2	Gau-New	0.1200	0.000864	0.5409
3	Lev-Mar	0.1183	0.001684	0.4166
4	Lev-Mar	0.1166	0.001682	0.3082
5	Lev-Mar	0.1166	0.0000246	0.3420
6	Lev-Mar	0.1155	0.001045	0.1696
7	Lev-Mar	0.1154	0.000177	0.2406
8	Lev-Mar	0.1150	0.000363	0.0774
9	Lev-Mar	0.1150	0.0000321	0.1449
10	Lev-Mar	0.1149	0.000105	0.0231
11	Lev-Mar	0.1148	0.0000156	0.0490
12	Lev-Mar	0.1148 (e1)	8.8068E-6	0.007633

The convergence criterion is satisfied.

From (e1), the badness-of-fit criteria are <0.15 and the graph (Figure 6.10) reasonably explains the data in two dimensions. From the graph we note that the body shops cluster as {A, C, F} and {B, D, E}. The researcher needs to further investigate the reason for this clustering. One should be careful not to find patterns when they do not exist.

6.15 Path Analysis

To study the causal relationships between variables, *path analysis* and *structural equation modeling* (SEM) are used. These are generalizations of multiple

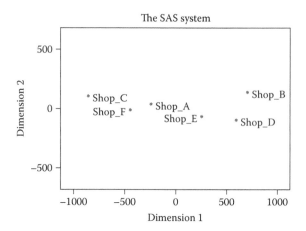

FIGURE 6.10
MDS output of body shops for repair costs.

regression in explaining the relationship. The independent variables are called *exogenous variables* and the dependent variables are called *endogenous variables*. In the multiple regression context, every variable is either exogenous or endogenous, whereas in path analysis, a variable can be both exogenous and endogenous. In path analysis, a variable may have a *direct or indirect effect* on another variable. Path analysis is a precursor to SEM and we will discuss this analysis in this section. For details regarding SEM, the interested reader is referred to Bollen (1989).

Path analysis was originally used in population genetics by Sewall Wright (1921) and for some time it was not widely used. Recently, sociologists, psychologists, economists, and political scientists are using this technique to explain the cause–effect relationships. In path analysis, several multiple regression equations are built in.

For conducting the path analysis one may need raw data on the variables or the variance–covariance matrix or correlation matrix. To get consistent estimates, the data are collected on a large number of units, for example, 200–300.

Suppose a researcher is interested in the price a person is willing to pay in buying his/her car. For this purpose the scientist collects data on home owners and gets responses on the age (V1), education in years (V2), annual income (V3), savings (V4), price of the home (V5), and price the respondent is willing to pay to buy a car (V6). One can take the age and education as exogeneous variables as they are not explained by other variables. The annual income depends on the individual's education and age. Here the endogeneous variable is annual income and is explained by the age and education level of the individual. The home price depends on the annual income of the individual and also the education level of the individual. Similarly, the savings may also depend on the annual income and education level. The price the individual is willing to pay for a car is dependent on the age, price of the home, and the savings. Let us suppose that the researcher collected the data on 300 individuals and formed the following variance and covariance matrix:

$$\begin{bmatrix} 25 & 3.6 & 247.5 & 198 & 39 & 60 \\ 3.6 & 16 & 198 & 86.4 & 36.4 & 36 \\ 247.5 & 198 & 22500 & 6480 & 3510 & 3000 \\ 198 & 86.4 & 6480 & 14400 & 5148 & 1080 \\ 39 & 36.4 & 3510 & 5148 & 16900 & 845 \\ 60 & 36 & 3000 & 1080 & 845 & 2500 \end{bmatrix}$$

The following program provides the necessary path coefficients and the error variances in prediction of the endogeneous variables.

```
data carprice(TYPE = COV);
_type_ = 'cov'; input _name_ $ v1-v6;
cards;

    v1    25        .        .        .        .        .
    v2    3.6      16        .        .        .        .
    v3    247.5   198    22500        .        .        .
    v4    198      86.4    6480    14400        .        .
    v5    39       36.4    3510     5148    16900        .
    v6    60       36      3000     1080      845     2500
    ;

proc calis cov data = carprice edf = 300;
Lineqs
  V3 = B1 V1 + B2 V2 + E1,
  V4 = B3 V2 + B4 V3 + E2,
  V5 = B5 V2 + B6 V3 + E3,
  V6 = B7 V1 + B8 V4 + B9 V5 + E4;
Std
  v1 v2 = 25 16,
e1 e2 e3 e4 = e_1 e_2 e_3 e_4; *The diagonal elements of the
  variance-covariance matrix are given for the exogeneous
  variables only;
run;
```

                              ***
                    The CALIS Procedure
  Covariance Structure Analysis: Maximum Likelihood Estimation

Fit function   0.2667
Goodness-of-fit index (GFI)   0.9213 (f9)

GFI adjusted for degrees of freedom (AGFI)   0.6693
Root mean square residual (RMR)   1019.1832
Parsimonious GFI (Mulaik, 1989)   0.3071
Chi-square   80.0120
Chi-square DF   5

Pr > Chi-square   < 0.0001
Independence model chi-square   227.93
Independence model chi-square DF   15
RMSEA estimate   0.2236
RMSEA 90% lower confidence limit   0.1820
RMSEA 90% upper confidence limit   0.2681
ECVI estimate   0.3554
ECVI 90% lower confidence limit   0.2804
ECVI 90% upper confidence limit   0.4764
Probability of close fit   0.0000
Bentler's comparative fit index   0.6477
Normal theory reweighted LS chi-square   76.9194
Akaike's information criterion   70.0120
Bozdogan's (1987) CAIC   46.4765
Schwarz's Bayesian criterion   51.4765
McDonald's (1989) centrality   0.8828
Bentler and Bonett's (1980) nonnormed index   -0.0569
Bentler and Bonett's (1980) NFI   0.6490
James, Mulaik, and Brett (1982) Parsimonious NFI   0.2163
Z-test of Wilson and Hilferty (1931)   7.4207
Bollen (1986) normed index Rho1   -0.0531
Bollen (1988) nonnormed index Delta2   0.6635
Hoelter's (1983) critical *N*   43

The CALIS Procedure
Covariance Structure Analysis: Maximum Likelihood Estimation
Manifest Variable Equations with Estimates

	$v3 = 8.3898*v1 +$	$10.4873*v2$	$+ 1.0000\ E1$		(f1)
Std Error	1.5900 B1	1.9875 B2			
t-value	5.2765	5.2765			(f2)

	$v4 = 0.2699*v3 +$	$2.0604*v2$	$+ 1.0000\ E2$		(f1)
Std Error	0.0455 B4	1.7077 B3			
t-value	5.9262	1.2065			(f2)

	$v5 = 0.1526*v3 +$	$0.3866*v2$	$+ 1.0000\ E3$		(f1)
Std Error	0.0521 B6	1.9551 B5			
t-value	2.9269	0.1977			(f2)

	$v6 = 0.0340*v4 +$	$0.0349*v5$	$+ 2.0764*v1 + 1.0000\ E4$	(f1)
Std Error	0.0233 B8	0.0214 B9	0.5600 B7		
t-value	1.4563	1.6274	3.7082		(f2)

```
                   Variances of Exogenous Variables
       Variable    Parameter  Estimate      Standard    t Value
                                            Error

       v1                     25.00000
       v2                     16.00000
       E1          e_1        18347 (f3)    1498        12.25
       E2          e_2        12473 (f4)    1018        12.25
       E3          e_3        16350 (f5)    1335        12.25
       E4          e_4        2309 (f6)     188.54979   12.25
       ***
```

```
                      The CALIS Procedure
        Covariance Structure Analysis: Maximum Likelihood Estimation
        Manifest Variable Equations with Standardized Estimates (f7)
```

$v3 = 0.2797*v1 + 0.2797*v2 + 0.9030\ E1$
    B1   B2
$v4 = 0.3373*v3 + 0.0687*v2 + 0.9307\ E2$
    B4   B3
$v5 = 0.1761*v3 + 0.0119*v2 + 0.9836\ E3$
    B6   B5
$v6 = 0.0820*v4 + 0.0911*v5 + 0.2088*v1 + 0.9664\ E4$
    B8   B9   B7
                         ***

```
              Correlations among Exogenous Variables
              Var1     Var2     Parameter     Estimate
              v1       v2                     0.18000 (f8)
```

In the output, the rows indicated by (f1) contain the regression coefficients of the exogenous variables. These regression coefficients are called *path coefficients*. We draw a graph showing a straight line with an arrow pointing to the endogenous variable and the start showing the exogenous variable (Figure 6.11). On this line, the regression (path) coefficient will be shown. In the rows (f2) the *t*-values to test the significance of the path coefficients are given. In the graph we put 1 or 2 stars on the path coefficient, depending on the significance of the coefficient at 0.05 or 0.01 levels. The exogenous variables will be connected by a curvy line with arrows on both sides and indicating the correlation between the exogenous variables. These correlations will be shown in the output at (f8). An arrow pointing toward the endogenous variable and beginning with the error variance given at (f3), (f4), (f5), and (f6) will be given and these quantities are the residual sum of squares in fitting the multiple regression equations.

There are several goodness-of-fit measures. In (f9), we showed the goodness based on the *goodness-of-fit index (GFI)*. The GFI deals with the error and reproducing the variance and covariance matrix and if this GFI is

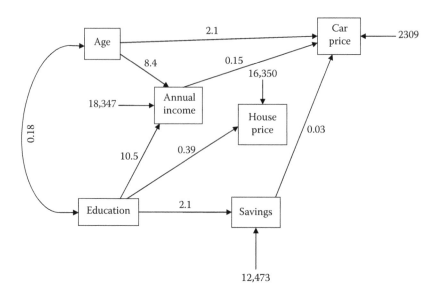

FIGURE 6.11
The path analysis for the car price.

greater than or equal to 0.9, the model is considered to be acceptable. In our problem this is 0.92 and our model is considered adequate. For other goodness-of-fit measures and structural equation modeling, the interested reader is referred to the *SAS manual*, Hoyle (1995), Loehlin (2004), and Bollen (1989).

6.16 Choice-Based Conjoint Analysis

Conjoint analysis is a tool to examine the preferences of the respondents in making a decision. The available products will be considered and subsets of these products are made. These subsets are known as *choice sets* and the respondents are asked to choose the product of their choice. In each of the choice sets "No choice" option will also be included. In making such decisions one has to pay more to get more benefits from the product, and people have to balance out the factors (usually called attributes in this context) in reaching a decision.

Suppose we have four brands of a product available and we show these products and ask the respondents which of those four brands they are willing to purchase or they do not buy any of these four brands. Suppose n respondents are asked and n_1, n_2, n_3, n_4, and n_0 be the number of respondents choosing one of the brands, 1, 2, 3, 4, or no choice. Usually, the responses considered for the four brands are $l_1 = ln(n_1/n)$, $l_2 = ln(n_2/n)$, $l_3 = ln(n_3/n)$, and $l_4 = ln(n_4/n)$. The model used for these l_1 to l_4 responses is

$$E(l_1) = \beta_1 + \beta_{1(2)} + \beta_{1(3)} + \beta_{1(4)}$$
$$E(l_2) = \beta_2 + \beta_{2(1)} + \beta_{2(3)} + \beta_{2(4)}$$
$$E(l_3) = \beta_3 + \beta_{3(1)} + \beta_{3(2)} + \beta_{3(4)}$$
$$E(l_4) = \beta_4 + \beta_{4(1)} + \beta_{4(2)} + \beta_{4(3)},$$

where β_i's are the *brand effects* and $\beta_{i(j)}$'s are the *cross effects* of the jth brand on the ith brand. In some problems, people may be interested in studying the contrast of the cross effects and of the *brand effects* and in other problems, they may be interested in estimating each of the cross effects and brand effects. In this case, the designs used are 3-designs with equal and unequal set sizes, and Raghavarao and Padgett (2005) provide some details of this method and we consider this briefly in Section 6.16.1.

Consider a new graduate looking for a job. The factors or attributes of interest to the graduate are salary, vacation time, opportunities for promotion, health benefits, and so on. If the graduate sees a position with all likeable attributes, he/she will definitely choose that job. On the contrary, if a job with low values of the attributes is available he/she may not take the job. In this decision making and in the actual situations, the prospective graduate has to give up on some benefits to choose others. This kind of situation will be examined in Section 6.16.2.

A new area of research which is expected to be useful is the mixture-amount designs and we will briefly discuss this in Section 6.16.3. The monograph by Raghavarao et al. (2010) discuss the design issues related to the choice-based conjoint analysis, and the interested reader is referred to their monograph for further details and some computer programs.

6.16.1 Availability Designs and Cross Effects

Suppose v brands of a product are available in the market and we want to study the brand effects and the cross effects. For this purpose we form subsets, called choice sets, for the v brands and present it to different prospective buyers (or panel) and ask them to give their preferred brand or will not buy any brand shown to them. The l_i's as indicated in the introduction of this section will be used to draw inferences on the brand effects and cross effects.

Sometimes one may be replacing an available brand by another brand and the researcher would like to know the impact of this change on a different brand. This will be answered by estimating the contrast of the cross effects. For example, if Brand 2 is replaced by Brand 3 and the researcher is interested in knowing the impact of this change on Brand 1, the interest is in estimating $\beta_{1(2)} - \beta_{1(3)}$. Such contrasts are estimated optimally by forming b subsets of the v brands, with k brands in each subset (choice set) such that

1. Every brand is in r choice sets
2. Every pair of brands is in λ_2 choice sets
3. Every three brands are in λ_3 choice sets

Such designs are called *3-designs*.

Suppose a store is planning to introduce three brands of a product in their store. Naturally, the three brands selected should produce maximum revenue. In this case, we need to estimate the individual brand effects and the individual cross effects. This is optimally done by using the 3-designs mentioned earlier where all the choice sets are not of equal size.

The results related to the construction and properties of the 3-designs with equal or unequal choice set sizes were discussed by Raghavarao and Padgett (2005).

With $v = 4$, the 3-design of choice set size 3 is the following:

$$\{A, B, C\}; \{A, B, D\}; \{A, C, D\}; \{B, C, D\}$$

These four choice sets will be used to make inferences on the contrasts of brands and brand cross effects.

With $v = 4$, the 3-design of choice set sizes 4 and 3 is the following:

$$\{A, B, C, D\}; \{A, B, C\}; \{A, B, D\}; \{A, C, D\}; \{B, C, D\}$$

These five choice sets will be used to make inferences on the individual brand and cross effects.

6.16.2 Pareto-Optimal Choice Sets

Suppose v attributes (factors) are included in a decision-making process and the ith attribute is at s_i levels. A profile of all attributes is a combination of the v attributes specifying the level used for each of the attributes. In this process, one profile dominates (or dominated by) another profile in a choice set, and such situations should be avoided to exclude the obvious choices or no choices. A *Pareto optimal choice set* is one in which no profile is dominated or dominates another profile. The forming of *choice sets* is of interest. The discussion of Pareto-optimal choice sets with less number of profiles was considered by Raghavarao and Wiley (1998) and Raghavarao and Zhang (2002) (also refer Raghavarao and Padgett, 2005). With $v = 4$, the Pareto-optimal choice sets for estimating the main effects are

$$T_1 = \{1000, 0100, 0010, 0001, \text{no choice}\}$$

$$T_2 = \{1110, 1101, 1011, 0111, \text{no choice}\}$$

Suppose the four attributes that a new graduate considers when looking for a job are salary ($40,000 = 1, $35,000 = 0), vacation time (3 weeks = 1, 2 weeks = 0), health benefits (provided = 1, not provided = 0), and promotion prospect (2 years = 1, 5 years = 0)). The first profile in the choice set T_1 implies that the job has got $40,000 salary with 2 weeks vacation time and no health benefits and promotion chances in 5 years. Using such choice sets one can model the main effects plan and estimate the significant main effects.

6.16.3 Mixture-Amount Designs

In the traditional choice-based conjoint analysis, when price is considered, it is used as a factor to construct the profiles for the choice sets. However, one can separate the amount and consider the allocation of the cost in some proportions for the other factors. Such designs are called mixture-amount choice-based conjoint designs and were discussed by Raghavarao and Wiley (2009).

Consider a tour package at different price levels as discussed in Section 5.19. The attributes of interest are lodging, boarding, and entertainment. There are some minimum expenses to be allocated to travel, lodging, boarding, and entertainment, and some discretionary money that can be allocated to the three attributes. Suppose the discretionary amounts are $300, $360, and $420. The discretionary amounts have to be allocated to boarding, lodging, and entertainment. A mixture design with three factors is the commonly used *simplex lattice designs*. This consists of 10 mixtures where the proportions allocated to boarding, lodging, and entertainment are as follows:

$$(1,0,0);\ (0,1,0);\ (0,0,1);\ (1/3,2/3,0);\ (2/3,1/3,0);\ (1/3,0,2/3);$$

$$(2/3,0,1/3);\ (0,2/3,1/3);\ (0,1/3,2/3);\ (1/3,1/3,1/3).$$

The model for the logit of the proportion of selected profiles to the proportion of no choice selection in each set will be modeled as

$$E\left(l_{X_1 X_2 X_3}\right) = \sum_{i=1}^{3} \beta_i X_i + \sum_{\substack{i,j=1 \\ i<j}}^{3} \beta_{ij} X_i X_j,$$

where X_1, X_2, and X_3 are the mixture proportions of the discretionary amount spent on food, lodging, and entertainment and $l_{X_1 X_2 X_3}$ is the log of the proportion of people choosing (X_1, X_2, X_3) to the proportion choosing no choice. In this model, there are six parameters, and six profiles are enough to estimate these parameters. In this model, we did not have the constant and quadratic terms because of the restriction that the sum of the proportions is 1.

However, Raghavarao and Wiley (2009) considered seven mixtures to discuss the choice-based conjoint analysis in seven choice sets as given in Table 6.11:

TABLE 6.11

Choice Sets of Three Mixture-Amount Profiles

Choice Set Number	Profile 1	Profile 2	Profile 3	Base Alternative
1	300,0,0	0,360,0	280,140,0	No choice
2	0,300,0	0,0,360	0,280,140	No choice
3	0,0,300	240,120,0	140,0,280	No choice
4	200,100,0	0,240,120	140,140,140	No choice
5	0,200,100	120,0,240	420,0,0	No choice
6	100,0,200	120,120,120	0,420,0	No choice
7	100,100,100	360,0,0	0,0,420	No choice

The entries in the profiles are the costs for the three attributes.

The modified mixture-amount model which will determine the optimum choice of the discretionary amount of spending and the allocation of that amount to the three attributes is calculated using the model

$$E(l_{ijkm}) = \alpha a_i + \beta a_i^2 + \gamma_1 a_i x_j + \gamma_2 a_i y_k + \delta_1 x_j + \delta_2 y_k + \delta_3 z_m$$
$$+ \delta_{12} x_j y_k + \delta_{13} x_j z_m + \delta_{23} y_k z_m,$$

where l_{ijkm} is the log of the proportion of people choosing (x_j, y_k, z_m) with discretionary amount a_i to the proportion of people choosing none of the three profiles. This model is motivated to determine the optimal discretionary amount, the interaction of this amount to the mixture levels, and the optimum mixture choices for the discretionary amount.

An artificial example and the analysis were given by Raghavarao and Wiley (2009). Similar designs can be constructed and analyzed as required.

6.17 Meta-Analysis

Researchers may want to combine the results of several studies (large or small) with similar characteristics to draw overall conclusions. This lumping of studies is known as *meta-analysis*. A good meta-analysis should include trials that are both published and/or not published. One should be careful in only obtaining results from trials published in the journals since they tend to be positively biased. The trials should not be lumped together to form one large data set. Instead, the results of each of the meta-analysis should be used separately, for example, effect size, *p*-values, and so on. The correlation coefficient and the standardized mean difference are the commonly used indexes for effect size. Pearson's *r* is an example of effect size that measures the relationship between the two variables. Cohen's *d* or Hodges' *g* are examples of the standardized mean difference. In order to get a good feel for the meta-analysis, the number of studies should also be reported, as well as the CI for the effect size. One often does a meta-analysis to obtain drug effects over a broad spectrum of patient populations. One should be careful not to base all conclusions on the meta-analysis.

Suppose we are comparing the effect of Drug A versus Placebo from different sites in a clinical trial. The significance of drug A can be determined at each site separately. If we want to combine the test results from all sites we use the CMH test. CMH test is a kind of meta-analysis of the studies from different sites.

Suppose k studies are made testing the significance of a null hypothesis and let $p_1, p_2, ..., p_k$ be the p-values of the studies at the k sites. We test whether the effect sizes produced at each site are homogeneous and if they are homogeneous we would want to combine all the results and test the significance of the combined data. We deal with this problem in the next two sections.

6.17.1 Homogeneity of the Effect Sizes

Let $p_1, p_2, ..., p_k$ be the p-values for a one-sided test and the homogeneity of the effect size is determined by testing the equality of the p-values under the null hypothesis. We achieve this in the following program by considering probits of the p-values and testing that the probits have 0 variance. Consider a study in seven sites with p-values given as

0.045, 0.59, 0.02, 0.24, 0.03, 0.01, 0.9.

```
data a; input pvalue@@; cards;
.045   .59  .02   .24   .03   .01   .9
;
data a1;set a; probit = probit(1-pvalue);
proc univariate noprint; output out = stats var = var n = k;
  var probit;
data stats;set stats; var = var*(k-1);
  pvalue = 1 - probchi(var,k-1);
keep pvalue; proc print;run;

   pvalue
   0.090748
```

The p-value of the output is more than $\alpha = 0.05$, and hence there is no evidence to conclude that the seven studies provide different effect sizes.

6.17.2 Combining the p-Values

When the k studies are homogeneous we combine the p-values to get a single p-value that gives an overall p-value to draw conclusions for the combined study at the k sites. This will be done by combining the p-values following the results of Fisher (1932). The following program provides the combined p-value for the data given in Section 6.17.1.

```
data a; input pvalue@@; cards;
.045   .59   .02   .24   .03   .01   .9
;
data a1;set a; logpi = log(pvalue);
proc univariate noprint; output out = stats sum = sum n = k;
  var logpi; data stats;set stats; chisq = - 2*sum;
  COMBPVALUE = 1 - probchi(chisq,2*k);
keep combpvalue; proc print;run;


  COMBPVALUE
  0.001820529
```

The combined p-value of 0.0018 is <0.05 and hence we conclude that by combining all the seven sites, the overall study is significant.

References and Selected Bibliography

Agresti, A. 1996. *An Introduction to Categorical Data Analysis*. New York, NY: Wiley.

Allison, P.D. 1995. *Survival Analysis Using the SAS System: A Practical Guide*. Cary, NC: SAS Institute.

Allison, P.D. 1999. *Logistic Regression Using the SAS System: Theory and Application*. Cary, NC: SAS Institute.

Altman, D.G. 1991. *Practical Statistics for Medical Research*. London: Chapman & Hall/CRC.

Altman, E.I., R.B. Avery, R.A. Eisenbeis, and J.F. Sinkey, 1981. *Application of Classification Techniques in Business, Banking and Finance*. Greenwich, CT: JAI Press.

Anderberg, M.R. 1973. *Cluster Analysis for Applications*. New York, NY: Academic Press, Inc.

Andersen, P.K. 1987. Conditional power calculations as an aid in the decision whether to continue a clinical trial. *Controlled Clinical Trials*, **8**: 67–74.

Armitage, P. and G. Berry, 1987. *Statistical Methods in Medical Research*, 2nd Edition. Oxford: Blackwell.

Bartlett, M.S. 1937a. Some examples of statistical methods of research in agriculture and applied biology. *J. Roy. Statist. Soc. Suppl.*, **4**: 137–183.

Bartlett, M.S. 1937b. Properties of sufficiency and statistical tests. *Proc. Roy. Soc. London*, **160A**: 268–282.

Basoglu, M., I. Marks, M. Livanou, and R. Swinson, 1997. Double-blindness procedures, rater blindness, and ratings of outcome: Observations from a controlled trial. *Arch. Gen. Psychiatry*, **54**: 744–748.

Basu, D. 1980. Randomization analysis of experimental data: The Fisher randomization test. *J. Amer. Statist. Assoc.*, **75**: 575–582.

Beck, J.R. and E.K. Shultz, 1986. The use of relative operating characteristic (ROC) curves in test performance evaluation. *Arch. Pathol. Lab. Med.*, 110: 13–20.

Begg, C.B. 1987. Biases in the assessment of diagnostic tests. *Statist. Med.*, **6**: 411–423.

Benjamini, Y. and Y. Hochberg, 1995. Controlling the false discovery rate: A practical and powerful approach to multiple testing. *J. Roy. Statist. Soc.*, **57B**: 289–300.

Bishop, Y., S.E. Fienberg, and P.W. Holland, 1975. *Discrete Multivariate Analysis: Theory and Practice*. Cambridge, MA: MIT Press.

Bland, M. 2000. *An Introduction to Medical Statistics*, 3rd Edition. Oxford: Oxford University Press.

Bloch, D. and H. Kraemer, 1989. 2×2 kappa coefficient: Measure of agreement or association. *Biometrics*, **45**: 269–287.

Bollen, K.A. 1989. *Structural Equations with Latent Variables*. New York, NY: Wiley.

Bowker, A.H. 1948. Bowker's test for symmetry. *J. Amer. Statist. Soc.*, **43**: 572–574.

Box, G.E.P. and D.R. Cox, 1964. An analysis of transformations. *J. Roy. Statist. Soc.*, **26B**: 211–246.

Breslow, N.E. 1974. Covariance analysis of censored survival data. *Biometrics*, **30**: 89–99.

Breslow, N.E. and N.E. Day, 1980. *Statistical Methods in Cancer Research, Volume I: The Analysis of Case-Control Studies*. IARC Scientific Publications, No. 32, Lyon, France: International Agency for Research on Cancer.

Brieman, L. 2001. Random forests. *Machine Learning*, **45**(1): 5–32.

Brieman, L., J. Friedman, R. Olshen, and C. Stone, 1984. *Classification and Regression Trees*. Belmont, CA: Wadsworth.

Bross, I. 1954. Misclassification in 2×2 tables. *Biometrics*, **10**: 478–486.

Bross, I. 1958. How to use Ridit analysis. *Biometrics*, **14**: 18–38.

Brownwell, K.D. and A.J. Stunkard, 1982. The double-blind in danger: Untoward consequences of informed consent. *Am. J. Psychiatry*, **139**: 1487–1489.

Carroll, R.J. 1998. Measurement error in epidemiologic studies, in *Encyclopedia of Biostatistics*, Vol. 4, Eds. P. Armitage and T. Colton. New York, NY: Wiley, pp. 2491–2519.

Cattell, R.B. 1965. Factor analysis: An introduction to essentials. *Biometrics*, **21**: 190–215.

Cattell, R.B. 1966. The scree test for the number of factors. *Multivariate Behav. Res.*, **1**: 245–276.

Cattell, R.B. 1978. *The Scientific Use of Factor Analysis*. New York, NY: Plenum.

Chatterjee, S. and B. Price, 1991. *Regression Analysis by Example*. New York, NY: Wiley.

Chaudhuri, A. and R. Mukerjee, 1988. *Randomized Response: Theory and Techniques*. New York, NY: Marcel Dekker.

Cicchetti, D.V. and T. Allison, 1971. A new procedure for assessing reliability of scoring EEG sleep recordings. *Am. J. EEG Technol.*, **11**: 101–109.

Cicchetti, D. and J. Fleiss, 1977. Comparison of the null distributions of weighted kappa and the C ordinal statistic. *Appl. Psychol. Meas.*, **1**: 195–201.

Cliff, N. 1988. The eigenvalue-greater-than-one rule and the reliability of components. *Psych. Bull.*, **103**(2): 276–279.

Cochran, W.G. and G.M. Cox, 1957. *Experimental Designs*, 2nd Edition. New York, NY: Wiley.

Cohen, J. 1960. A coefficient of agreement for nominal scales. *Ed. Psych. Meas.*, **20**: 37–46.

Cohen, J. 1968. Weighted kappa: Nominal scale agreement with provision for scaled disagreement or partial credit. *Psych. Bull.*, **70**: 213–220.

Collett, D. 1994. *Modelling Survival Data in Medical Research*. London: Chapman & Hall.

Collett, D. 2003. *Modelling Binary Data*, 2nd Edition. London: Chapman & Hall/CRC.

Conover, W.J. 1980. *Practical Nonparametric Statistics*, 2nd Edition. New York, NY: Wiley.

Cook, T.D. and D.L. DeMets, 2008. *Introduction to Statistical Methods for Clinical Trials*. Boca Raton, FL: Chapman & Hall.

Cook, R.D. and S. Weisberg, 1982. *Residuals and Influence in Regression*. New York, NY: Chapman & Hall/CRC.

Cox, D.R. and E.J. Snell, 1989. *The Analysis of Binary Data*, 2nd Edition. London: Chapman & Hall.

Cox, D.R. and A. Stuart, 1955. Some quick tests for trend in location and dispersion. *Biometrika*, **42**: 80–95.

D'Agostino, R.B. 1998. Propensity score methods for bias reduction in the comparison of a treatment to a non-randomized control group. *Statist. Med.*, **17**: 2265–2281.

Damaraju, L. 2009. Screening variable to determine binary responses to maximize the asymptotic relative efficiency. *JP J. Biostat.*, **3**(3): 215–224.

Damaraju, L. and D. Raghavarao, 2005. Statistical inferences accounting for human behavior. *Metrika*, **62**(1): 65–72.

Davis, C.S. 2002. *Statistical Methods for the Analysis of Repeated Measurements*. New York, NY: Springer.

Davison, M.L. 1983. *Multidimensional Scaling*. New York, NY: Wiley.

Delucca, P. and D. Raghavarao, 2000. Effect of investigator bias on the power and level of Wilcoxon Rank-Sum test. *Biostatistics*, **1**: 107–112.

Delucca, P., D. Raghavarao, and S. Altan, 1999. Effect of investigator bias on the power and level of the two sample Z-test. *Journal of Biopharmaceutical Statistics*, **9**: 279–288.

Der, G. and B.S. Everitt, 2006. *Statistical Analysis of Medical Data Using SAS*. Boca Raton, FL: Chapman & Hall/CRC.

Desu, M.M. and D. Raghavarao, 1990. *Sample Size Methodology*. Boston, MA: Academic Press.

Desu, M.M. and D. Raghavarao, 2004. *Nonparametric Statistical Methods for Complete and Censored Data*. Boca Raton, FL: Chapman & Hall/CRC.

DeWoody, K.L. and S. Altan, 2001. *Matrix Designs in Stability Studies in Recent Advances in Experimental Designs and Related Topics*, Eds. S. Altan and J. Singh. Huntington, NY: Nova Science Publishers, pp. 87–94.

Diggle, P.J., K.Y. Liang, and S.L. Zeger, 1994. *Analysis of Longitudinal Data*. Oxford: Clarendon Press.

Dillon, W.R. and M. Goldstein, 1984. *Multivariate Analysis: Methods and Applications*. New York, NY: Wiley.

Ding, Y. and D. Raghavarao, 2008. Hadamard matrix methods in identifying differentially expressed genes from microarray experiments. *J. Statist. Plan. Inf.*, **138**(1): 47–55.

Dobson, A.J. 2001. *An Introduction to General Linear Models*. London: Chapman & Hall.

Dorfman, R. 1943. The detection of defective members of a large population. *Ann. Math. Statist.*, **14**: 436–440.

Draper, N.R. 1963. Ridge analysis of response surfaces. *Technometrics*, **5**: 469–479.

Draper, N.R. and H. Smith, 1981. *Applied Regression Analysis*, 2nd Edition. New York, NY: Wiley.

Du, D.-Z. and F.K. Hwang, 1993. *Combinatorial Group Testing and Its Applications*. Singapore: World Scientific.

Duncan, D.B. 1975. *t* Tests and Intervals for Comparisons Suggested by the Data. *Biometrics*, **31**: 339–359.

Dunn, O.J. and V.A. Clark, 1974. *Applied Statistics: Analysis of Variance and Regression*. New York, NY: Wiley.

Dunnett, C.W. 1955. A multiple comparisons procedure for comparing several treatments with a control. *J. Amer. Statist. Assoc.*, **50**: 1096–1121.

Dunsmore, I.R. 1974. The Bayesian predictive distribution in life testing models. *Technometrics*, **16**: 455–460.

Dunteman, G.H. 1989. *Principal Component Analysis*. Newbury Park, CA: Sage.

Durbin, J. and G.S. Watson, 1950. Testing for serial correlation in least squares regression, I. *Biometrika*, **37**: 409–428.

Efron, B. 1971. Forcing a sequential experiment to be balanced. *Biometrika*, **58**: 403–417.

Efron B. 1979. Bootstrap methods: Another look at the jackknife. *Ann. Statist.*, **7**: 1–26.

Efron, B. 1982. *The Jackknife, the Bootstrap and Other Resampling Plans*. Philadelphia: SIAM.

Efron, B. and R. Tibshirani, 1993. *An Introduction to the Bootstrap*. New York, NY: Chapman & Hall/CRC.

Everitt, B.S. 1984. *An Introduction to Latent Variable Models*. London: Chapman & Hall.

Everitt, B.S. 1995. The analysis of repeated measures: A practical review with examples. *The Statistician*, **44**: 113–135.

Everitt, B.S. and G. Dunn, 2001. *Applied Multivariate Data Analysis*. London: Arnold.

Federer, W.T. and F. King, 2007. *Variations on Split Plot and Split Block Experiment Designs*, 2nd Edition, Hoboken, NJ: Wiley.

Fisher R.A. 1932. *Statistical Methods for Research Workers*, 4th Edition. London: Oliver and Boyd.

Fleiss, J.L. 1981. *Statistical Methods for Rates and Proportions*, 2nd Edition. New York, NY: Wiley.

Fleiss, J.L. and J. Cohen, 1973. The equivalence of weighted kappa and the intraclass correlation coefficient as measures of reliability. *Ed. Psych. Meas.*, **33**: 613–619.

Fleiss, J.L., J. Cohen, and B.S. Everitt, 1969. Large-sample standard errors of kappa and weighted kappa. *Psych. Bull.*, **72**: 323–327.

Freeman, D.H. 1987. *Applied Categorical Data Analysis*. New York, NY: Marcel Dekker.

Freund, R.J. and R.C. Littell, 1991. *SAS System for Regression*, 2nd Edition. Cary, NC: SAS Institute Inc.

Freund, R.J., R.C. Littell, and P.C. Spector, 1986. *SAS System for Linear Models*. Cary, NC: SAS Institute Inc.

Friedman, L.M., C.D. Furberg, D.L., De Mets, 1998. *Fundamentals of Clinical Trials*, 3rd edition, New York, NY: Springer-Verlag.

Frison, L. and S.J. Pocock, 1992. Repeated measures in clinical Trials: Analysis using mean summary statistics and its implications for design. *Statist. Med.*, **11**: 1685–1704.

Fruchter, B. 1954. Introduction to Factor Analysis. New York, NY: Van Nostrand.

Fuller, W.A. 1987. *Measurement Error Models*. New York, NY: Wiley.

Gehan, E.A. 1965. A generalized Wilcoxon test for comparing arbitrarily singly censored samples. *Biometrika*, **52**: 203–223.

Geller, N.L. and S.J. Pocock, 1987. Interim analysis in randomized clinical trials: Ramifications and guidelines for practitioners. *Biometrics*, **43**: 213–223.

Gower, J.C. 1967. A comparison of some methods of cluster analysis. *Biometrics*, **23**: 623–637.

Graybill, F.A. 1969. *Introduction to Matrices with Applications in Statistics*. Belmont, CA: Wadsworth.

Greenacre, M.J. 1984. *Theory and Applications of Correspondence Analysis*. London: Academic Press.

Hahn, G.J. and W.Q. Meeker, 1991. *Statistical Intervals: A Guide for Practitioners*. New York, NY: Wiley.

Hand, D.J. 1981. *Discrimination and Classification*. New York, NY: Wiley.

Hartigan, J. A. 1975. *Clustering Algorithms*. New York, NY: Wiley.

Hedges, L.V. and I. Olkin, 1985. *Statistical Methods for Meta-Analysis*. San Diego, CA: Academic Press.

Hochberg, Y. and A.C. Tamhane, 1987. *Multiple Comparison Procedures*. New York, NY: Wiley.

Hoerl, A. and R. Kennard, 1970. Ridge regression: Biased estimation for nonorthogonal problems. *Technometrics*, **12**: 55–67.

Hoffman, D.L. and G.R. Franke, 1986. Correspondence analysis: Graphical representation of categorical data in marketing research. *J. Mark. Res.*, **23**: 213–227.

Horton, N.J. and S.R. Lipsitz, 2001. Multiple imputation in practice: Comparison of software packages for regression models with missing variables. *Amer. Statist.*, **55**: 244–254.

Hosmer, D.W. and S. Lemeshow, 1999. *Applied Survival Analysis: Regression Modelling of Time To Event Data*. New York, NY: Wiley.

Hosmer, D.W. and S. Lemeshow, 2000. *Applied Logistic Regression*, 2nd Edition. New York, NY: Wiley.

Hoyle, R.H. 1995. *Structural Equation Modeling: Concepts, Issues, and Applications*. Thousand Oaks, CA: Sage.

Huber, P.J. 1981. *Robust Statistics*. New York, NY: Wiley.

Hunter, J.E. and F.L. Schmidt, 1990. *Methods of Meta-Analysis: Correcting Errors and Bias in Research Findings*. Newbury Park, CA: Sage.

Jackson, J.E. 1991. *A User's Guide to Principal Components*. New York, NY: Wiley.

Jennison C. and B.W. Turnbull, 2000. Group Sequential Methods with Applications to Clinical Trials. Boca Raton, FL: Chapman & Hall/CRC Press.

Johnson, R.A. and D.W. Wichern, 1998. *Applied Multivariate Statistical Analysis*, 4th Edition. Upper Saddle River, NJ: Prentice-Hall.

Jonckheere, A.R. 1954. A distribution-free k-sample test against ordered alternatives. *Biometrika*, **41**: 133–145.

Jones, B. and M.G. Kenward, 2003. *Design and Analysis of Cross-Over Trials*, 2nd Edition. London: Chapman & Hall/CRC.

Kalbfleisch, J.D. and R.L. Prentice, 2002. *The Statistical Analysis of Failure Time Data*, 2nd Edition. New York, NY: Wiley.

Kalish, L.A. and C.B. Begg, 1985. Treatment allocation methods in clinical trials: A review. *Statist. Med.*, **4**: 129–144.

Kaufman, L. and P.J. Rousseeuw, 1990. *Finding Groups in Data: An Introduction to Cluster Analysis*. New York, NY: Wiley.

Kennard, R.W. 1971. A note on the C_p statistic. *Technometrics*, **13**: 899–900.

Klecka, W.R. 1980. *Discriminant Analysis*. Beverly Hills, CA: Sage.

Kleinbaum, D.G. 1994. *Logistic Regression: A Self-Learning Text*. New York, NY: Springer-Verlag.

Kleinbaum, D.G. 1996. *Survival Analysis: A Self-Learning Text*. New York, NY: Springer-Verlag.

Krishnamoorthy, K. and D. Raghavarao, 1993. Untruthful answering in repeated randomized response procedures. *Can. J. Statist.*, **21**: 233–236.

Kruskal, J.B. and M. Wish, 1978. *Multidimensional Scaling*. Beverly Hills, CA : Sage.

Lachin, J.M. 2000. *Biostatistical Methods: The Assessment of Relative Risks*. New York, NY: Wiley.

Lachin, J.M. 2005. A review of methods for futility stopping based on conditional power. *Statist. Med.*, **24**: 2747–2764.

Lachin, J.M., J.P. Matts, and L.J. Wei, 1988. Randomization in clinical trials: Conclusions and recommendations. *Control. Clin. Trials*, **9**(4): 365–374.

Lagakos, S.W. 1988. Effects of mismodelling and mismeasuring explanatory variables on tests of their association with a response variable. *Statist. Med.*, **7**: 257–274.

Lakshmi, D. 1995. *Inferences in the Presence of Misclassification Errors*. Unpublished Ph.D. Dissertation, Temple University.

Lakshmi, D.V. and D. Raghavarao, 1992. A test for detecting untruthful answering in randomized response procedure. *J. Statist. Plan. Inf.*, **31**: 387–390.

Lakshmi, D.V. and W.K. Smith, 1993. Comparing proportions in the presence of false positive and false negative instrument sorting errors. *Biometrics*, **49**: 639–641.

Lan, K.K.G. and D.L. DeMets, 1983. Discrete sequential boundaries for clinical trials. *Biometrika*, **70**: 659–663.

Lan, K.K.G. and J. Wittes, 1988. The B-value: A tool for monitoring data. *Biometrics*, **44**: 579–585.

Landis, J.R. and G.G. Koch, 1977. The measurement of observer agreement for categorical data. *Biometrics*, **33**: 159–174.

Lawless, J.F. 1982. *Statistical Models and Methods for Lifetime Data*. New York, NY: Wiley.

Lawley, D.N. and A.E. Maxwell, 1971. *Factor Analysis as a Statistical Method*. New York, NY: American Elsevier Publishing Company.

Lee, E.T. and J.W. Wang, 2003. *Statistical Methods for Survival Data Analysis*, 3rd Edition. New York, NY: Wiley.

Lehmann, E.L. 1998. *Nonparametrics: Statistical Methods Based on Ranks*. Upper Saddle River, NJ: Prentice-Hall.

Levene, H. 1960. *Robust Tests for Equality of Variance in Contributions to Probability and Statistics*, Ed. I. Olkin. Palo Alto, CA: Stanford University Press, pp. 278–292.

Littell, R.C., R.J. Freund, and P.C. Spector, 1991. *SAS System for Linear Models*, 3rd Edition. Cary, NC: SAS Institute Inc.

Littell, R.C., G.A. Milliken, W.W. Stroup, and R. Wolfinger, 1996. *SAS System for Mixed Models*. Cary, NC: SAS Institute Inc.

Little, R.J.A. and D.B. Rubin, 2002. *Statistical Analysis with Missing Data*, 2nd Edition. New York, NY: Wiley.

Loehlin, J.C. 2004. *Latent Variables Models: An Introduction to Factor, Path, and Structural Analysis*, 4th Edition. Mahwah, NJ: Lawrence Erlbaum Associates.

Loh, W. and Y. Shih, 1997. Split selection methods for Classification Trees. *Statistica Sinica*, **7**: 815–840.

Long, J.S. 1983. *Confirmatory Factor Analysis*. Beverly Hills, CA: Sage.

Louviere, J.J., D.A. Hensher, and J.D. Swait, 2007. *Stated Choice Methods: Analysis and Application*. UK: Cambridge University Press.

Mallows, C.L. 1973. Some comments on C_p. *Technometrics*, **15**: 661–675.

Mallows, C.L. 1995. More Comments on C_p. *Technometrics*, **37**: 362–372.

Mantel, N. 1963. Chi-square tests with one degree of freedom: Extensions of the Mantel–Haenszel procedure. *J. Amer. Statist. Assoc.*, **58**: 690–700.

Marquardt, D.W. and R.D. Snee, 1975. Ridge regression in practice. *Amer. Statist.* **29**(1): 3–20.

McCullagh, P. 1980. Regression models for ordinal data. *J. Roy. Statist. Soc.*, **42B**: 109–142.

McCullagh, P. and J. Nelder, 1989. *Generalized Linear Models*, 2nd Edition. London: Chapman & Hall.

Milliken, G.A. and D.E. Johnson, 1984. *Analysis of Messy Data, Volume I: Designed Experiments*. New York, NY: Chapman & Hall.

Morrison, D.F. 1976. *Multivariate Statistical Methods*, 2nd Edition. New York, NY: McGraw-Hill.

Myers, W.R. 2000. Handling missing data in clinical trials: An overview. *Drug Information Journal*, **34**: 525–533.

Myers, R.H. and D.C. Montgomery, 1995. *Response Surface Methodology*. New York, NY: Wiley.

Nagelkerke, N.J.D. 1991. A note on a general definition of the coefficient of determination. *Biometrika*, **78**: 691–692.

O'Brien, P.C. and T.R. Fleming, 1979. A multiple testing procedure for clinical trials. *Biometrics*, **35**(3): 549–556.

Pocock, S.J. 1977. Group sequential methods in the design and analysis of clinical trials. *Biometrika*, **64**: 191–199.

Pocock, S.J. 1983. *Clinical Trials: A Practical Approach*. New York, NY: Wiley.

Pocock, S.J. and R. Simon, 1975. Sequential treatment assignment with balancing for prognostic factors in the controlled clinical trial. *Biometrics*, **31**: 103–115.

Punj, G. and D.W. Stewart, 1983. Cluster analysis in marketing research: Review and suggestions for application. *J. Mark. Res.*, **20**: 134–148.

Raghavarao, D. 1971. *Constructions and Combinatorial Problems in Design of Experiments*. New York, NY: Wiley.

Raghavarao, D. 1988. *Exploring Statistics*. New York, NY Marcel Dekker.

Raghavarao, D. and L.V. Padgett, 2005. *Block Designs: Analysis, Combinatorics and Applications*. Singapore: World Scientific.

Raghavarao, D. and J.B. Wiley, 1998. *Estimating Main Effects with Pareto Optimal Subsets. Australian and New Zealand J. Statist.*, **40**: 425–432.

Raghavarao, D. and J.B. Wiley, 2009. Conjoint measurement with constraints on attribute levels: A mixture amount model approach. *Int. Statist. Rev.*, **77**: 167–178.

Raghavarao, D. and D. Zhang, 2002. 2^n Behavioral experiments using pareto optimal choice sets. *Statistica Sinica*, **12**: 1085–1092.

Raghavarao, D., J.B. Wiley and P. Chitturi, 2010. *Choice-Based Conjoint Analysis: Models and Designs*. Boca Raton, FL: Chapman & Hall.

Rao, C.R. 1964. The use and interpretation of principal component analysis in applied research. *Sankhya*, **26A**: 329–358.

Rosenbaum, P.R. and D.B. Rubin, 1983. The central role of the propensity score in observational studies for causal effects. *Biometrika*, **70**: 41–55.

Rosenberger, W.F. and J.M. Lachin, 2002. *Randomization in Clinical Trials: Theory and Practice*. New York, NY: Wiley.

Rubin, D.B. 1976. Inference and missing data. *Biometrika*, **63**: 581–592.

Rubin, D.B. 1987. *Multiple Imputation for Nonresponse in Surveys*. New York, NY: Wiley.

Schiffman, S.S., M.L. Reynolds, and F.W. Young, 1981. *Introduction to Multidimensional Scaling: Theory, Methods, and Applications*. New York, NY: Academic Press.

Sharma, S. 1996. *Applied Multivariate Techniques*. New York, NY: Wiley.

Shoukri, M.M. and V.L. Edge, 1996. *Statistical Methods for Health Sciences*. Boca Raton, FL: CRC Press.

Silverman, B.W. 1986. *Density Estimation for Statistics and Data Analysis*. New York, NY: Chapman & Hall.

Snedecor, G.W. and W.G. Cochran, 1989. *Statistical Methods*, 8th Edition. Ames, IA: Iowa State University Press.

Steel, R.G.D. and J.H. Torrie, 1980. *Principles and Procedures of Statistics*, 2nd Edition. New York, NY: McGraw-Hill.

Steel, R.G.D., J.H. Torrie, and D. Dickey, 1997. *Principles and Procedures of Statistics: A Biometrical Approach*, 3rd Edition. New York, NY: McGraw-Hill.

Stokes, M.E., C.S. Davis, and G. Koch, 1995. *Categorical Data Analysis Using the SAS System*. Cary, NC: SAS Institute Inc.

Terpstra, T.J. 1952. The asymptotic normality and consistency of Kendall's test against trend, when ties are present in one ranking. *Indag. Math.*, **14**: 327–333.

Timm, N.H. 2002. *Applied Multivariate Analysis*. New York, NY: Springer.

Tukey, J.W. 1949. One degree of freedom for nonadditivity. *Biometrics*, **5**: 232–242.

Tukey, J.W. 1977. *Exploratory Data Analysis*. Reading, MA: Addison-Wesley.

Van der Heijden, P.G.M. and J. de Leeuw, 1985. Correspondence analysis used complementary to loglinear analysis. *Psychometrika*, **50**: 429–447.

Walter, S. and R. Cook, 1991. A comparison of several point estimators of the odds ratio in a single 2×2 contingency table. *Biometrics*, **47**(3): 795–811.

Warner, S.L. 1965. Randomized response: A survey technique for eliminating evasive answer bias. *J. Amer. Statist. Assoc.*, **60**: 63–69.

Weisberg, S. 1985. *Applied Linear Regression*, 2nd Edition. New York, NY: Wiley.

Welch, B.L. 1951. On the comparison of several mean values: An alternative approach. *Biometrika*, **38**: 330–336.

Westfall, P.H., R.D. Tobias, D. Rom, R.D. Wolfinger, and Y. Hochberg, 1999. *Multiple Comparisons and Multiple Tests Using the SAS System*. Cary, NC: SAS Institute Inc.

Wolf, F.M. 1986. *Meta-Analysis: Quantitative Methods for Research Synthesis*. Beverly Hills, CA: Sage.

Wright, S. 1921. Correlation and causation. *J. Agri. Res.*, **20**: 557–585.

Yates, F. 1933. The analysis of replicated experiments when the field results are incomplete. *Emp. J. Exp. Agr.*, **1**: 129–142.

Young, F.W. 1987. *Multidimensional Scaling: History, Theory, and Applications*. Hillsdale, NJ: Lawrence Erlbaum Associates.

Zelen, M. 1971. The analysis of several 2×2 contingency tables. *Biometrika*, **58**: 129–137.

Index